The Child in His Family

CHILDREN AT PSYCHIATRIC RISK

VOLUME 3

YEARBOOK OF THE INTERNATIONAL ASSOCIATION FOR CHILD PSYCHIATRY AND ALLIED PROFESSIONS

EDITOR-IN-CHIEF—E. JAMES ANTHONY, M.D. (U.S.A.)

CO-EDITOR—CYRILLE KOUPERNIK, M.D. (FRANCE)

The Child in His Family

CHILDREN AT PSYCHIATRIC RISK

VOLUME 3

Edited by

E. JAMES ANTHONY, M.D.
St. Louis, Missouri, U.S.A.

and

CYRILLE KOUPERNIK, M.D.
Paris, France

*With editorial assistance from Colette Chiland,
Paris, France*

Editorial Board

*Gerald Caplan, M.D. (U.S.A.)
R. Corboz, M.D. (Switzerland)
Lionel Hersov, M.D. (England)
E. Irvine, A.P.S.W. (England)
Reimer Jensen, Cand. Psych. (Denmark)
Stanislau Krynski, M.D. (Brazil)
Jon Lange, M.D. (Norway)
Serge Lebovici, M.D. (France)
Reginald S. Lourie, M.D. (U.S.A.)
Joseph Marcus, M.D. (Israel)
Winston S. Rickards, M.D. (Australia)
Albert J. Solnit, M.D. (U.S.A.)*

A WILEY-INTERSCIENCE PUBLICATION

JOHN WILEY & SONS, New York • London • Sydney • Toronto

Library of Congress Cataloging in Publication Data:

Anthony, Elwyn James.
    Children at psychiatric risk.

    (The Child in his family, v. 3) (Yearbook of the
International Association for Child Psychiatry and Allied
Professions, v. 3)
    "A Wiley-Interscience publication."
    Based on the proceedings of two international study
groups (Bled, Yugoslavia, 1972 and Dakar, Senegal, 1973);
also a precongress publication for the 1974 Philadelphia
congress of the International Association for Child Psychiatry and Allied Professions.
    1. Vulnerable children (Psychiatry)—Congresses.
2. Preventive psychiatry—Congresses. 3. Child psychiatry—Congresses. I. Koupernik, Cyrille, 1917–
joint author. II. Title. III. Series. IV. Series:
International Association for Child Psychiatry and
Allied Professions, Yearbook, v. 3.
    [DNLM: 1. Child psychiatry—Congresses. 2. Family—
Congresses. 3. Parent-child relations—Congresses.

WINN705E v. 3 1972 / WS350 C5363 1972–73]
RJ499.A1C42   vol. 3   [RJ47]   618.9′28′9008s
ISBN 0-471–03228–X   [618.9′28′905]   74–6169

Printed in the United States of America
10 9 8 7 6 5 4 3 2 1

To *FRANCES,* for her tolerance, patience, and loyalty over these strenuous editorial years

Contributors

Claudine Amiel-Tison, Associate Professor, Intensive Care Unit, Maternité Port-Royal, Paris, France

E. James Anthony (M.D.), Blanche F. Ittleson Professor of Child Psychiatry, Director, Division of Child Psychiatry, Washington University School of Medicine, St. Louis, Missouri, U.S.A.

Tolani Asuni (M.A., M.D., D.P.M., F.R.C.Psych., F.N.M.C.Psych.), Professor of Psychiatry and Medical Superintendent, Faculty of Health Sciences, University of Ife, Neuro-Psychiatric Hospital, Aro-Abeokuta, Nigeria

Bertram S. Brown (M.D.), Director, National Institute of Mental Health, Rockville, Maryland, U.S.A.

Colette Chiland (M.D., Ph.D.), Professor of Clinical Psychology at the Université René Descartes (Sorbonne), and Psychiatrist at the Association de Santé Mentale du 13° arrondissement de Paris, Paris, France

Donald J. Cohen (M.D.), Associate Professor of Pediatrics and Psychiatry, Yale University School of Medicine and The Yale University Child Study Center, New Haven, Connecticut, U.S.A.

Theodore B. Cohen (M.D.), Chairman, Vulnerable Child Workshop, American Psychoanalytic Association, Narberth, Pennsylvania, U.S.A.

Henri Collomb (M.D.), Professeur de Psychiatrie, Faculté de Médecine et de Pharmacie de Dakar, Dakar, Sénégal, West Africa

James P. Comer (M.D.), Associate Professor of Psychiatry, Yale Child Study Center and Associate Dean, Yale Medical School, New Haven, Connecticut, U.S.A.

René Diatkine (M.D.), Professeur Associé de Psychiatrie de l'Enfant à la Faculté de Médecine de Genève, Directeur-Ajoint, Centre Alfred BINET, Paris, France

Sibylle K. Escalona (Ph.D.), Professor of Psychiatry (Psychology), R. F. Kennedy Center for Research in Mental Retardation and Human Development, Albert Einstein College of Medicine, New York, New York, U.S.A.

vii

Norman Garmezy (Ph.D.), Professor of Psychology, University of Minnesota, Minneapolis, Minnesota, and Clinical Professor of Psychiatry (Psychology), School of Medicine, University of Rochester, Rochester, New York, U.S.A.

Michael J. Goldstein (Ph.D.), Professor of Psychology, University of California, Los Angeles, Los Angeles, California, U.S.A.

Ernest A. Haggard (Ph.D.), Professor of Psychology, Department of Psychiatry, The Abraham Lincoln School of Medicine, University of Illinois at the Medical Center, Chicago, Illinois, U.S.A.

Lionel A. Hersov (M.D., M.R.C.P., F.R.C.Psych., D.P.M.), Consultant Physician, Children's and Adolescents' Department. The Bethlem Royal Hospital and The Maudsley Hospital, London, England

Elizabeth E. Irvine (M.A.), Retired, Formerly Reader in Social Work, University of York, York, England

Reimer Jensen, Professor, The Royal Danish School of Educational Studies, Copenhagen, Denmark

Joan Berlin Kelly (Ph.D.), Senior Staff Psychologist, Department of Psychiatry, Mt. Zion Hospital and Medical Center, San Francisco, California, and Co-Principal Investigator, Children of Divorce Research Project, Community Mental Health Center, Marin County, California, San Rafael, California, U.S.A.

Cyrille Koupernik (M.D.), Membre Associé, Collige de Médecine de Hôpitaux de Paris, Paris, France

T. Adeoye Lambo (M.B., Ch.B., M.D., F.R.C.P., D.P.M.), Deputy Director-General, World Health Organization, Geneva, Switzerland

Jon Lange (M.D.), Medical Director, Department of Child Psychiatry, Ullevål Sykehus, Oslo, Norway

Serge Lebovici (M.D.), Professeur Associé de Psychiatrie de l'Enfant à l'Université de Paris 6 Pitié-Salpêtrière, Directeur, Centre Alfred BINET, Paris, France

Gloria F. Leiderman (Ph.D.), Associate Director and Head Psychologist, Peninsula Children's Center, Palo Alto, California, U.S.A.

P. Herbert Leiderman (M.D.), Professor of Psychiatry, Stanford University School of Medicine, Stanford, California, U.S.A.

Reginald S. Lourie (M.D., Med., Sc.D.), Professor, Child Health and Human Development, Psychiatry and Behavioral Sciences, George Washington University Medical School, and Director, Department of Psychiatry, Children's Hospital of the District of Columbia, and Medical Director, Hillcrest Children's Center, Washington, D.C., U.S.A.

Joseph Marcus (M.D.), Director, Department of Child Psychiatry and Development, Jerusalem Mental Health Center (affiliated Hebrew University-Hadassah Medical School), Jerusalem, Israel

Alexandre Minkowski (Professeur), Chef de Service, Service de Médecine Néonatale Hôpital Port-Royal, and Professeur de Neonatologie, Centre de Recherches de Biologie du Développement Néonatal, Paris, France

Henry B. M. Murphy (M.D., Ph.D.), Professor, Department of Psychiatry, McGill University, Montreal, Canada

Adewale Omolulu (F.R.C.P.I., F.M.C.P.H., D.P.H., D.C.H.), Professor of Nutrition and Director, Food Science and Applied Nutrition Unit, University of Ibadan, Ibadan, West Nigeria

Sally Provence (M.D.), Professor of Pediatrics, Director, Child Development Unit, Yale University Child Study Center, New Haven, Connecticut, U.S.A.

Lee N. Robins (Ph.D.), Professor of Sociology in Psychiatry, Washington University School of Medicine, St. Louis, Missouri, U.S.A.

Eliot H. Rodnick (Ph.D.), Professor of Psychology, University of California, Los Angeles, Los Angeles, California, U.S.A.

Leon E. Rosenberg (M.D.), Professor of Human Genetics, Pediatrics and Medicine, Chairman, Department of Human Genetics, Yale University School of Medicine, New Haven, Connecticut, U.S.A.

Michael Rutter (M.D., F.R.C.P., F.R.C.Psych., D.P.M.), Professor of Child Psychiatry, Institute of Psychiatry, London, England

John J. Sigal (Ph.D.), Research Director, Associate Professor, Institute of Community and Family Psychiatry, Jewish General Hospital, and Department of Psychiatry, McGill University, Montreal, Canada

Albert J. Solnit (M.D.), Sterling Professor of Pediatrics and Psychiatry, and Director, Child Study Center, Yale University, New Haven, Connecticut, U.S.A.

Colin M. Turnbull (D.Phil.), Professor of Sociology and Anthropology, Virginia Commonwealth University, Academic Center, Richmond, Virginia, U.S.A.

Simone Valantin, Maître Assistant de Psychologie, Université de Paris, Paris, France

Judith S. Wallerstein (M.S.W.), Lecturer, School of Social Welfare, University of California, Berkeley, Berkeley, California, and Principal Investigator, Children of Divorce Research Project, Community Mental Health Center, Marin County, California, San Rafael, California, U.S.A.

Foreword

Of the many urgent needs that challenge us in the field of mental health, perhaps none outranks the long-standing priority of developing improved preventive techniques. A recent biometric report prepared by the National Institute of Mental Health showed that in 1971 there were more than 2.7 million admission episodes to mental health facilities in the United States. An additional estimated million or more individuals sought help from private practitioners, neighborhood health centers, and nonpsychiatric hospitals. Fortunately, we were able to assist a great many of these individuals to cope with their problems and to maintain healthy and vigorous lives. Still, in terms of economic costs alone, these statistics and the lives they represent are critical. Even more significant is the incalculable human cost of illness and psychiatric distress to the afflicted individuals, their families, and friends.

I do not trace the history of psychiatric research to illustrate the solid advances our profession has made toward the effective treatment of mental and emotional disorders. Yet no matter how effective modern management of mental illness may appear, we are continually forced to realize that treating acute disorders remains a holding action. Through the development of improved therapies and medications, more efficient utilization of manpower resources, and the increasing availability of services, we are approaching a point at which we are able to meet the immediate needs of many persons. The ultimate answer, however, lies in a fuller understanding of the origins and causes of mental illness, followed by comprehensive intervention and prevention programs. Through research, the accomplishments as well as the tentative explorations add to our knowledge base and are a prelude to more sophisticated questions, refined hypotheses, and substantive gains.

The Child in His Family: Children at Psychiatric Risk provides an amalgam of research in areas related to mental health that appears to signal a new and promising trend in psychiatry and medicine. The emergence of what has come to be termed the high risk approach to studies of normal and abnormal development exemplifies the evolution of our knowledge and capabilities. It is painstakingly built on the accumulated findings of years of study for clues to the pathogenesis of various disorders. In this context, the term risk is now being applied to yet unknown vulnerable populations for mental and physical disorders. The promise of the strategy is manifold. It provides a means for investigators to sidestep what has traditionally been an often insurmountable barrier—the problem of distinguishing *cause* from *consequence* of illness. New paths, though long and arduous, are being opened for planning and implementing intervention programs.

In a broad sense, the concept underlying the study of children at psychiatric risk is the root of the entire NIMH child mental health research program. Several years ago when I became director of the NIMH one of my first acts was to establish child mental health as the Institute's number one, across-the-board priority. Within weeks, an ad hoc committee was set up to review the NIMH research, training, and service programs for children and youth. The group was requested to make specific recommendations that could be implemented immediately, as well as set long range objectives. The committee's final report did provide specific and realistic suggestions that have become in many ways the goals of the Institute's child program. The child priority has provided a conceptual platform from which we are able to both analyze and assess our considerable efforts previously in this area and to proceed toward new goals.

With respect to populations who are apparently at some level of psychiatric risk, another figure from the report cited earlier is warranted. Of the total number of admissions episodes to facilities, more than one third represent persons under 24 years of age. We must ask ourselves how many of these young people and their families could have been spared the tolls of distress and agony they were forced to pay.

The reduction of psychiatric risk and the prevention of disorder is implicit in all research. Within NIMH programs and in our cooperative efforts with the World Health Organization and collaborating research facilities around the world, the issues of psychiatric risk and prevention are basic. Often we do not attempt to define or single out the vulnerable child, but have supported research directed toward identification of the biochemical, physiological, and psychosocial risks to children.

In specific areas—for example, the child at risk for schizophrenia—some of the basic issues in high risk studies have been tentatively identified. A series of studies, led in large part by the early work of the Danish investigators Sarnoff Mednick and Fini Schulsinger, have been initiated within the last 10 or 15 years. A high risk strategy can be employed in these studies with an increasingly sophisticated design and purpose. However, as we move into the area of general psychiatric risk for a population at large—that is, foregoing reliance on genetically based samples often employed in schizophrenia-related investigations—the research task becomes as diffuse as the issues in question. We not only have to discern what constitutes risk, but also must identify the consequences of risk. It has been estimated that 10 to 20 percent of the children in a general population require attention for emotional disturbance, retardation, speech disorders, or other behavioral disorders. These diagnostic categories are marked by overlap and vagueness, and, to be very direct, the best option open to researchers is to cover all fronts. Therefore, research on pre- and postnatal care, infant stimulaton and deprivation, stress in school, adolescent lifestyles, and college activities are all pertinent to issues of psychiatric risk.

This book provides an open-ended and multidimensional discussion of risk factors. The breadth of its definition of risk greatly enhances its usefulness to any one of the disciplines represented here. Merely by focusing on the existence of risk factors, the book raises the consciousness of researchers, particularly those who may be less familiar with the high risk concept or its wide applicability. Because it is an emerging area of study, the high risk field is singularly open to cross-fertilization of ideas and input. The extensive selection of papers on the assessment of risk factors gives some measure of the scope of this undertaking. It is encouraging to note that just as the demands of the high risk approach disregard traditional disciplinary and theoretical lines, so has the response of the international research been open and innovative. Scientists of diverse persuasions have been quick to grasp that the high risk research strategy offers a unique opportunity to test etiological hypotheses. The list of contributors indicates the confluence of theoretical orientations and cultural perspectives the field has attracted.

This surge of interest in high risk studies raises issues that the researcher, and even more, the clinician and administrator, face regularly. As we begin to deal with psychiatric disorders prospectively rather than retrospectively, we must attune ourselves to the potential effects on children of our classifications and labeling and to our influence as researchers on children's lives. For our purposes, labels and various descriptors are diagnostic tools, but they can also be used to control access to health service and educational systems and thus exert a powerful influence on the courses of development open to individuals. It is an issue appropriately included in this book, since it is one of the ethical considerations that must underlie our efforts in this area.

The concept of psychiatric risk implies much more than a research protocol or strategy. It encompasses not only a range of crucial ethical issues but also methodological ones, and must be measured in years of human growth and development as well as in abstract portions of a longitudinal project.

In this respect, all of us—whether medical or psychological professionals, teachers or parents—share a mutual concern in the child at psychiatric risk. He is every child and the risk to him is hidden in the world he inherits from us. This book constitutes a valuable research tool in its consolidation of knowledge and in the signposts it provides for future efforts. More importantly, it highlights an issue of crucial human concern to all peoples of the world.

BERTRAM S. BROWN, M.D.
Director
National Institute of Mental Health

Preface

Let us count the many features that make this a most unusual book. First, it represents an initial attempt to explore, in depth and breadth, the clinical phenomena associated with psychiatric risk and vulnerability and to reveal the expanding dimensions of this comparatively new field to the mental health practitioner with the intention of alerting him to the real prospect of primary prevention. It could and should orient him to the importance of both prophylaxis and treatment in the total approach to optimal psychological functioning.

Second, the book is unusual in the way that it has been built up. Most of it evolved from the proceedings of two international study groups that met in 1972 in Bled, Yugoslavia, to consider the basic risks involved in heredity, constitution, reproduction, and early life experience, and in 1973 in Dakar, Senegal, to study the environmental risks concerned with growing up in rapidly developing societies.

However, since not all the recognized specialists of so-called risk research could be called upon to attend these meetings and present the fruits of their work, a final section in the book was set aside to include them, thus justifying the claim of this volume to be comprehensive. It is the first time that this significant new area has been brought together in its entirety.

A third unusual feature will be evident in the *site visits* and *discussions* that are reported. It was deemed important for the success of the study group meeting that the visiting experts obtain first-hand impressions of the local condition before they tried to adapt their knowledge to it. A further corrective experience was derived from the interchanges between the visiting and local specialists, which not only did much to reduce the incidence of hasty generalizations but also made it more possible to differentiate between particular and universal phenomena. With this undertaking as a model, we hope that transcultural discourse will eventually become a recognized mode for investigating the many facets of developmental psychopathology across the world. It should help to cure the parochialism that is such a disturbing aspect of national academies where universal statements about child rearing often stem from no further than the immediate backyard.

The fourth and last feature may be unusual to other associations but not to the International Association for Child Psychiatry and Allied Professions. In this association, participants at the congresses have been prepared, since 1966, with a special congress book that has attempted to summarize the knowledge in the field. Volume 3 of the International Yearbook series will perform this function for the 1974 *Philadelphia Congress on the Vulnerable Child,* but its range of contributions is such that it should establish itself as a source and resource book on risk for many years to come.

A special mention must once again be made of the work of Mrs. Martha Kniepkamp who has already convoyed Volumes 1 and 2 of the International series through the many pitfalls of preparation of manuscripts, proofreading, and indexing that lie between the inception of a book and its publication. To all this she brings a diligence and a reliability that have been a constant solace to the two editors. She has made herself an almost indispensable part of the Yearbooks and we are extremely grateful to her.

E. JAMES ANTHONY, M.D.
CYRILLE KOUPERNIK, M.D.

St. Louis, Missouri
Paris, France
March 1974

Contents

Contents

The Child in His Family

Children at Psychiatric Risk

Volume 3

THEORY FOR A NEW FIELD

Introduction: The Syndrome of the Psychologically Vulnerable Child

E. James Anthony, M.D. (U.S.A.)

In 1927 Cimbal [7] gave a vivid description of certain children who manifested what he termed *Lebensfeigheit*, which can be roughly translated as cowardliness with respect to living. They were strikingly apprehensive and "always afraid of everything." Fear seemed to be a permanent and pervasive attribute with nothing specific about it. Every element in the environment could become an object of fear irrespective of the child's experience. The children rarely raised their voices above a whisper and seemed to be "afraid of their own shadows." As infants they were perturbed by the unfamiliar and tended to have tempestuous "stranger reactions," and throughout childhood they avoided novelty in all forms. They grew up to become constricted adults who were timid, undecisive, and somewhat withdrawn. Once they found a niche for themselves, they tended to remain there for a lifetime.

These are children who not only look vulnerable and have always looked vulnerable but are, in fact, vulnerable. They are vulnerable to almost minimal departures from the expectable, and they tend to protect themselves by encapsulating themselves in the environment. This self-protective and counterphobic attitude and behavior may work as long as the environment is relatively safe, and, to use Freud's expression [12], as long as these individuals are not exposed to "too searching a fate."

These children therefore look and behave vulnerably from the very beginning of life and possibly, if we were better acquainted with prenatal functioning, from before birth.

Hartmann [14] felt that it was necessary to assume that the child was born with "a certain degree of preadaptiveness," meaning that it was already in a rudimentary way equipped with an apparatus of perception, memory, motility, and other primary autonomous functions of the ego and thus prepared for dealing with reality even before it had experienced reality. The second factor determining the degree of vulnerability of the infant was the so-called protective barrier against stimuli, a theoretical construct put forward by Freud as a probable antecedent of later defense mechanisms. Bergman and Escalona [4] used the concept of a "thin" protective barrier in accounting for the unusual sensitivities of children as a result of which there is a precocious ego development. It is this latter outcome that conduces to a high degree of vulnerability with impaired resistance. According to Hartmann [14], the deficiencies in the primary autonomous ego functions render the individual vulnerable to the development of serious mental disorder.

The third theoretical factor, as advanced by Anna Freud [11] in the genesis of vulnerability, was the capacity to postpone and control discharge in response to stimulation, and she regarded this as one of the essential features of the human ego from its very beginning. A fourth factor, put forward by Buhler [5] on both observational and theoretical grounds, was the presence of a "primary positive response" of the infant to the world outside alongside the primary negative ones, and there is some evidence to link these positive attitudes to the positive object relationships developing later. There is also evidence to attest that there are wide variations among infants with respect to these postulated structures and functions as a constitutional "given." In addition, the impact of deprivation or trauma in this earliest period may significantly interfere with their further evolution and thereby lead to an increase in vulnerability. There is no doubt that both hereditary and environmental factors work together, in differing proportions under different circumstances, to decide on the ultimate vulnerability of the individual. Freud [12] was fairly convinced that defenses have a hereditary core, and it would be logical to assume that this was equally true for vulnerabilities of the defense system.

Various infant studies have added to our knowledge of constitutional vulnerability. Making use of a startle response and an oral test, Fries and her associates [13] categorized infants into three normal and two pathological, congenital activity types. She used the term "congenital" because she regarded constitution as a joint product of the action of genes, intrauterine influences, and birth experiences. These early activity patterns were viewed as biological forerunners of later reactions to difficulties, predisposing the child to certain defense and escape mechanisms which, in turn, made him vulnerable to particular neuroses or symptom formations. On the basis of her investigations, she concluded that the two extreme types—the excessively quiet and the excessively active—appeared to be more vulnerable to psychological illness. This "constitutional complex" has been found to be stable over a period of 30 years, uniquely permitting predictions made in infancy to be tested successfully in adult life.

In the Menninger study, Heider [15] viewed the degree of vulnerability in infancy as a resultant of factors related to equipment, to so-called management processes, meaning the ways in which the child handles himself in the case of stress, and to environment for the relationship between the individual's functional pattern and the influences affecting him, chiefly that of his mother during the infantile period. A significant relationship was found between the level of vulnerability in infancy and at the preschool ages, and there was a slight tendency for vulnerability to increase over this period, although this may have been an artifact of the study. The vulnerable infant was less robust, less energetic, less active, less interested, less trustful, and less likely to be part of a good mother-child relationship. His general incompetence could stem from a low sensory reactivity because of congenitally raised or defensively raised thresholds and low motor activity, which might also be congenitally determined or defensively determined in the shape of escape or withdrawal.

The well-known investigation by Thomas, Chess, Birch, and Hertzig [20] also focused on congenital differences in infants, and they have tried to relate these predispositions for "primary reaction patterns" to later normal or abnormal behavior. Of their nine categories, the activity level, threshold, intensity of reaction, mood, and distractibility were especially discriminatory with respect to individual differences. It seemed that in terms of the total pattern, each infant was unique. It was found that neither the temperament of the child nor the parental characteristics alone had independent influence on the child's development, but the two sets of factors worked together interdependently. Although children evincing an amodal pattern on intensity, adaptability, regularity, and mood were more vulnerable, all of them developed behavior disorders because of the modifying influence of the parental reaction.

Babies have been observed to differ widely in the strength of their tendency to startle or show avoidance reactions to unpleasant stimuli. This tendency for anxiety or generalized fearfulness is clearly a predisposition possessed by all infants, but it is likely, as Diamond [8] suggests, "to be established as a lasting disposition if it is given frequent exercise in this period." During this initial period of instability, the infant seems particularly vulnerable to the hazards of care and to contact with the mothering one. Sullivan [18] spoke of the "fear-like state" that could be induced in the infant either by trauma or by contact with an emotionally disturbed mother. Her anxiety could induce anxiety in the infant through the interpersonal process of empathy. This meant that the mental health of the mother in relation to her baby was of crucial importance in the development of his sensitivity to frightening experiences. In his schema of development Erikson [9] also emphasized the significance of the mother: "The amount of trust derived from earliest infantile experiences does not seem to depend on absolute quantities of food or demonstrations of love but rather on the quality of the maternal relationship." For him, basic mistrust in this period was the essence of all subsequent vulnerabilities. The trust and confidence are generated in the infant by the "good enough" management of the mother who is able to establish a mutual communication that allows the baby to "read" the meaning of her behavior and to inform her through its behavior. Escalona [10] has spoken of "the esthetic pleasure of watching perfect mothering" as evidenced in the way the mother knows just how her baby likes to be bathed, the speed at which to feed him and how much to put on the spoon, the position in which he likes to sleep, and whether rocking or patting is more effective. The baby is gratified by the mother's skillful ministrations, and the mother is gratified through his positive response to her.

The vulnerable constitution may manifest itself as much in structure as in function. Walker [21] in a study of nursery school children correlating somatotype and the teacher's rating of behavior found that ectomorphic types were generally the problem children about whom the parents complained because they were shy, sensitive, irritable, unfriendly, nervous, fearful, and anxious, all of which would predispose them to the subsequent development of internalizing syndromes of the anxious, depressive, phobic, and obsessional varieties. The importance of physique in relation to adjustment was recognized 35 years ago by Burt [6], who found no correlations between thinness and inhibition, and 20 years later Davidson and his associates in Parnell's laboratory [17] found a significant association in 7-year-olds between ectomorphy and a constellation of behaviors made up of anxiety, restlessness, fussiness, and conscientiousness. The same connection was followed into adolescence by Parnell [17], who discovered that ectomorphic students with poor muscular development and below average in fat were six times more likely to seek psychiatric help than other somatotypes.

Along with primary action and reaction patterns, temperament and body build was a significant relationship to vegetative functioning. Wenger [22] described the *S* child (sympathetic predominant) as emotionally unstable, tense, restless, impulsive, overactive, insecure, and dependent on affection and approval from others, some of which would place him among the vulnerable group of children.

Finally, in the context of hormonal development, Tanner [19] found evidence to link late maturation with maladjustment, feelings of inadequacy and rejection, and a sense of not belonging to the group. These late maturers also tended to be predominantly ectomorphic.

These various theoretical ideas and investigations into constitution, summarized and discussed by Anthony [1], build up a picture of the vulnerable individual in the making, whose snowballing development through infancy, childhood, and adolescence is punctuated by crisis and catastrophe as vulnerable periods of transition are reached. It is often difficult to decide unequivocally whether the mother has let the child down by failing to inculcate basic trust and confidence because of deficiencies in her "holding" capacity and preoccupation with her infant, or whether the infant's constitutional deficiencies would tax the resources of the average mother. That the pair are mismatched is generally very obvious to the observer. If one adds to this poor environmental conditions and inadequate social and cultural opportunities, conditions of risk are set up that make it even more difficult for the vulnerable individual to emerge unscathed at the other end of childhood.

Nevertheless, the environment may be as benign and as expectable as one could wish, and the vulnerable child will still succumb. Within a bad environment where the average child will survive and the "invulnerable" one will flourish, [2] the vulnerable child is very likely to break down completely. He is the prototype of the "glass doll" in the analogy used by Anthony [3]. In Table 1 the relationships between risk, vulnerability, and disorder are brought together in various combinations. The hypervulnerable individual may become disordered in spite of a good environment, and the "invulnerable individual" remains unaffected in spite of a bad environment. This has emerged as an important finding in the seven-year research conducted by Anthony on the children of psychotic parents.

It is not surprising to the clinician that the vulnerable child begins to become chronically dissatisfied with his environment, to envisage it as threatening or depriving, and constantly to find fault with the

Table 1   Relationship of Risk, Vulnerability, and Disturbance

	High Risk	Low Risk
High Vulnerability	(1) HR, HV	(3) LR, HV
Low Vulnerability	(2) HR, LV	(4) LR, LV

	High Risk	Low Risk
Disturbed	(1) HR, D	(3) LR, D
Nondisturbed	(2) HR, ND	(4) LR, ND

	High Vulnerability	*Low* Vulnerability
Disturbed	(1) HV, D	(3) LV, D
Nondisturbed	(2) HV, ND	(4) LV, ND

people and things within it. His whole picture of the world is colored by disturbing experiences outside that seem to be to a large extent products of distorting tendencies within the individual. A striking example of this can be seen in the work of one of the most vulnerable and creative people in the world of literature. Kafka [16] transposed his intense feelings of vulnerability into his writing. All through his life he was keenly aware that he did not perceive and experience the same world that others did and that the distortion and destruction were essentially inside him. This idea that the environment was average and expectable and that people were average and expectable until his own vulnerable self intruded on them haunted his imagination for most of his life. It was like a perpetual affliction.

Kafka recalled as a child opening his eyes after a short sleep in the middle of the day, and while still drowsy, hearing his mother calling down from the balcony to someone else in a natural tone saying: "What are you doing, my dear; it's so hot." A woman answered from the garden: "I'm having tea outside." They spoke comfortably, unselfconsciously, and as though this were what anyone would expect [16]. For Kafka, the child, fearful and knowing his fear, this was what the world was like, quiet and predictable, until his mind set to work on it. In this sense the vulnerable child creates his own risks and generates his own fearfulness. He becomes, as Cimbal [7] describes him, perpetually afflicted with *Lebensfeigheit*. The world is forever transformed, or to put it in Kafka's words: "I am, as it were, specially appointed to see the phantoms of the night."

References

1. Anthony, E. J. The behavior disorders of childhood, in *Carmichael's Manual of Child Psychology*, Vol. II, P. H. Mussen, Ed. John Wiley & Sons, New York, 1970.
2. Anthony, E. J. The syndrome of the psychologically invulnerable child. In this volume.
3. Anthony, E. J. A risk-vulnerability-intervention model for children of psychotic parents. In this volume.
4. Bergman, P. and Escalona, S. K. Unusual sensitivities in very young children. *The Psychoanalytic Study of the Child*, Vol. 3/4. International Universities Press, New York, 1949.
5. Buhler, C. The reality principle. *Amer. J. Psychother.*, 8 (1954).

6. Burt, C. The analysis of temperament. *Brit. J. Med. Psychol.*, 17 (1938), 158–188.
7. Cimbal, W. J. O. *The Neuroses of Childhood in Relation to Bedwetting. (Die Neurosen des Kindesalters).* Urban & Schwartzenberg, Berlin, 1927.
8. Diamond, S. *Personality and Temperament.* Harper and Row, New York, 1957.
9. Erikson, E. H. *Childhood and Society.* Norton, New York, 1950.
10. Escalona, S. Emotional development in the first year of life, in *Problems of Infancy and Childhood*, M. Senn, ed. Josiah Macy Foundation Publications, New York, 1953.
11. Freud, A. *The Ego and the Mechanisms of Defense.* International Universities Press, New York, 1936.
12. Freud, S. Analysis terminable and interminable, in *Collected Papers*, Vol. 5. Hogarth Press, London, 1950.
13. Fries, M. E. and Woolf, P. J. The influence of constitutional complex on developmental phases, in *Separation-Individuation*, J. McDevitt and C. Settlage, Eds. International Universities Press, New York, 1971.
14. Hartmann, H. *Essays on Ego Psychology.* International Universities Press, New York, 1964.
15. Heider, G. M. Vulnerability in infants and young children. *Gen. Psychol. Monograph*, 73 (1966), 1–216.
16. Kafka, F. *Beschreibung eines Kamfes.* Der Heizer, Berlin, 1906, p. 183.
17. Parnell, R. W. Physique and mental breakdown in young adults. *Brit. Med. J.*, 1, (1957), 1485–1490.
18. Sullivan, H. S. *The Interpersonal Theory of Psychiatry.* Norton, New York, 1953.
19. Tanner, J. M., The morphological level of personality. *Proc. R. Soc. Med.*, 50 (1947), 301–303.
20. Thomas, A., Chess, S., Birch, H., and Hertzig, M. E. A longitudinal study of primary reaction patterns in children. *Comprehen. Psychiat.* (1960), 103–112.
21. Walker, R. N. Body build and behavior in young children. *Monogr. Soc. Res. Child Devel.*, 27:3 (1962), 1–94.
22. Wenger, M. A. Study of the significance of measures of autonomic balance. *Psychosom. Med.*, 9 (1947), 301.

Normality as a Concept of Limited Usefulness in the Assessment of Psychiatric Risk

Serge Lebovici, M.D. and René Diatkine, M.D. (France)

The Concept of Normality

The distribution of psychiatric facilities in the community confirms
the impression that the section of the population seeking professional
help is not the same as that requiring specialized treatment. Indeed,
it by no means presents a comprehensive picture of cases that may be
called pathological. Conversely, to speak of normality in connection
with children who do not draw attention to themselves is to run the
risk of overlooking hidden pathology.

Psychiatric practice with children has afforded us the opportunity
of viewing both "normal" and pathological symptoms (the latter
being likely to pass completely undetected); we address ourselves
first to the concept of normality with the hope not only that we may
cast some light on the psychiatric risks in so-called normality, but also
that we will raise sufficient doubts about the correctness of gauging
these risks according to standards used for assessing pathology where
the part played by so-called cerebral factors often seems to be
overstressed.

The word normality comes from the Latin *norma*, meaning square (the instrument), and hence something at "right angles": the *normal* person is one who is and behaves as expected.

The definitions of normality should not, nowadays, correspond to those of health or mental health in particular, whether one has in mind adjustment and the ability to adjust, or aptitude for happiness, since what is often meant by a normal individual is one who is average, or who shows no signs of anomaly. The idea of *norm* (biological, statistical, or moral), cannot and therefore should not be applied directly to the field of mental health.

Similarly, we must bear in mind that unusual behavior is not necessarily abnormal and, conversely, that frequently encountered behavior is not necessarily normal. From this standpoint, many epidemiological studies of general populations have disclosed a considerable incidence and prevalence of psychiatric symptoms, without helping, however, to determine the range and limits of morbidity.

On the strength of these studies, one might be tempted to dispense with precise boundaries of pathology in spite of the fact that this would inordinately extend the domain of psychiatry.

In the same context, the distinction made between child psychiatric disorder and maladjustment (particularly pronounced in France in the operation of official programs) tends to assign certain learning difficulties to the field of psychiatry. It seems to us that these should not be classified under "specific disorders of development" as is done in certain nosologies of childhood mental disorders. Dyslexia, dysphasia, dysgraphia, and the like, can just as well be caused by deficiencies in the cultural background or educational management; on the other hand, they can equally be expressions of disturbance in mental functioning, aggravated by the experience of failure and the reactions of parents and teachers to this.

Thus to define the conditions of risk in child psychiatry, we have to raise questions regarding the notions of normality and abnormality since it cannot be taken for granted that a precise definition of these concepts will be put to good operational use in medical practice. With children, particularly, treatment is justified as much by concern for possible future developments as for the present status. The detection of disturbance in its early stages belongs as much to the field of prevention as to the specialty of child psychiatry.

To distinguish between the physiological and the pathological in medicine is generally not easy [1]. For example, an inflammatory reaction is normal in certain conditions of physical insult, and its absence would give cause for alarm. The association of insult and inflammation, on the other hand, does define a pathological fact.

In speaking of normality and illness in this context one is making certain about the life process and its transience or permanence. In psychiatry, similarly, Goldstein [4] has stated that to behave sanely is to behave in an orderly manner, but that recovery may be marked by the establishment of a new order. In dealing with mental pathology, one should respect these neo-organizations that do not necessarily correspond to the norms of the particular culture to which the child and his family belong. For instance, as regards the specific learning disturbances already mentioned, the practice of reeducation should not lead to a demand that the child conform to normal as defined by performance on standard developmental tests.

These examples, which could be multiplied, indicate that the predicament of "not being well," whether applying to the child or to his family, may be harmfully overextended. It would include both those who are "not normal" and those who are "not happy." In fact, the need to seek professional help is determined more and more by social and cultural factors, for example, the level of sophistication of referring agencies, rather than by any actual potential in the patients for change.

All this points to the danger latent in a purely nosological and descriptive point of view based on the traditional medical model. No description, whether symptomatic or syndromatic, is qualified to define the normal child simply by the absence of these so-called morbid entities. The diagnosis of health should not be based solely on the absence of ill-health.

The Contribution of Psychoanalysis

Psychoanalysis has made an essential contribution to this problem. According to Freud, the experiences of early relationships and early conflict are responsible for organizing the mental functions, and pathological conditions are not attributable simply to regressions or to nonorganizations arising from the early life conditions and the structures that define them. Instead, it is postulated that every disorder produces a reorganization of the ego, stemming from conflicts and their expression in fantasy, from instinctual cathexes and their distribution, and, finally, from the functioning of the various agencies within the psyche. The Jacksonian model of pathological disintegration and the corresponding antithesis of normal and pathological is here replaced by the hypothesis of organizations intended to preserve the ego and the inner reality, whatever the processes involved. For this reason, it is not possible to compare the disorganization of a function in an adult with the maturational difficulties of a child, and one would not expect to find in the child antecedents of adult mental disorders in their earliest or mildest forms.

Language disturbances, for example, may be traced to maturational difficulties, but they cannot be related to specific retardation. Closely linked to the deficiencies that brought them about, they develop on their own in various directions corresponding to the various stages of development through which they proceed, before finally becoming vital organizations in mental functioning.

In such cases, one must try to estimate the repercussions of these specific disturbances, and it does not make sense to say of a child that he is normal apart from the specific difficulties he is undergoing. Reeducation, when attempted, is also likely to fail owing to associated inhibitions, or else to lead to the appearance of mental symptoms, if it threatens the secondary gains derived from the instrumental difficulty.

The point being made is that psychiatric risk is not definable in terms of simple maturational problems that generate pathology. From this standpoint, there are no basic or primary or maturational disorders, at least not in our own psychiatric experience. To accept such hypotheses would be tantamount to assuming a notion of development controlled by an embryology of behavior without taking ecological factors into account. This is quite contrary to the viewpoint that functional modalities themselves operate on the organization of the functions.

The structural school of American psychoanalysis, stemming from the work of Hartmann, has differentiated the processes of maturation from a form of development in which external factors act conjointly with inherent equipment. Perhaps one should go one step further than this school's inclusion of both maturation and nonconflictual mental functioning within the developmental scheme, and postulate that even though the modalities of individual reactions are partly determined by natal or perinatal tendencies, their future is shaped by organizations that have their own destiny apart from the events that contributed to their genesis, and would seem to follow a pattern of repetitive behaviors.

In short, psychiatric risk is not limited to instrumental deficiency or to cerebral disorders, whether anatomical or functional. Moreover, when a child is taken to the psychiatrist because of an uneasiness (especially on the part of the family) that his condition has aroused, there is no relationship between the gravity of the symptoms and the concern about it.

Here again we believe that the findings of psychoanalysis are of great value in delimiting the field of psychopathology. In postulating the equivalence of infantile neurosis and transference neurosis, especially in the cases of *Little Hans* and of the *Wolf-man*, Freud has shown us that disorders in children are not destined to last, but that they are determining elements of mental disorders in adults through the organization of successive structures that do not exclude (quite the contrary) the disappearance of the initial symptoms. The neurosis of the wolf-man appears, for instance, as an avatar of an infantile neurosis that had developed in two stages, and had seemed to be cured when the child was 10 years old. In adulthood, the complex condition of this patient did not reproduce the archaic disorders that had occurred when he was a child, but the initial disorders would have alerted the present-day child psychiatrist to the importance of phobic displacements and obsessional reaction formations. He would have been able to evaluate the importance of transient neurotic solutions shaped by the interplay of drives and countercathexes, and to have made some surmises concerning the potential for ego development.

Two Psychoanalytic Points of Views

Here, however, two divergent opinions come to light. Psychoanalysts of the Kleinian persuasion believe that the "genetic continuum" places fantasied object-relationships in the struggle between the life and death instincts and consequently within the framework of the splitting of the good and bad objects, which generates a deep-seated ambivalence within the mental system and determines a "normal" psychotic position, and that neurotic states are simply a providential working through of this position. This viewpoint attaches no importance whatsoever, at least in principle, to actual experiences, and inclines to an ahistoric point of view which would call for (or justify) the treatment of all children, if such a thing were possible.

Anna Freud, on the contrary, suggests—like Hartmann and his disciples—that "normal and pathological development" be taken into account [3]. She accepts the idea that intrapsychic conflicts are inevitable but considers it necessary to predict possible sequels with great caution: she does not admit that such sequels are the raw product of instinctual conflicts. For her, it is a question of evaluating their working through. From our side we would add that one should try to measure the ability of the child to organize new operations or, put differently, to estimate the weight of the internal inhibitory factors. The appearance or disappearance of symptoms takes on its full meaning only in relation to these processes.

Following the same line of argument, progression and regression cannot be considered in quite the same way. Both these movements introduce conflicts that can operate in different directions, and in turn induce new conflicts. Certain conflictual structures lose their organizing power and maintain themselves in a dangerous state of stability that becomes repetitive. Activity (or behavior) becomes restricted without necessarily producing perceptible symptoms. This can be better understood by studying the vicissitudes of object-relations as described by psychoanalysis. Starting from an initial ambivalence, a decisive step is taken when the mother, invested with birth feeling before she has been separately perceived, ceases to be just a functional object that satisfies or fails to satisfy the child's needs and becomes a differentiated object permanently and unquenchably desirable. She remains both good and bad. Having broken out from the functional unity of maternal care, the child must repair it in terms of his primary anxieties. The mother lays the foundations of the ego, of the notions of here and there and of presence and absence, and organizes the first symbolic meanings. Meanwhile, the child acquires a sense of self and the feeling of continuity.

His fantasies allow him some relief from the catastrophic

experience of absence, giving it a meaning that necessarily includes the role of the father and makes the organization inevitable. It is these various fantasies that link the struggle against depression with cognitive schemas.

This fundamental situation allows us to assess the potential for further development, however substantial the initial deficiencies, the functional disorders, or even the brain damage. Depending on these factors, as well as on the quality of relational experiences, the child may have to restrain his activities and to organize his mental life in pathological ways. In the more fortunate cases, the strength of the object cathexes, taken in conjunction with a rich early experience, will allow him to overcome the contradictions of his ambivalence and to organize a range of enhancing activities that eventually lead to the differentiated identifications involved in the evolution of the oedipal conflict.

It is not our intention here to contrast in detail psychoses (in which mental representation is poorly constructed or not constrained at all because of the failure in object relationships) with neuroses (in which the occurrence of inevitable conflicts during the elaboration of the thinking process may cause phobic displacements and reaction-formations that are ineffective in controlling drives and open the way to obsessional symptoms). We must, however, consider the possibility of assessing the influence of these symptoms on mental functioning.

Such an appraisal is particularly difficult to make during the latency period when, for instance, methodical and clean children organize reaction formations that consolidate into defense mechanisms and eventually into character traits; on the other hand, the outcome may take a more benign course toward sublimation.

We did not intend to survey the problems arising in connection with the emergence of various forms of mental disorder in the child during the course of his development but only to indicate, on the basis of a brief discussion of neurotic and psychotic organizations, that the recognition of symptoms in themselves by no means enables us to circumscribe the field of psychiatric intervention. It has also been necessary to emphasize that preventive work, based on a careful evaluation of the risk threatening the child, should not be concerned only with the distinction between normal and pathological.

The patterns of mental functioning that have established

themselves in the course of the child's development and that are still
subject to various changes until adulthood continue to play a role
during the entire lifetime of the individual. From this point of view,
the concept of normality is of no help in estimating the precariousness
of these organizations. Every child must find his own equilibrium
in accordance with his early relationships and his natural endowment,
and an understanding of the developmental potential of this
equilibrium is needed if one hopes to measure the psychiatric risks
involved.

Some Current Studies on the Assessment of Risk

Many studies have demonstrated the difficulty of estimating the
degree of risk. We mention here only those in which we have
participated. In one particular investigation (not yet completed)
on two samples of 6-year-old children (now 18 years old) who have
been followed for the last 12 years, only 17 out of 66 were free of
symptoms [2]. The symptom count was based on an interview with
either the child or his parents. A certain number of the children
may have presented transitory symptoms. Like many other
investigations, this one also demonstrated the very small percentage
of those who could be called "mentally healthy." In another study a
representative sample of the population seen in consultation at the
Alfred Binet Center in Paris was matched against a subgroup of the
population not seen in consultation, and the same frequency of
neurotic symptoms was found in both groups.

Many of these current studies tend to show that risk can be
assessed in terms of two types of data: one concerned with social and
cultural factors and the other with the organization of mental
functioning. Sociocultural inequalities are manifest in our societies
and follow-up studies have demonstrated the risk potentials of this
fact. Earlier studies pointing to the vulnerability of mental
functioning include one made in St. Louis, Missouri [6] suggesting
that "academic progress is an index of mental health" and that poor
performance on intelligence tests could be a "distress symptom in the
child" [2]. In France clinical evidence suggests that it is more
difficult for the child of a workman to learn to read than for the child
of an intellectual, supporting the conclusion that risk is a function
of the familial and social environment and, as such, warrants

interpersonal and psychological intervention.

We also have means of judging which children should be treated and which not, based on the study of their mental functioning. This means not only being able to predict, for example, whether a child will recover from his neurosis, but it also allows us to form an opinion of his developmental potential and of his ability to work through his conflicts and to use the inevitable regressions without serious disorganization. What is more, a neurotic organization, when sufficiently flexible, would support the hope that the child will solve his difficulties on an intrapsychic level rather than act them out or somatize them.

Of course follow-up studies only give a feeble echo of what it is possible to learn from longitudinal studies, but they do suggest that predictive error is greater for apparently favorable cases, whereas the factors that prompt us to diagnose "high risk" are easy to evaluate, more accurately forecasted, and more indicative of irreversible conditions.

A Working Hypothesis

A hypothesis has been formulated that warrants further exploration. A twofold problem arises in this connection: to explain the inception and the maintenance of certain difficulties, it has become customary to draw on the concept of "minimal brain dysfunction." In such cases, the historical evidence of significant perinatal difficulties has led to the assumption that the child is at higher psychiatric risk and that therefore the only useful action to be taken is to adopt widescale preventive obstetrical measures as a purely preventive policy. However, it should be equally realized that even when organic damage or dysfunction has already occurred therapeutic measures are still of great importance and efficacy. The brain-damaged child also has an environment to live in and development to undergo.

The hypothesis of minimal brain dysfunction (MBD) does not seem to have the exploratory and predictive power to define and demarcate the risk aspects in child psychiatry. Furthermore, there is a tendency to view pathology in dichotomous fashion so that manifestations are either organic or functional. Assuming that such an entity as MBD does exist, the most helpful way of understanding

it is through its repercussions on mental functioning, and it is a
mistake to isolate, investigate, and treat it as a separate entity. In
the absence of a complete workup in every case, the hypothesis
postulating that MBD plays a major etiological role in the causation
of a variety of psychiatric disorders could lead to the launching of
complex research programs with the aim of discovering vulnerable
children by contrasting them with those supposed to be normal. This
distinction would result in specific directions for treatment, through
drugs, for example. This methodological approach has merely the
appearance of being scientific, and is in reality simplistic and
shortsighted. Moreover, central nervous system investigations tend to
produce equivocal and controversial findings. Above all, a program
of this nature carries the additional risk of isolating, on rather
questionable grounds, children who may be in danger of overzealous
investigation and sorely in need of treatment.

On the other hand, there are cases where the evidence strongly
suggests the existence of MBD, which is bound to weigh heavily on
the psychological development of the child affected, and it is
therefore very logical to deal with the problem of obstetrical risk by
the appropriate preventive measures. What we have been saying in
no way dispenses with the institution of basic precautions. We are
stressing the fallacy of setting up normality against abnormality
without concluding that children suffering from these disorders
should also be treated for all the risks to which they are exposed.
Here, once again, the psychic repercussion of the disorder, as well
as the way in which it is caught up in relational experiences and in
mental development, should caution against the making of sharp
distinctions between preventive and therapeutic action. Studies of
the subsequent history of premature babies, for instance, seem to
show that departments specializing in premature care take insufficient
notice of what is known concerning the importance of the early
mother-child relationship. Only very recently have some units been
giving attention to the facilitating sensory contact between mother
and child to mitigate the aftereffects of a medically enforced
deprivation that must be held partly responsible for the fragility of
these children in later years. Since prematurity carries with it the
risk of mental difficulties, it would also be well to apply, in suitable
cases, methods of therapy that are not one-sided but have multilateral
aspects allowing the integration of data concerning the body image

as well as the organization of the self through a reparatory relationship.

Conclusion

We have discussed the notion of normality in the evaluation of psychiatric risks that threaten the child. This did not seem useful on the one hand because the absence of symptoms does not necessarily mean that all is well, and on the other because the recognition of psychopathological disturbances certainly does not depend, in the case of children, on the presence of manifest symptoms or of observable anomalies. We feel that all children must overcome the consequences of the primary ambivalence affecting their psychological life at its inception and the desires that go along with it. In every case, development depends on the child's innate endowment as well as on vicissitudes in his relationships. The risk is therefore greater when the child lacks the support of a family to provide the necessary instruments of socialization or when some deficiency or accident of birth hinders his development.

We have especially tried to point out the danger of studying these problems from a one-sided point of view, which could well lead to false conclusions based on unproven hypotheses or to the isolation of their meaning, conducing to a relative neglect of mental functioning, a topic that warrants patient inquiry, combined methods of therapy, and cautious conclusions.

References

1. Canguilhem, C. *The Normal and the Pathological.* Presses Universitaires de France, Paris, 1966.
2. Chiland, C. *The Six-Year-Old Child.* Presses Universitaires de France, Paris, 1971.
3. Freud, Anna. *Normality and Pathology in Childhood Assessments of Development.* International Universities Press, New York, 1965.
4. Goldstein, K. *Organism.* Beacon Press, Boston, 1963.
5. Prole, L. *Mental Health in the Metropolis.* McGraw-Hill, New York, 1962.
6. Stringer, L. A. Academic progress as an index of mental health. *J. Social Issues,* 15 (1959), 16–29.

Some Paradoxes Connected with Risk and Vulnerability

Colette Chiland, M.D., Ph.D. (France)

In the double-entry table constructed by Anthony [1], in which high and low risk are connected with maximal and minimal vulnerability, two categories seem especially pertinent to this presentation: children at high risk who seem relatively immune, and children at low risk who prove to be very vulnerable. An attempt is made here to understand and illustrate these two paradoxical outcomes from data drawn from a longitudinal study of 66 children selected at random from the general population, and from clinical material obtained in the practice of child psychiatry [5, 6, 8].

Two problems will be considered:

Predictable risks for groups exposed to similar predicaments and amenable to statistical investigation.

Unpredictable vulnerabilities that are a function of individual susceptibilities.

Predictable Risks

There are two main risks in a Western culture that threaten the child: the risk of becoming psychiatrically disturbed, and the risk of

23

failure at school. There is, of course, a certain amount of overlapping of the two categories.

School failure is sometimes the consequence of other psychological difficulties and sometimes the earliest manifestation of psycho-pathology. It is seldom possible to establish a direct relationship between school failure and adult mental disorder. More frequently, school failure is followed by lack of success in the employment field.

School achievement, on the other hand, can be closely linked to the child's psychic organization, to the psychic organization of his parents, to the structure of the family relationships, to the social-cultural status of the family, and to the structure of the school. On the elementary school level, success is of course largely a function of the intellectual level of the child; but given an equal intellectual level, success becomes a function of the *sociocultural level of the parents*. At the time the child begins school his intellectual level also depends on his past history in relation to the sociocultural status of his family. For the child coming from an inferior sociocultural level, the risk is appreciable that his learning to read will be delayed, and when this happens a snowballing of academic difficulties is likely, if no special intervention is made, for the rest of his school years. Even with vigorous intervention the lag is difficult to reduce.

These facts have been noted on a large scale in the United States, where the problems raised by the Blacks, the Puerto Ricans, the Mexican-Americans, and other minorities, are particularly dramatic; and they have also been investigated in England [9] and in France [7]. Schools in their present structure function well, or reasonably well, for children of middle- and upper-class families, but they often only exaggerate the handicap of those who come from the lower classes (with the exception of a few gifted and invulnerable individuals). Without the teachers' awareness, and usually contrary to their conscious wishes, the school system helps to maintain the social stratification of the society. The preliminary stage in prevention requires that the teachers be made consciously aware of this situation, which would then be followed by a series of interventions within the school, dealing with its organization and the teacher training programs. It is a surprising fact that within the same country with the same uniform educational system there can be both very good and very bad schools [10].

The problem, however, goes beyond the school, and nothing can evolve if the community does not feel concerned, as Comer [9] points out, and beyond the immediate community there is the larger political question: To what extent should the school play a compensatory role in equalizing social inequalities? Unless something of this is done, the situation will continue to exact its price in juvenile delinquency, in the production of mediocre and incompetent adults, and in psychosomatic and mental disorder.

What, then, are the sociocultural factors that put the child at risk for school failure? On intelligence tests in which verbal ability plays an important role, the testable intelligence of these children is inferior (which, of course, does not exclude the presence of superior intelligences among them), but even when they are on an equal intellectual level there is less chance for it to be turned to scholarly account. This undoubtedly has something to do with language development, as Bernstein [3] has shown. In a working-class milieu, the child is spoken to only in the context of actions to be performed, and there is very little occasion for the use of narrative language or metalanguage.

This attitude with regard to language, the absence of linguistic play, of parent-child playfulness, and of interest in cultural objects is a facet of what de Lauwe [12] calls working-class preoccupation behavior—job insecurity, reduced time at home, uncomfortable and overcrowded housing conditions, and so forth.

The child's upbringing and the care he receives in infancy depend on these same detrimental living conditions. The lower the socioeconomic level, the more frequently are infants hospitalized for illness and the greater the need to place children in residential homes and other institutions. When the level of intelligence that has been recorded at 6 years is found to fall in later childhood, frequent milieu changes in the first 6 years of life are common [7].

Even if one maintains that intelligence, at least in its operational form—concrete thinking—is partly independent of language (Piaget's thesis is that operational thinking is rooted in action and not in language), those environmental conditions that stimulate the development of language are frequently found to be, at the same time, stimulating the development of concrete operational thinking, and this is even more strongly the case with abstract thinking.

One could subscribe to the thesis that children who fail at school and show a decreasing testable intelligence are actually less intelligent that their successful peers only by classroom criteria. In terms of manual ability and natural lore that they will eventually acquire— the farmer's knowledge of nature or the fisherman's knowledge of the sea—they would come out largely ahead of the "intellectuals." It is a fact that the scale of values of our society is not the only one possible, but it is also a fact that these children, probably irreversibly after a certain age (10 to 12 years?), have lost the possibility of attaining a certain mode of mental functioning, which implies a better level of operational thinking, of language quality, and of fantasy. That means at least an impoverishment of mental life, but the question remains open as to whether this also entails a greater risk of mental illness; there is some evidence that this might be so [7].

At the level of secondary school, the risk of failure is linked to other conditions, in which the equilibrium of family relationships (the psychopathology of parent and child) is disturbed, but the risk of mental disorder is more in evidence.

Socioeconomic difficulties may increase the likelihood of psychopathology, but the risk is not as directly dependent on them as is elementary school failure. The conditions of psychopathological risk appear more difficult to define given the present state of our knowledge. The relationship is not a linear one between the fragility of endowment, anomalies of intrafamilial communication, such as the "double-bind," and the occurrence of neuroses, psychoses, and character disorders. In response to minimal pathology in parents, within the bounds of normal variation one sometimes sees major disturbances in the children. One cannot attribute everything or nothing to biological factors, everything or nothing to the psychopathology of the parents. The psychoanalytic viewpoint calls attention to the specific role of the subject, to his instincts, and to his defensive organization.

To quote Winnicott: "The child's illness belongs to the child— A child may find some means of healthy growth in spite of environmental factors, or may be ill in spite of good care" [14]. In our longitudinal study no family was without its hardships; however, the most threatening to the security of the child were the chronicity or repetitiveness of physical and mental illness in the parents or conflict between the parents. Nevertheless, families change in time for better or worse, and parents who are good parents at one stage of a child's life may not be good at another stage, and families may be favorable for one type of child and not for another.

Unpredictable Vulnerabilities

It is known that the intellectual impairment in a child with cerebral palsy is not proportional to the extent of the neurological lesions ascertained. There is even more reason, outside the field of evident organic illness, for forecasting to be difficult. Macroscopic factors manifest themselves, but the factors that protect or render the child more fragile are often microscopic and fugitive, or so that observation is difficult.

The children of psychotic parents are deemed to be at risk, but, as Winnicott pointed out, there may be mitigating circumstances. At stages of development, these parents can meet their children's needs. The most pernicious factor, according to Winnicott, is the unpredictability of mood changes [14]. In a recent work Lebovici [11] found that the open recognition by all of the parental illness as an accepted fact is a protective factor for the child, who would be in greater danger living with unrecognized borderline parents.

Unfortunately not all indisputably psychotic parents are under care, or even recognized as ill. In our longitudinal study, 3 out of the sample of 66 children (Nicolas, Paulette, and Berthe) had mothers with incontestable psychoses; 2 of the 66 had been seen by a psychiatrist (Nicolas' mother was schizophrenic and Paulette's mother delusional, but neither was under treatment). On making a home visit the social worker was horrified by the appalling conditions in which these children lived. Berthe's mother was unwed and suffered from delusions of reference. She had never consulted a psychiatrist and was not officially recognized as ill, and, as a consequence, there was no one in contact with the home to protect the child.

These three children were not suffering from childhood psychosis. Nicolas had been diagnosed as prepsychotic at the age of 6 years and this was confirmed at age 11. The two others fell within the normal range at age 6; at most one was struck by Berthe's silliness in spite of a near normal intelligence and a satisfactory school record. Over the years, however, small signs have suggested the existence

of breaks;[1] at 12 and 13 years, Berthe and Paulette began to
participate in the delusions of their mothers and one might predict
that a few adverse circumstances would lead to the development
of an adult psychosis. These children could have been considered
invulnerable; no one would have thought of bringing them for
psychiatric consultation, and an anamnesis taken at an adult age
would not have disclosed a disturbed childhood. It was the chance
participation in the longitudinal study that brought them to clinical
notice.[2]

The identification and full recognition of the parent's peculiar
behavior as an "illness" undoubtedly helps the child to come to terms
with it and protect himself from it, this being as true here as in other
family difficulties in which "secrets" and "skeletons in the closet"
operate harmfully. Some children become psychotic because they
have been compelled to live in a network of ambiguous family
relationships. Lebovici has reported a case (unpublished) in which
the child calls her unwed mother, who nurses her, "sister" and her
maternal grandmother "mother." We have encountered cases in our
practice in which massive learning difficulties resistant to remedial
teaching and psychotherapy, and inexplicable by any psychometric,
linguistic, or organic findings, have appeared to be significantly
related to the father's analphabetism, experienced as extremely
shameful and kept successfully hidden from the children.

CASE OF A

A Parisian, who had failed to learn to read at school, was the father of 12
children, 9 boys and 3 girls. The mother had attended secondary school. The 3
girls had no school problems, but all the boys were dyslexia. It suggested a sex-
linked genetic problem, but careful investigation disclosed that identification
with the father was at the root of the situation. The parents then decided to
reveal the father's "secret" and after this was done, the children (with the
exception of one child) made dramatic progress and succeeded in achieving
their professional apprenticeship. The matter was, of course, more complex
than this brief resumé would indicate: for example, the mother's choice of
marital partner was also involved.

---

[1] Anthony has described these "micropsychotic episodes," as well as childhood *folie à
deux*, in some detail [2].
[2] Anthony has referred to the curious fact that the disturbances of these high risk children are often undetected during childhood and attributes this to the "camouflaging"
by the environment. He has also pointed to the child's need to know about the
illness [2].

CASE OF B

A very intelligent worker who had learned to read but was unable to write except phonetically. He was so ashamed of this that he developed phobic behavior; refusing to drive a car because if involved in an accident he would be unable to fill out the necessary papers; refusing union responsibilities at the factory in spite of his keen questions because his "condition" would be discovered. His wife was under orders to destroy all messages that he wrote to her immediately after reading them. Only after he underwent intensive psychotherapy were the learning difficulties of the two children, a girl and a boy, resolved.

Children are particularly vulnerable to anything that discredits the parental image, and the earlier this occurs, the more detrimental it is to the construction of the ego ideal, an essential ingredient in intellectual development and school success.

The different children in a family may react very differently— to the same handicapping situation.

CASE OF FAMILY S

The parents were immigrants and unable to speak French well, and therefore unable to help their children in their school work. By 6 years, the daughter had mastered a very pure French, already knew how to read, and was a year ahead of her class in school, while her brother was backward both in reading and writing.

CASE OF FAMILY J

A girl and her brother were abandoned by their mother when they were, respectively, in their first and third years. They were placed successively in several foster homes before being taken in by an aunt and uncle two years later. The boy is failing at school, steals and runs away, while the girl, in spite of a mediocre intelligence (IQ: 88) and language difficulties, has done paradoxically well in school and is thriving. Working to her advantage is her capacity for attracting affection everywhere she goes, which has allowed her to obtain more attention and care than her brother in the same circumstances of deprivation.

These examples could be multiplied almost indefinitely and contrasted with cases in which children with every opportunity and talent have failed lamentably. One such case was the boy who had the highest intelligence quotient of all the children in our longitudinal study (IQ: 135). After a satisfactory beginning in elementary school, he began to fail academically and to show marked neurotic, masochistic, and self-defeating behavior.

Conclusion

All data from our study and practice lead us to conclude that
at the present state of our knowledge we are better able to define
situations of risk for the child than to identify the elements of
vulnerability or invulnerability. At best, we recognize them after the
fact, having observed a paradoxical resistance to stress or a
disconcerting fragility within an overtly satisfactory context.

When one studies a sample from the general population, one
comes up with numerous individuals who have experienced the same
stresses as patients and have emerged relatively unscathed. This leads
us to conclude that the critical factor determining vulnerability or
resilience to risk is not the risk itself but rather the relationship
between the risk and the person in terms of his psychobiological
makeup, his past history, his individual characteristics, and so forth.

What follow-up studies have shown is that only a relatively few
children whose childhood disturbances have necessitated psychiatric
care and major therapeutic measures (e.g., special boarding schools)
become mentally ill as adults. A majority find a niche in life at a
socioprofessional level that is inferior to what their intellectual ability
and sociocultural background would lead one to expect—mental
impoverishment in place of mental illness [4, 13].

What we now know, contrary to what was long thought, is that
the childhood of mentally ill adults has not been "silent," or
psychologically uneventful. The pathological manifestations were
simply not recognized, or were hidden or distorted in the
recollections of the parents. When a less biased report is available,
say from a former schoolmate, a history of peculiar episodic behavior
or personality traits usually can be obtained.

Excluding the patent psychoses of childhood, for which the
prognosis remains ominous, the most disruptive disorders are not
always the most dangerous for the future. Certain mildly neurotic
symptoms, such as phobias, are being regarded as almost part of
normal development, and in these times it would be almost
impossible to find a child who has grown up asymptomatically.
Among the 66 children in our longitudinal sample only one could be
said to even approximate to this ideal and she was by no means the
most interesting psychologically [7].

Much remains to be learned before we discover what, on different levels (biological, historical), causes vulnerability and before we know "the natural history of mental illnesses."

As we learn more on different levels, from the biological to the historical, about the complete "natural history" of mental illness from infancy to old age, we might reach a point when we can say something definite about the perplexing co-problems of vulnerability and invulnerability.

References

1. Anthony, E. J. The syndrome of the psychologically invulnerable child. In this volume.
2. Anthony, E. J. A clinical evaluation of children with psychotic parents. *Amer. J. Psychiat.*, 126 (1969), 2.
3. Bernstein, B. B. A sociolinguistic approach to socialization, in *Direction in Sociolinguistics*, J. Gumperz and D. Hymes, eds. Holt, Rinehart and Winston, New York, 1942.
4. Cahn, R. et al. Follow-up study of maladjusted children. *Sauvegarde de l'Enfance*, 16 (1961), 7–8, 521–602.
5. Chiland, C. School failures in the first grade. *Psychol. Francaise*, 9 (1964), 1, 15–26.
6. Chiland, C. et al. Epidemiological data from a follow-up study of school children. *Bull de E'I.N.S.E.R.M.*, 21 (1966), 3, 455–466.
7. Chiland, C. *The Six-Year-Old Child and His Future*. Presses Universitaires de France, Paris, 1973.
8. Chiland, C. Daily practice and research in relation to a follow-up study. *L'Information Psychiat.*, 49 (1973), 7, 671–675. 1973.
9. Comer, J. The black child in school. In this volume.
10. Douglas, J. W. B. *The Home and the School*. MacGibbon and Kee, London, 1964.
11. Lebovici, M. *Living with a psychotic parent*. Doctoral Thesis, Paris, 1973.
12. de Lauwe, C. *The Daily Life of Working Class Families*. Editions du E.N.R.S., Paris, 1956.
13. Robins, L. N. *Deviant Children Grow Up*. Williams and Wilkins, Baltimore, 1966.
14. Winnicott, D. W. The effect of psychotic parents on the emotional development of the child, in *The Family and Individual Development*. Tavistock, London, 1965.

Intervention Programs for Children at Psychiatric Risk; The Contribution of Child Psychiatry and Developmental Theory

Sibylle K. Escalona, Ph.D. (U.S.A.)

Child psychiatry as a profession, and child development as a science, have responded to social pressure and to overwhelming human need by focusing attention (not for the first time) on what we may have to offer, by way of programs or at least guidelines for programs, to reduce the incidence of pathology and maldevelopment in segments of the population that generate more than their share of developmental deviations. The two most relevant so-called target populations—those thought to be in greatest need of intervention—are the very poor and those children who display at birth or in early infancy deficits in the central nervous system (CNS), or other vital organic spheres. Nor are these two high risk groups independent of one another. It is among the poor that paranatal complications, prematurity, and "minimal brain dysfunction" (an umbrella term for diffuse and mild CNS deviations often associated with behavioral and developmental pathology) are the most frequent. There can be no doubt that untold numbers of potentially normal and able children become the victims of depriving, brutalizing, or wholly insufficient life conditions and grow up as damaged, unduly limited, or manifestly sick individuals. Mental ill health and its prevention are surely among the most important public health issues of our time.

To say that intervention on behalf of children at psychiatric and developmental risk is important and desirable is not equivalent to saying that our knowledge, theories, and techniques enable us to achieve the goal. Both child psychiatry and child development have reason to be wary. Earlier attempts to apply psychiatric knowledge preventively, in the areas of child rearing and education, have met with scant success. The same is true for the proscriptions and prescriptions based on other developmental theories such as parent guidance based on Arnold Gesell's work and child-rearing practices based on J. Watson's version of learning theory (which now has a renaissance in early childhood educative practices based on operant conditioning).

When inferences derived from psychodynamic or academic theory were translated into policies or procedures involving child-rearing techniques, they remained largely ineffective. Breast feeding, delayed and lenient weaning and toilet training, an emphasis on providing affection and close contact, and a host of other mental hygiene teachings did not prove of help to troubled mothers, nor did they reduce the incidence of childhood maladjustment. By the same token, children reared on strict schedules, children rewarded for desirable actions only, children taught and trained in close conformity to normative standards developed for each age level, all continued to produce their share of developmental failures. Each wave of authoritative advice on child-rearing "ideology," insofar as parents did in fact adopt recommended practices, did affect the manner in which children adapted and developed to some extent and may have affected the focal areas of conflict and developmental difficulty,[1] but was regularly followed by widespread disenchantment and a swing in the pendulum of both expert and public opinion to the opposite extreme.

At first glance it would appear that the combination of clinical experience and conceptual articulation of the etiology of psychiatric illness, along with the skills involved in effective therapeutic intervention and a theory of personality development that articulates the special needs, phase-specific conflicts, and capacities of children

[1] For instance, in the United States the so-called permissive era of child rearing during the 1950s brought a reduction in the incidence of feeding disturbances but an increase in sleep disorders and some other symptoms.

do provide the information needed to identify high risk populations and to develop preventive intervention programs to minimize or counteract the risk. Moreover, psychoanalysis was the first psychological theory to recognize what has since been confirmed by both biological and psychological research: experience during the formative early years is decisively important for later personality development. Therefore preventive and remedial efforts would logically be directed at children still young enough to be at risk and not yet impaired or damaged in their functioning.

Closer scrutiny of what is implied in such a statement raises serious questions. The identification of groups or populations who are at psychiatric risk is not a simple matter. Retroactive study, whether in the form of individual case studies or in more systematic clinical research, has shown beyond a doubt that particular life stresses, deprivations, frustrations, and traumata during the preschool years are significantly related to later psychiatric illness or deviant impaired development. Among psychiatric patients, as well as among persons showing learning failure, psychosocial pathology, and other overt malfunctioning, the incidence of maternal psychopathology, of family disruption, of separation and loss at crucial times, of neglect, conflict, isolation, of harsh, punitive, or inappropriate child-rearing practices and many other malign features is greater than in so-called normal, that is, unselected populations. The same applies to risk factors of an intrinsic sort. Controlled studies have left no doubt that groups of children showing cognitive deficit and/or social/emotional pathology differ from the population at large in that a disproportionally larger number were premature, experienced paranatal complications, or showed ambiguous diffuse indications of neurological dysfunction in infancy. *Retrospectively,* the association between biological risk factors and many environmentally determined social and psychological risk factors has been demonstrated.

However, *prospective* studies—the effort to predict on the basis of identified risk factors a greater frequency of developmental deviations and psychopathology—have not fared as well. The fact is that none of the specific high risk factors, such as child-rearing practices, family disruption, psychopathology of parents, and the like, predict later psychopathology. The very same traumatic events or deficits that do produce maladaption and illness in those who become patients are also found among large numbers of normal individuals, who, for reasons we have yet to learn, sustain these risks without significant impairment of personality development. In other words, knowing the child-rearing practices of parents, and knowing that events potentially disruptive or traumatic have occurred, does not predict the developmental outcome for the child.

This discrepancy between results obtained from retrospective and prospective investigations is not limited to environmental and specifically psychiatric risks. For instance, prematurity, minor neurological deviations, and paranatal complications are widely recognized as high risk factors in relation to cognitive and overall development. Yet when such high risk babies are longitudinally studied and examined at later school age, they do not differ significantly from normal control groups either in intelligence or in the incidence of pathology [1].

The work of Bowlby [2] and Bowlby and Ainsworth [3] on the effect upon young children of abrupt separation from the mother is a good example. Bowlby, Spitz, and many others showed that such separation nearly always leads to massive disruption, regression, failure to learn, and symptoms akin to those of depression—the symptomatology observed is so severe that lasting and irreversible damage to personality development was assumed. Yet when school-age children who had in common the experience of early separation / hospitalization were examined, these children functioned well both cognitively and socially. There was a slightly greater incidence of minor adjustment problems in this group as compared to the control, but severe psychopathology had not occurred as the result of early separation. In other words, manifest psychopathology in early childhood does not necessarily predict later maladjustment.

Anna Freud, on the basis of rich clinical experience, came to the same conclusion and specified the manner in which the unforeseeable events during important later phases of development will determine the resolution of earlier conflicts and imbalances, or the failure of such resolution [4, 5]

The term high risk implies the expectation that the presence of specific identifiable attributes of the environment or the organism greatly increases the probability that psychopathology will occur. In the psychiatric and psychological domain such an expectation is contradicted by all available research data.

Yet there is one relationship between early life conditions and developmental outcome that is incontrovertibly established. Severe and chronic poverty does lead to a far higher incidence of psycho-social and cognitive impairment and pathology than is found in other socioeconomic strata. (At least in industrial societies, the only setting for which the information is available.) This relationship has been confirmed in prospective and other varieties of controlled investigation.

In all respects normal development is threatened by being born and reared under poverty conditions. However, even this unquestionable fact leaves unresolved two issues of great importance. First, while the incidence of cognitive deficit, maladaption, and psychiatric illness is higher among the poor, the prediction is statistical and not case-specific. No one has yet succeeded in predicting which individuals among the high risk population defined by low socioeconomic status will show deviant developmental outcome, and which individuals will survive intact. Much less can we predict the kind or the severity of later pathology for individuals in such a population. Second, we do not know at what ages or developmental time spans poverty conditions critically interact with the child's functioning. Recent research suggests that, except for the greater incidence of neurological and other physical disabilities, socioeconomic status does not significantly contribute to either cognitive or social and emotional maldevelopment during the first two years of life [6, 7].

Since we do not know with clarity which components of life in poverty affect what aspects of personality development or when these malignant effects occur, the only "intervention" logically supported by the facts is to eliminate poverty as such—a social goal so obviously desirable that scientific justification is irrelevant. Implementation of the changes needed to approach this goal clearly falls beyond the range of psychiatric competence.[2]

Another implication of the general premise that psychiatry can at present devise effective intervention programs is that we know enough about viable normal and optimal conditions for personality development to do so. Psychiatric understanding of children's needs and of their development largely derives from experience with the manifold ways and multiple determinants of maldevelopment. To

---

[2] It is the author's personal belief that appropriate action within the body politic has greater promise in relation to preventive psychiatry than does neutralizing accommodation to the "risks" generated by the status quo.

place positive intervention efforts on this basis is not dissimilar to the notion that a wholesome diet can be prescribed once poisonous foods have been identified. In the past mental health advice has indeed partaken of this quality. It stressed the avoidance of noxious influences more than elucidation of supportive and facilitating conditions and actions in their place. Or else, what was recommended as strengthening and supportive was defined as the near-opposite of the noxious. If too little body contact between mother and baby, or the impersonal mode of feeding via a propped bottle can be harmful, breast feeding and high levels of tactile stimulation were recommended; if early harsh toilet training is detrimental, then great delay and an absence of social pressure for bowel control became the model. To remain with the nutritional analogy, it was as though once the ill effects of starvation diets were known, the goal became to overfeed. Nonclinical branches of developmental theory also have failed to focus on normal processes of personality development, and on the necessary and sufficient conditions on which it rests. In addition to developmental sequences with respect to certain part functions, and to isolated aspects of learning, perception, and cognition, all we do know with certainty is that children can and do develop normally—though differently—under widely different conditions of existence.

Turning now to a conceptual analysis of the terms high risk and intervention, and relating these to one model of child development, will prove that the difficulties mentioned do not lie with our understanding of personality development (incomplete though it is) but rather with a failure to logically and consistently apply the theory to concrete issues. Furthermore, when an interactional model of child development is taken seriously, our hard-won understanding of how children grow, of the threats and obstacles to normal personality development, and of responsive therapeutic intervention are relevant to the issue of preventive and/or supportive efforts in behalf of endangered children.

To begin with, the term high risk derives from a conceptual model alien to all psychodynamic theories in that it is a statement of probability. As such it must be based on actuarial data; at very least it requires statistical information concerning the expected frequency of a phenomenon in normal populations, as contrasted to the frequency of the same phenomenon in selected populations. The severity of risk is then a function of the difference between the two frequencies. For significant psychosocial and psychiatric pathology such actuarial data do not exist, nor is it self-evident what the appropriate "normal population" from which expected frequencies could be derived would be, if for no other reason than that different cultures and different societies do not judge normalcy versus aberration by the same criteria. In this context the term intervention refers to programs to be administered to "target populations," on the assumption that certain experiences or certain procedures will benefit all recipients.

Both notions address themselves to what a group or a population has in common, disregarding differences in external circumstances or in the individual's response to them. Just as children without families, poor children, or those born prematurely are selected for their communalities, so perceptual cognitive stimulation, group experience, or child-rearing advice to parents is delivered in essentially the same manner to all. Definitions and programs of this sort are entirely appropriate and impressively effective in many areas of public health when they arise within an epidemiological frame of reference. For instance, mass inoculation proved its merit despite the fact that in rare instances the individual response to the vaccine is malign. It must be remembered that not only actuarial data but scientific comprehension of the relevant biochemical and physiological phenomena were needed to mount this medical intervention program.

In contrast, psychiatric theory and developmental psychology, insofar as they deal with total personality development, are of an entirely different sort. This theory came about through the detailed, essentially qualitative study of individuals, and of the infinitely varied complex settings that shape their lives. General psychological and developmental principles and regularities were derived and distilled on this basis, and then in turn applied to individuals, further observations leading to changes and refinements in the theory. The conceptual models so evolved find confirmation and refutation not through actuarial data, not through prediction and stringent experiment, but through the convergence of many strands of evidence in the same direction, through their explanatory power, and through effectiveness in application to concrete life situations. The prototype of this variety of theory building in its most advanced form is the theory of evolution, which followed the same pattern and only very late in its development began to permit limited experimental test. It is occasion for neither wonder nor chagrin that a *direct* translation of psychiatric understanding into probabilistic and epidemiological systems is ill fated.

Nonetheless, theories of child development arrived at in this manner require independent and objective confirmation before they can become the basis for social action that will affect the lives of children and their families. It behooves us to develop a theory that is compatible with *all* known facts of relevance, be they experimental, epidemiological, pedagogical, or simple commonsense observations. As a step in that direction, the author has elsewhere suggested a model of the developmental process that is compatible with both clinical and more general developmental facts [8]. The central issue is how we are to understand the interaction between environmental and intrinsic, constitutional and maturational factors as both determine developmental outcome. We know that there is no specific and constant relationship between any group of environmental factors or of biological intrinsic characteristics and a particular developmental consequence, but we know also that all relevant characteristics of the environment and of the child organism can and do alter development and its outcome; thus it is necessary to include with our conceptual scheme something about the pathways through which these external and internal determinants enter the develop- mental process. In brief it is proposed that it is not the objective environmental facts, nor the special dispositions and capacities of the organism that—even in aggregate—predict for an individual child personality characteristics, defense structure, learning patterns, vulnerabilities, and whether or not normal adaptation will be achieved. By virtue of both organismic and acquired characteristics each child selectively perceives, interprets, and processes all of the objective real features of the particular environment to which he must adapt. Conversely, lability of the central nervous system, high or low levels of sensitivity or reactivity, cognitive, sensory or motoric deficits, or any other characteristic of the child, will affect him differently depending on the demands, challenges, supports, and requirements provided by the social and physical environment.

The missing link or intermediate variable between extrinsic and intrinsic determinants, on the one hand, and developmental course and outcome, on the other, is the concrete constellation of experience patterns; that is, the manner in which whatever forces and conditions prevailing at any time affect the event structures, the perceptions, feelings, meanings, and most of all the actual content, intensity, and sequencing of immediate experience. The consequence of interposing an *intervening variable* between that which determines experience patterns (the aggregate of extrinsic and intrinsic factors) and the experience patterns themselves is that the issue of how the child will be affected by what befalls him and by his own characteristics is not viewed as the mathematical resultant of all relevant inner and outer factors but as the outcome of complex reciprocal processes between these factors. We therefore look for consistent and in principle predictable relationships between experience patterns and developmental outcomes.

Before tracing the consequences of such a model for the task of identifying high risk populations and of developing intervention programs, one example may clarify the implications. The syndrome of infantile autism has universally been found associated with (and, indeed, partially defined by) the absence of normal reciprocal patterns of social and affective mutual responsiveness between the infant and his mother (or mother surrogate). For many years the antecedent—the "cause" for this illness—was searched for in the personality characteristics of the mother. Mothers of autistic children were found to be distant, cold, somehow incapable of providing for intimate and highly attuned contacts with their children. Decades of clinical investigation forced recognition of the fact that autism occurs in families where the mother's mode of functioning in no way corresponds to such an image. Closer observation also showed that often it is the baby who is unable to respond normally to appropriate and even exquisite maternal care. Finally, organic pathology could be detected in some patients and was suspected in many more. Controversy between the "organic" and "psychogenic" view concerning the etiology of infantile autism continues, with solid evidence on both sides.

In our developmental model the facts in no way contradict each other. If we assume that the lack of a reciprocal, affectionate, animated social bond between infant and mother-person is the critical experience deficit, leading to infantile autism or other psychopathology, all facts confirm the invariant link between this experiential variable and subsequent symptomatology. However.

a lack of normal mother-baby interaction may come about largely because the infant is incapable of providing his share of the interaction (the organic view); it may occur because of mother's inability to relate normally to the baby (the psychogenic view); or it may come about as infants vulnerable on this score are matched to mothers who have more than ordinary difficulty in responding to their babies, and cannot sufficiently accommodate to the "difficult" and relatively unresponsive baby. Regardless of how this came about, wholly inadequate human interactions in infancy lead to concurrent and subsequent childhood psychopathology.

To the degree that we know or can discover such links between significant constellations of experience patterns at various age levels and their impact on critical components of developmental progress, we are in a position to specify who is at risk, what the risk consists of, and at least approximately how great the risk. The evidence for the existence of risk factors would then come from an appraisal of a child's functioning at a given time and in a given setting, not from the absence or presence of predetermined environmental or organismic conditions. For instance, to use an example in the foreground of current thinking, a toddler surrounded by appropriate toys and action opportunities and by responsive caretakers is—in terms of his experience—not receiving rich perceptual and social "stimulation" if in fact he does not attend to or explore the objects or engage in the expected varieties of social interchange with other people. Conversely, a surprising number of infants and toddlers from objectively impoverished family environments prove to be active, exploratory, well-developing youngsters who are able to derive sufficient stimulation from transactions with the perceptual and action opportunities that remain in the absence of toys, didactic games, and excursions to the park.[3]

The recognition that the same external circumstances and events may have widely different significance for different individuals and at various developmental stages is axiomatic in the realm of clinical psychiatry. It is also part and parcel of all so-called dynamic or holistic theories of child development. All that the interactional

---

[3] The same cannot be said, or at least is reported far less often for somewhat older children from precisely the same milieu. At later preschool ages and beyond, experience patterns probably critical for cognitive and certain aspects of personality development may not be within the range of what a life style dictated by severe chronic poverty can provide.

model of development as sketched above attempts to do is to carry the implications of this recognition into the areas of preventive applied child psychiatry as well as into the logical structure of research designed to validate developmental theory.

Where does all this leave us with respect to our contribution to the social problem of how best to safeguard the development of children who are in fact at psychiatric risk?

1. Certain extreme conditions that constitute a risk factor are readily identified and agreed upon. They include children without families, children grossly neglected or abused, children reared in a setting of chronic severe poverty, and children who display significant specific deficit or abnormality involving the central nervous system and/or the sensorium.

An interactional model of child development, as well as clinical experience, suggests that systematic intervention programs applied in much the same manner to all children in such populations should be limited to remedial social and medical procedures that decrease or remove the intrinsic or environmental stress condition. That is, for infants without families a setting providing fairly stable and highly personal contacts with one or a few caretakers (in family day care, foster care, or appropriately designed group settings) is needed. Those grossly neglected or abused similarly require removal to a less threatening and reasonably stable environment. Those suffering from neurological or other bodily impairment require medical supervision and access to remedial treatment programs. And any and all actions that improve housing, employment, nutrition, and any other tangible hardship due to poverty will indirectly counteract the root of so much evil.

However, interventions directed at altering the attitudes and child-raising techniques of parents, or interventions aimed at providing stimulation, or any programmed sequence of experiences presumably growth promoting for all, will have to be tentative, experimental, subject to careful evaluation, certainly for children below the age of 3 or 4 years. In short, such efforts would be viewed and presented not as solutions implemented on a large scale but as field studies designed to provide much needed information about early development.

2. Instead of massive efforts to alter the life experience of young children in certain predetermined ways, the interaction paradigm suggests that preventive efforts in behalf of potentially endangered children consist chiefly of the early identification of overt developmental deviations, and remedial intervention as dictated by the nature of the aberration. On the assumption that adequate

adaptation and developmental progress at any one phase of childhood leaves
the individual better prepared to take the next developmental step and that
significant malfunctioning during a given developmental period is likely to leave
the child more vulnerable to stresses yet to come, it is reasonable to focus interventions on those members of the high risk group who are in fact exhibiting
developmental difficulty.

In practice, this means screening devices, diagnostic facilities, and
most important, services offering social, educative, psychiatric,
medical, and whatever other supports may be required to meet the
specific needs of children at various ages beset by particular
developmental problems. In these areas both the skills and the
specialized knowledge of child psychiatrists and of child development
specialists are relevant, if not yet fully adequate.

3. If the aim is to detect developmental difficulties as they arise, and to provide
whatever kind of intervention is appropriate to those identified as in need of
help, and believing also that screening and remedial services for high risk
populations as conventionally defined must have high priority, there remains
the vital issue of evolving appropriate developmental services.

In accordance with our model, and indeed in accordance with
clinical experience, we do not expect that all available modes of
remedial or corrective intervention will be equally effective. Again,
the source and nature of the difficulty, the particulars of the child's
(and the family's) past and present experience, will provide clues
as to whether support and guidance to the parents, direct work with
the child, educative, medical, psychotherapeutic, or purely environmental manipulations may be most appropriate. Last but not least, if
the focus is on healthy personality development (rather than mere
competence in the performance of cognitive or social skills), present
knowledge makes it difficult to distinguish between universal
developmental needs and cultural variations, all of which are equally
viable from a developmental and social point of view, though some
of these patterns may not conform to the values held by the
professionals who render service. Knowing that the strength and
validity of human relationships within and beyond the family are the
single most important factor supporting personality development
during childhood, and that the integrity of such relationships is
linked to pervasive yet highly personal sets of values, expectations,
and goals developed within subcultures, we should recognize the
danger of disrupting intrafamily equilibrium if the remedial

intervention is based on assumptions and goals alien to the recipient of the service. Manipulation of the powerless by those with power is an inherent danger in all programs affecting people's lives. Preventive psychiatric efforts need to avoid both the appearance and the reality of invading the right of families to maintain their own style of life and of child rearing—as long as their choices do not demonstrably damage the child's development.

In summary, the implications of what has been said are that the only high risk population that is defined by actuarial criteria refers to children reared in severe and chronic poverty. Moreover, psychiatric risk cannot presently be defined in terms of either specific environmental or biological variables, except for extreme instances. However, manifest and overt developmental deviation and/or malfunctioning in itself constitutes a risk factor. Those who, at any stage of childhood, fail to thrive and fail to achieve the developmentally appropriate patterns of personal, social, or cognitive functioning are necessarily at a disadvantage when confronted with the requirements, opportunities, and stresses encountered in later childhood and maturity.

Hence programs leading to the identification of developmental disorders as soon as they appear, accompanied by a whole range of services prepared to meet the special needs of these children, constitute an approach that makes best use of the skills that psychiatric, psychological, and other childhood specialists now possess. Such programs are adapted to the theory of personality development based on a dynamic and structural interaction model. They allow families, communities, and agencies who care for children to select the kind of help they can accept and avoid the danger of externally imposed change and the social climate of manipulation or coercion that can evoke. Finally, such programs require practitioner and scientist alike to gather relevant experience and information on which to build a more complete and effective understanding of behavior and development.

References

1. Sameroff, A. J. and Chandler, M. D. Reproductive risk and the continuum of caretaking casualty, in *Review of Child Development Research*, Vol. 4. F. D. Horowitz, M. Helherington, S. Scarr-Salapatek, and G. Siegel, Eds. University of Chicago Press, Chicago, 1974.

2. Bowlby, J. *Maternal Care and Mental Health*. WHO Monograph Series No. 2, Geneva, 1951.
3. Bowlby, J. Ainsworth, M., Boston, M., and Rosenbluth, D. The effects of mother-child separation—A follow-up study. *Brit. J. Med. Psychol.*, 29 (1956), 211–247.
4. Freud, A. Child observation and prediction of development. *Psychoanalytic Study of the Child*, Vol. XIII. International Universities Press, New York, 1958.
5. Freud, A. *Normality and Pathology in Childhood*. International Universities Press, New York, 1965.
6. Golden, M. and Birns, B. Social class and cognitive development in infancy. *Merrill-Palmer Quarterly*, 14:2 (1968).
7. Birns, B. and Golden, M. Prediction of intellectual performance at three years from infant test and personality measures. *Merrill-Palmer Quarterly*, 18: 1 (1972).
8. Escalona, S. *The Roots of Individuality*. Aldine, Chicago, 1968.

A Theory of Adaptation and the Risk of Trauma

Ernest A. Haggard, Ph.D. (U.S.A.)*

Those who work with children generally agree that terms like adaptation and trauma designate important aspects of experience and behavior and also refer to states which, for practical purposes, can be identified and described without much difficulty. Theorists tend to differ, however, as to how to conceptualize the behavior phenomena we call "adaptation" and "trauma." The differences among theorists' views probably stem from differences in their implicit or explicit assumptions about the determinants of human behavior. These differeing assumptions lead to different theoretical formulations which, in turn, lead to different notions of how such concepts or states as adaptation and trauma should be understood and, if necessary, dealt with.

Theorists' acceptance or rejection of two assumptions seems to account for many of the contradictions in how they view human behavior in general and adaptation and trauma in particular. One assumption has to do with whether the effects of the stimuli, drives, and so on, which appear to initiate and maintain behavior are essentially linear, additive, and independent, or whether they tend

* This work was supported in part by a Research Career Program Award (MH-K6-9415) from the U.S. Public Health Service, grant G69-465 from the Foundations' Fund for Research in Psychiatry, and an award from The Grant Foundation.

to be nonlinear and patterned. The second assumption has to do with whether the determinants of behavior can be separated meaningfully into those which are internal or external to the individual or whether they must always be considered in concert (with more than lip service to their inseparability). At the risk of gross oversimplification, these two assumptions will be considered briefly.

The First Assumption. The conceputalization of behavior exclusively in quantitative terms which are linear and additive has many attractions, one of which holds out the promise of enabling one to reduce and describe seemingly complex phenomena in terms of a limited number of simple dimensions. Thus one may speak of degrees of adaptation (or trauma), or of adaptation and trauma as being at opposite poles of a single dimension. The reliance on linear conceptualizations also leads one to assume that, over time, the same dimensions—and the relationships among different ones—will tend to remain relatively stable. This type of conceptualization of human behavior probably is derived from the theories of "classical" (not "modern") physics.[1] In contrast to this approach, theorists such as Freud, Erikson, and Piaget emphasize the interdependence and nonlinear aspects of behavioral determinants, especially as the individual passes through a series of phases or stages on the path from infancy to maturity.[2]

The Second Assumption. It has long been customary to distinguish between, and to deal separately with, the inner and outer determinants of human behavior (e.g., "drives" versus external stimuli). This distinction probably is based on the fact of man's skin —the boundary or interface between his body and the world in which he lives. But it does not follow that this boundary should be used in attempting to conceptualize the determinants of man's behavior, just because it is useful in distinguishing his physical being from his environment. In fact, it is likely that many of the classical

[1] See Becker [1] for an analysis of how the eighteenth-century philosophers changed the substantive but not the formal aspects of their theories of man and his world.
[2] The nonlinearity of most (if not all) bodily processes is taken for granted, but because we are accustomed to thinking in linear terms we transform (to try to make linear) the indices of bodily processes so that they conform to our customary ways of thinking and our systems of arithmetic and data analysis [2]. See also Piaget's [3] discussion of the roles of systems and structures in the conceptualization of human behavior.

"problems" that have plagued theorists (e.g., nativism versus environmentalism) stem from this unnecessary and inappropriate distinction.

In the discussion which follows emphasis is placed on two propositions: first, the determinants of behavior depend in part on the individual's stage of physical and psychological development and, second, in conceptualizing behavior the individual cannot be considered apart from his environment context.[3] More specifically, a behavioral system will be outlined and used to discuss some aspects of adaptation and trauma, including a consideration of effects of changes over the individual's life cycle and various status changes, and to speculate about how one might forestall or ameliorate such maladaptive states as trauma.

A Behavioral System

Aspects of this system were summarized in connection with a survey of literature on situations in which individuals underwent "experimental isolation" in laboratories, or periods of extended isolation in nature, and as a consequence of these experiences showed a variety of perceptual, cognitive, emotional, and related behavioral disturbances [5].[4] For our purposes here this summary can be quoted in part, as follows:

> This system has three major components: A, the energetics of behavior; B, the structures and schemata, innate or acquired, that organize and regulate behavior, overt or covert; and C, the environmental context in which the behavior occurs.
>
> The A, B, and C components are, of course, familiar constructs.[5] For example, the A component corresponds in general to what has been called primary or basic drive, id, impulse, urge, or motivational state. The B component, which

---

[3] To say that both the inner and the outer determinants must be considered simultaneously with respect to any behavioral event or episode is to state in somewhat different terms Lewin's [4] contention that behavior is a funtion of the person and his environment.

[4] Man's often bizarre experiences and behaviors under conditions of isolation, especially when such conditions are unfamiliar to him, indicate his (greatly underestimated) dependence on his usual environment for the maintenance of his "normal" or customary behavior patterns. See also Zubek [6] for a survey of the literature on the sensory and perceptual deprivation studies.

[5] The major components of this system are presented in the form of abstract symbols such as A's, B's, and C's in order to avoid the verbal entanglements that would arise if the concepts and terms referred to by these symbols were used, since they differ in meaning and usage from one theoretical orientation to another.

involves the means by which the individual interacts with his environment (e.g., perception, learning, memory, thinking, and overt response) has been referred to by such terms as mind, self, and ego, and various constructs (e.g., associations, central integrations, cell assemblies, engrams, memory traces, psychic structures, and schemata) have been inferred to account for the development and nature of the B component. The C component refers to parts or all of the total environmental stimuli, reality, field or context, including the cultural, social, and physical aspects of it, and to which the "individual" (i.e., the A and B components must relate in one way or another. Although these three components are not quite coordinate and the boundaries between them are not quite clear, it is essential to keep in mind that the three components must be considered in concert and as aspects of a conceptual unity.

The behavioral system involving the A, B, and C components rests on certain general assumptions or propositions, such as:

1. At birth the normal infant possesses the constitutional structures necessary for survival in a benign and supportive environment. This assumption implies the existence of those primitive B structures and/or schemata which permit at least minimal articulation (or adaptation) between the A and C components which are normal for neonates.

2. Along with the rapidly developing neurophysiological structures, new schemata develop to facilitate new ABC articulations under increasingly complex but relatively specifiable A and C conditions. In the human being, the system initially is dominated primarily by the A component (i.e., the infant is "practically all id"), but with time the B component develops in relation to an increasingly complex C component, so that (relative to A) B and C come to play increasingly important roles in determining behavior. Along with the intrinsic differences in the properties of individuals' A, B, and C components, with time increased definition develops between the A and B and the B and C components and the relationships among them, so that individuals will differ with respect to their AB, BC, and ABC definitions and relationships.

3. Particular B schemata "have their roots" in both the particular A and C components existing at the time such B schemata are developed. Subsequently, particular B schemata will be activated if the associated A's and C's exist and are sufficiently imperative. (Haggard [5] pp. 444–446)

The following propositions also pertain to states such as adaptation and trauma:

4. Although the infant comes "equipped" with some behavior patterns that reflect rudimentary B schemata (sometimes called instincts), they are modified over time as they articulate between the developing A component and the characteristics of the C component (e.g., lower or middle class, urban or rural) to which the individual is exposed and learns to adapt.

5. New B schemata develop in accordance with "the laws of learning," which involve, for example, the nature and strength of

the A's (e.g., the strength of one or more "drives"), the nature and stability of the existing B schemata,[6] and various spatial and temporal patternings of the C component (e.g., strength and timing of the conditioned and unconditioned stimuli in classical conditioning.

6. With time, and as the individual becomes "socialized," the B schemata serve to "bind"[7] the A component with respect to particular C contexts, with aspects of the C component serving to support or reinforce the B schemata. Consequently, if important aspects of C are lost (as in isolation and bereavement), B will be weakened, and a "nonsocialized" expression of A may occur (ref. 5, pp. 458–462).

7. With respect to the articulation of the A, B, and C components (i.e., adaptation), the development of B schemata (i.e., new learnings) sometimes go awry. This may happen in two ways. First, B schemata may be developed which fail to articulate effectively between the A and C components, hence do not bind A sufficiently; in that particular respect the individual's behavior is not "socialized."[8] Second, B schemata may be developed which bind A effectively—but too well, in the sense of not being normally amenable to modification as subsequent changes occur in the A's and C's.[9]

8. In general, the behavioral system loses plasticity over the course of its life span, partly because the energies of the A component wane with time and partly because of the availability of existing B schemata, which are appropriate to the C conditions with which the individual has become familiar.[10]

---

[6] What and how much an individual can learn at any time will depend in part on his prior experience history. This is particularly apparent when he has suffered a marked deprivation of "normal" experiences [7–9].

[7] Murphy [10] used the term canalization to describe this process.

[8] This condition may exist when, for example, the individual is expected to acquire B's before he is developmentally ready to and/or because the C component lacks the stable "objects" whose presence otherwise would facilitate the development of the B schemata that would be required to bind A.

[9] Such B *schemata* (or learnings) typically occur when A and/or C components are so strong or dominant that they "overwhelm" B. On the level of overt behavior one usually describes the results of such B schemata as fixated or stereotyped responses, which are highly resistant to extinction or relearning. On the covert level such B schemata may account for the differences between the superego and the ego, in that the former is assumed not to be amenable to modification as a result of the customary ABC articulations but tends to be modified only on an appropriate reinstatement of the ABC conditions (or surrogates of them) which existed when the maladaptive, relatively unmodifiable, B schemata were initially established.

[10] Except for periods of strong motivation or arousal, the main exception to this generalization occurs during puberty, which, among other things, involves the resurgence and refinition of the A component.

Thus adaptation generally involves articulation among the A, B, and C components at any given time. But the fact that a state of adaptation exists does not designate the nature of the three components or of the specific interrelationships among them. For example, adaptation may exist for an infant who is hungry, is able to take food, and has access to an appropriate food source—but for an adolescent, a young adult, or an elderly person, adaption can differ enormously in terms of the definitions and interrelationships among the three components. Conversely, a state of stress may be said to exist within the system—with the potential risk of trauma— when at least one of the components does not articulate well with the others (i.e., when the system fails to "get it all together"). Thus trauma may result when, under particular C conditions, the B schemata cannot bind or regulate A (e.g., uncontrolled anger), or when C is sufficiently foreign or threatening, so that the individual (AB) is not able to deal adequately with it (e.g., in extremt isolation, or in battle).

These propositions will be elaborated with respect to the effects of changes or continuities over the life cycle and various changes in status or other conditions. In doing this, the discussion of the life cycle emphasizes the characteristics of the A and B components and the AB relationships; the discussion of status changes emphasizes effects of changes in the C component and the relation of the existing A and B components, and their relationships to such changes.[11] No attempt is made to be thorough and systematic; rather, representative conditions and studies are cited to indicate some of the factors that may result in states of adaptation or of trauma in terms of the behavioral system that was outlined earlier.

The Life Cycle

Perhaps man's greatest resource for adapting to himself and the world in which he lives is the extent of his "time-binding" ability. It not only enables him to develop cultures, with all their diversity and richness, but it also enables him to build upon and profit from his own experiences as an infant, as a child, as an adolescent, and as an adult. By and large his prior experiences later serve to his

---

[11] The distinction between these two emphases corresponds in general to the proposition that adaptation (or stress or trauma) can result from predominately "intrapsychic" or "external" sources. See also Haggard [5], pp. 462–465.

advantage, insofar as they prepare him for dealing with future events—but this is not always the case. In the absence of a benign teleology, it frequently happens that what the individual learns early in life may restrict or even preclude later adaptation.

One way that early learning tends to interfere with later adaptations lies in the discontinuity, or incompatibility, of what an individual is taught as a child and how he is expected to act as an adult. For example, in our culture it has been common to train young children to nonaggressive and nonsexual as preadolescents, but with the expectation that they will be aggressive (or at least assertive) and sexual as adults [11]. It can be assumed that the more frequently and traumatically the young child is trained to be nonaggressive and nonsexual, the more difficult it will be for him to adapt later to the adult roles of assertiveness and sexuality.

Another way that early learnings may interfere with later adaptations occurs when the early learnings themselves are maladaptive. One relevant example is found in a study of poor and good work adjustment in adults (defined in terms of whether an individual was able both to use his skills effectively and to find satisfaction in his work). As children, the poorly adjusted individuals tended, for example, to identify with unstable and immature adults, to experience strong feelings of rejection, to develop strong antagonisms toward their parents and rivalries with their siblings, and to be deeply ambivalent toward their early home situation. The well-adjusted individuals showed a pattern of early home experiences and reactions which, in general, was the reverse of the pattern for their poorly adjusted counterparts [12]. As adults, the individuals in both groups apparently carried the modes of adaptation that they had learned as children into their adult work situations, especially with respect to how they related both to themselves and to other individuals.[12]

---

[12] Essentially the same phenomenon of generalizing inappropriately from one individual (e.g., the father) to another (e.g., the boss) occurs in many other situations. In terms of the behavioral system outlined earlier, one can hypothesize that for the individuals in the poorly adjusted group, the *AB* relations (e.g., ambivalence, anxiety, or even revenge) they developed as children with respect to one aspect of *C* (their father, as both a person and as an authority figure) were reactivated (see proposition 3) in the work situation, especially if the boss resembled the father in appearance as well as in the role of authority figure. In psychoanalytic or other psychotherapeutic situations the term "transference often is used to designate this phenomenon, especially when particular "internalized" aspects of *C* (e.g., of the father) are involved.

Some early learnings which initially are adaptive may inadvertantly
turn out to be maladaptive. For example, in a study of a class of
high-achieving children who were observed and tested from the third
grade through high school [13] many faltered in their schoolwork
for a time when pubertal changes occurred. Furthermore, some of
the "best" students seemed to be faced with an awesome decision:
to yield their very superior level of academic achievement or to
yield the prospect of psychosexual maturity. Generally speaking, this
decision had to be made by those students who with a vengeance had
focused their major interest in life on intellectuality and academic
achievement. It appears that several children who chose intellectuality
rather than suffering the temporary disorganizations of adolescence
remained in a psychological-intellectual latency period and came to
resemble those "intellectuals" who excel as critics of others' work
while remaining essentially sterile as scholars.[13]

Although behavioral plasticity decreases with age, the extent of
man's ability to adapt to different environmental contexts is
indicated by the wide variety of cultures that exist and to which
infants adapt.[14] Bombard [15] also suggests that, other things equal,
children are more likely to weather a crisis situation than adults are.[15]

[13] These generalizations are based on systematic observations and interviews, and on
intelligence, achievement, and personality tests on all of the children. Although the
propositions discussed here are not based on statistical tests of the data, such tests
were made in a similar study of college freshmen [14] with compatible findings. In
terms of the proposed behavioral system, it can be assumed that some of the children
had developed rigid and highly effective *B* schemata in association with a
prepubertal *A* component (which included latent anger toward those who had pushed
them excessively to achieve academically, and which emerged as a keen critical and
competitive attitude toward their fellow students and teachers, and often their
parents as well). With the onset of puberty, and the consequent redefinition of the
A component, some of the children apparently chose to maintain (or were afraid not
to maintain) the prepubertal *AB* relation rather than developing new ones in
association with the changing *A* component, because to do so would have interfered
too much with their current high level of academic achievement. (The average
performance for the group as a whole on standardized achievement tests—the 50th
percentile for them—corresponded to the 95th percentile on the national norms.)
[14] With respect to linguistic skills, for example, it is said that every normal infant
spontaneously makes all the speech sounds that are used in all the languages spoken
by man. By middle childhood, however, much of this plasticity is lost, so that most
individuals will speak a second language (i.e., one not native to them) with a
discernible accent.
[15] In commenting on the sinking of the Titanic, Bombard wryly observed, "When the
first relief ships arrived, three hours after the liner had disappeared, a number of
people had either died or gone mad in the lifeboats. Significantly, no child under the
age of ten was included among those who had paid for their terror with madness and
for their madness with death. The children were still at the age of reason" (p. x).

However, by the time an individual reaches advanced age new adaptations may be difficult, to say the least. In a study of elderly persons' entering a home for the aged, Lieberman [16] found that the typically high first-year mortality rates "apparently are related to the impact of institutionalization on the aged but are not related to average age on admission or to the number of chronically ill persons admitted" (p. 515). In general, elderly persons prefer to maintain or reinstate those *C* conditions that are familiar and in which they are comfortable—that is, for which appropriate *B* schemata exists—so that they do not have to make major new adaptations.

Since behavioral plasticity facilitates adaptation, it is regrettable that all individuals lose some of their adaptive potential as they grow older. But individuals within any cultural group differ with respect to how rapidly they "age" in this sense. In addition to possible genetic or other physical determinants (e.g., illness or tissue damage), individuals differ in behavioral plasticity in part because of the experences they have undergone. For example, children who experience "favorable" home conditions retain a greater degree of adaptability than children who have suffered early traumatic emotional experiences, or been reared under a high degree of stress, or under minimally stimulating environmental conditions, or been deprived of maternal care. Correspondingly, the members of some sociocultural groups retain a greater degree of behavioral plasticity than others. For example, individuals reared in urban settings tend to be much more adaptable to new situations, especially those involving complex social interactions with strangers, than do their counterparts reared in families who live essentially in geographic and social isolation [17, 18]. Since the isolates learn to relate primarily to members of their family until they go to a small boarding school at age 7, they not only develop exceptionally close ties with the members of their own family, but they also lack the urban child's range of casual experiences with a wide variety of other persons. In other words, individuals born and reared on an isolated farm, as compared with those born in an urban setting, lack the opportunity to develop the "psychic mechanisms" (*B* schemata) that would enable them to relate easily to others.[16]

---

[16] Social isolates have remarked that after they have lived, say, 35 years on an isolated farm, they are not able to live comfortably in towns or cities where they would have to relate constantly to other persons.

Status Changes

The term status changes is used to refer to alterations in one or more aspects of C, the environmental context. But since the A, B, and C components are interdependent, changes in C can be expected to effect changes in the characteristics of the coexisting A and B components—which could, in turn, alter the psychological and physiological functioning of the behavioral system.

Some of the psychological effects following changes in the C component have already been noted, such as the changes associated with the experimental isolation studies. Another example is the likelihood of an infant's depressive reaction following the prolonged absence of his mother [19]. Physical illness in an adult also may result from the loss of a loved one [20] as well as from the run-of-mill life changes which add to the general "wear and tear" of the system [21, 22]. Although any change in the C component presumably taxes the behavioral system to some extent, effects of changes in C appear to be most profound when the loss of "cathected objects" is involved, that is, the loss of those aspects of the environmental context which matter most to the individual (Haggard [5], pp. 458-462).

On a broad cultural scale, disruption of the familiar world and habitual ways of relating to it may have a disorganizing effect on behavior and, in turn, increase the likelihood of stress and trauma. The disruptions that accompany war, with their effects on mores and behavior, are a case in point. In this connection, it may be that the asocial and demoralized behavior that characterizes the "mountain people" [23] stems as much from their loss of homeland, and hence their traditional way of life, as from the scarcity of food in the arid land they now occupy.[17]

One aspect of a change in the C component which may influence the adaptation of the individual (in the sense of making him more vulnerable to stress and trauma) involves changes in the historical-cultural-psychological atmosphere in which he lives. At one time— say, in the Middle Ages—Western man presumably was secure in his knowledge of what he could depend upon, both in this world and in the next. But much of this certainty has been lost following

---

[17] It is not difficult to note similarities between the disintegration of the culture of the mountain people and corresponding effects when Native Americans were confined to reservations and African Negroes were uprooted and forced to work the plantations in America.

a series of events, including the Renaissance, the Reformation, the Age of Reason, the Industrial Revolution, and the rise of science and technology (which have culminated in "the bomb"). And meanwhile man has suffered a series of ego-deflating losses: for example, following Copernicus, the loss of his place in the center of the universe; following Darwin, his uniqueness among living creatures; and following Freud, his rationality as the guiding force of his inner life and his behavior. Such events as these have contributed to the erosion of what once were the eternal verities of Western culture and now, in an atmosphere in which few uncertainties exist, it is hardly surprising that many individuals experience the anxiety of uncertainty [24]. It is characteristic of the current intellectual and esthetic expressions of our time, whether in literature, the theater, or in art, to reflect such uncertainty[18] or even the "absurd" nature of man's experience, insofar as it does not relate in any understandable way to a sense of meaning and order in one's world [26] and hence in one's life.

What To Do About Stress and Trauma?

If adaptation involves the articulation of the *A*, *B*, and *C* components, then stress occurs when, for some reason, the components do not articulate adequately. But because the three components are interdependent, and each of them is subject to change (sometimes fortuitously), everyone experiences stress from time to time. If the stress is intense and/or prolonged enough, trauma (which indicates a functional breakdown of the system) will result.

The conditions that encourage and also alleviate stress and trauma may be grouped into two broad classes. One class has to do with the relatively short-term states of stress and trauma that result when one or more of the components fail to articulate fully with the others. This class of phenomena frequently reflects an individual's difficulty in managing his behavior effectively in a

---

[18] Marriott [25], for example, in discussing art around the turn of the present century, observed that "some artists, like Rousseau, stayed in Paris but inhabited a strange world of their own. France was changing rapidly, enormous technological advances were taking place—trains, airplanes, derigibles, balloons, suggesting the telescoping of time and space. There are no airplanes in the paintings of Picasso and Braque; instead there are suggestions of the breaking up of traditional ideas of time and space."

threatening environmental situation.[19] The other class of phenomena has to do with stress and trauma that continue over a substantial period of time, and involves a threat to the individual's psychological and physical well-being. The alleviation of this type of stress or trauma calls for the change of established behavior patterns as well as change of methods for dealing with particular events.

One way to minimize short-term stress is to prepare the individual ahead of time so that he will not be caught off-guard by abrupt and unexpected events, and by his reactions to them.[20] As an example of the benefits of such preparation, Glasserman [28] found that when children about to have eye surgery were fully informed of the nature of the operation and what to expect when their eyes were bandaged, and could talk with other children who had recently undergone and recovered from the operation, they experienced substantially less stress—and trauma—than children who underwent the operation without this preparation.

Sometimes events produce disquiet or even stress not because they are in any way threatening to the individual but because they fail to support previously established habits, expectancies, or other modes of adaptation. It is probably for this reason that McLuhan [29] suggested that an internationally televised Roman Catholic mass "might be able to stabilize the 'psychic lives' of (Church) members disturbed by the changes of Vatican II" (p. 49). As discussed earlier, the reinstatement of a cathected aspect of the *C* component can be expected to support the *B* schemata as they articulate with aspects of the *A* component.

It is not always possible, however, to effect changes in the *B* and *C* components, as described in the preceding examples, to minimize stress and the risk of trauma. But it is frequently possible to effect

---

[19] For example, in connection with a survey of the psychological causes and results of stress, it was observed that "A person is able to act realistically and effectively in such a situation only if he knows the nature and seriousness of the threat, knows what to do, and is able to do it" (Haggard [27], p. 448).

[20] This procedure, by developing the needed *ABC* articulations (symbolically if not actually), tends to preclude excessive stress or trauma when the "real" stress-producing situation occurs. In some situations, such as preparation for battle, the training may involve a gradual approximation of the risks of battle, because "Realistic training under realistic conditions of stress is a necessary procedure if many individuals are not to become psychiatric casualties when confronted by actual danger. In fact, one observer believes that 'shell shock' is nothing but insufficient training" (Haggard [27], p. 447).

a "fit" between the characteristics of an individual's *A* and *B* components and the requirements and gratifications associated with his environmental context:

> A person may adjust successfully to some situations, even though he is a misfit in others. For example, an accident-prone individual might be placed to advantage in a commando or paratroop unit, where he could satisfy his tendency to find excitement in risk—but not aboard a submarine. Again, an individual whose only point of vulnerability is a dread of being alone should not necessarily be disqualified for submarine duty, because the occasion which would arouse his anxiety would not exist in this situation. On the contrary, his need for group support may even facilitate his adjustment as a submarine. (Haggard [27], p. 456)

Although most individuals shun situations involving short-term stress, it is not at all uncommon to find them persisting in specific habits, or in a general way of life, that increases the likelihood of the ultimate stress and trauma. The use, or the excessive use, of stimulants and other drugs are too familiar examples of this phenomenon. It is ironic, furthermore, that whereas many individuals can learn to deal rather effectively with specific instances of short-term stress, their success in dealing with long-term stress of this sort often comes with great difficulty.

The behavior patterns involved in long-term stress tend to be intractable because all three components and their interrelationships must be involved and must be modified for the behavior change to be "successful"—that is, durable.[21] However, the likelihood of changing maladaptive behavior patterns is reasonably good under certain circumstances. For example, if an individual is motivated enough (the *A* component) to seek aid and support voluntarily from an organization such as Synanon or Alcoholics Anonymous (the *C* component), and to learn something of others' problems and the sources of his own (the *B* component), and to participate in those activities that are directed toward helping others as well as himself to change his own behavior, while also learning to control his craving for the drug (*A-B* interactions), the likelihood of a durable behavior

---

[21] In this connection Etzioni [30] cites a wide range of maladaptive or otherwise less than adequate behaviors which prove to be resistant to change. In those instances where only one component is involved, little if any evidence exists of important adaptive change. For example, to know and fully appreciate the effects of smoking cigarettes (the *B* component) is hardly sufficient to break "the habit," or to be exposed to improved educational opportunities (the *C* component) may not result in improved academic achievement [31].

change is reasonably good. But to speak of behavior changes that involve the articulation of all three components and their interactions is to speak of what usually is called the socialization process. In both instances, extensive changes in the three components to eliminate maladaptive behavior and the socialization process in children are similar in the extent to which the individual must learn to master both his inner life and his behavior in an environmental context.[22] Furthermore, the goal is the same in each of these cases: to maximize adaptation and thus minimize the risk of stress and trauma.

References

1. Becker, C. L. *The Heavenly City of the Eighteenth-Century Philosophers* Yale University Press, New Haven, 1932.
2. Haggard, E. A. On the application of analysis of variance to GSR data: I. The selection of an appropriate measure. *J. Exp. Psychol.*, 39 (1949), 378–392.
3. Piaget, J. *Structuralism*. Basic Books, New York, 1970.
4. Lewin, K. Behavior and development as a function of the total situation, in *Manual of Child Psychology*, L. Carmichael, Ed. John Wiley & Sons, New York, 1946, pp. 791–844.
5. Haggard, E. A. Isolation and personality, in *Personality Change*, P. Worchel and D. Byrne, Eds. John Wiley & Sons, New York, 1964, pp. 433–469.
6. Zubek, J. P. Behavioral and physiological effects of prolonged sensory and perceptual deprivation: A review, in *Man in Isolation and Confinement*, J. E. Rasmussen, Ed. Aldine, Chicago, 1973, pp. 9–83.
7. Bowlby, J. *Maternal Care and Mental Health*. World Health Organization, Geneva, 1951.
8. Thompson, W. R. Early Environment—Its importance for later behavior, in *Psychopathology of Childhood*. P. H. Hoch and J. Zubin, Eds. Grune & Stratton, New York, 1955, pp. 120–131.
9. Riesen, A. H. Stimulation as a requirement for growth and function in behavioral development, in *Functions of Varied Experiences*, D. W. Fiske and S. R. Maddi, Eds. Dorsey, Homewood, Ill., 1961, pp. 57–80.
10. Murphy, G. *Personality: A Biosocial Approach to Origins and Structure*. Harper, New York, 1947.
11. Benedict, R. Continuities and discontinuities in cultural conditioning. *Psychiatry*, 1 (1938), 161–167.

---

[22] Although children do not submit easily to all aspects of the socialization process, adults who set out to "resocialize" themselves probably find the task much more difficult than children do. Adults suffer at least two disadvantages that children do not have: a relative decrease in behavioral plasticity and the constant availability of previousy developed *B* schemata and *AB* relationships, which, although latent, provide a ready alternative to the new behavior patterns. The term regression is used when the previously established behavior patterns recur and, with respect to the current environmental context (*C*), are judged to be maladaptive.

12. Friend, J. G. and Haggard, E. A. Work adjustment in relation to family background. *Appl. Psychol. Monogr.* 16, Stanford University Press, 1948, pp. 1–150.
13. Haggard, E. A. Socialization, personality, and academic achievement in gifted children. *School Review,* 65 (1957), 388–414.
14. Haggard, E. A. Personality dynamics and intellectual achievement, in *Achievement in the College Years: A Record of Intellectual and Personal Growth,* L. Murphy and E. Raushenbush, Eds. Harper, New York, 1960, pp. 116–133.
15. Bombard, A. *The Voyage of the Heretique.* Simon and Schuster, New York, 1953.
16. Lieberman, M. Relationship of mortality rates to entrance into a home for the aged. *Geriatrics,* 16 (1961), 515–519.
17. Haggard, E. A. and von der Lippe, A. Isolated families in the mountains of Norway, in *International Yearbook of Child Psychiatry, The Child in His Family,* Vol. I, John Wiley & Sons, New York, 1970, pp. 465–488.
18. Haggard, E. A. Some effects of geographic and social isolation in natural settings, in *Man in Isolation and Confinement,* J. E. Rasmussen, Ed. Aldine, Chicago, 1973, pp. 99–143.
19. Spitz, R. A. Hospitalism: An inquiry into the genesis of psychiatric conditions in early childhood, in *The Psychoanalytic Study of the Child,* Vol. I. A. Freud, H. Hartmann, and E. Kris, Eds. International Universities Press, New York, 1945, pp. 53–74.
20. Parkes, C. M. The first year of bereavement. *Psychiatry,* 33 (1970), 444–467.
21. Gunderson, E. K. E. and Rahe, R. H., Eds. *Life stress and Illness.* Charles C. Thomas, Springfield, Ill., in press.
22. Levi, L., Ed. Stress and distress in response to psychosocial stimuli. *Supplement No. 528 to Acta Medica Scandinavica,* 191 (1972), 1–166.
23. Turnbull, C. M. *The Mountain People.* Simon and Schuster, New York, 1972.
24. Tillich, P. *The Courage to Be.* Yale University Press, New Haven, 1952.
25. Marriott, C. Impressionism to cubism in 9 minutes. The Art Institute of Chicago. Film produced for The Art Institute of Chicago by Mike Gray Associates, 1973.
26. Nostrand, H. L. French culture's concern for relationships: Relationism. *Foreign Language Annals,* 6 (1973), 469–480.
27. Haggard, E. A. Psychological causes and results of stress, in *Human factors in undersea warfare.* National Research Council, Washington, D.C., 1949, pp. 441–461.
28. Glasserman, M. R. La psicoprofilaxis quirúrgica: Una técnica de prevención. *Acta Psiquiát. Psicól. Amér. Lat.,* 15 (1969), 239–244. See also Glasserman, M. R. y Sluzki, C. E. Psicoprofilaxis quirúrgica: Una investigación acerca de su efectividad. *Acta Psiquiát. Psicól. Amér. Lat.,* 15 (1969), 261–264.
29. McLuhan, M. McLuhan predicts televised liturgy. *Montreal Gazette,* June 9, 1973, p. 49.
30. Etzioni, A. Human beings are not very easy to change after all. *Saturday Review: The Society,* June 3, 1972, pp. 45–47.
31. Coleman, J. S., Campbell, E. Q., Hobson, C. J., McPartland, J., Mood, A. M., Weinfeld, F. D., and York, R. L. *Equality of Educational opportunity.* U. S. Government Printing Office, Washington, D.C., 1966.

THE BLED CONFERENCE

The Bled Conference* On Genetic-Constitutional and Early Childhood Factors in Risk

Meeting of The International Study Group on "Children at Psychiatric Risk" at Bled, Yugoslavia, July 24-28, 1972

PARTICIPANTS

CHAIRMAN:	E. James Anthony, M.D.,** *President International Association for Child Psychiatry and Allied Professions*
CO-CHAIRMAN:	Serge Lebovici, M.D.
SESSIONAL CHAIRMAN:	Reginald Lourie, M.D.
RAPPORTEUR:	Albert Solnit, M.D.
LOCAL ORGANIZERS IN YUGOSLAVIA:	Maja Beck-Dvorzak, M.D. Eduard Klain, M.D.

INVITED SPEAKERS

Norman Garmezy, Ph.D.
Sally Provence, M.D.
Michael Rutter, M.D.
Leon Rosenberg, M.D.
Julius Richmond, M.D.
A. Minkowski, M.D.**
Herbert Leiderman, M.D.

*Sponsored by the National Institute of Mental Health, the Grant Foundation, and the Commonwealth Fund.

**Also presented a paper.

OFFICIAL DISCUSSANTS

Joseph Marcus, M.D.**
Stanislau Krynski, M.D.
Winston Rickards, M.D.
Elizabeth Irvine, M.S.W.**
Reimer Jensen, Cand. Psych.
Jon Lange, M.D.
Lionel Hersov, M.D.**

ORGANIZERS OF THE INTERNATIONAL CONGRESS OF CHILD PSYCHIATRY AND ALLIED PROFESSIONS, 1974

Herman Belmont, M.D.
Herman Staples, M.D.
Sylvia Brody, Ph.D.
Norman Lourie, M.S.W.
Theodore B. Cohen, M.D.

PARTICIPANTS FROM YUGOSLAVIA

Nada Anić
Maja Beck-Dvoržak, M.D.
Petar Erak, M.D.
Eduard Klain, M.D.
Anica Kos-Mikus, M.D.
Vojin Matić, M.D.
Karlo Pansini, M.D.
Savka Morić-Petrović, M.D.
Branko Poljak, M.D.
Ljubiša Rakić, M.D.
Milica Vlatković-Prpić, M.D.

Director of Grant Foundation

Philip Sapir

Introduction: Risk and Mastery in Children from the Point of View of Genetic and Constitutional Factors and Early Life Experience

Lionel A. Hersov, M.D., M.R.C.P.,
F.R.C. Psych., D.P.M. (England)

"Risk" and "mastery" are two important but apparently disparate concepts. Risk has different connotations, one active as in "risk taking," the other passive in the sense of being "at risk." Mastery on the other hand clearly includes the notion of activity power and control. "At risk" is primarily a statistical concept in epidemiology applied to groups or population samples, whereas mastery refers to a psychological process in an individual. The aim of this paper is to discuss the relation of these two concepts to each other in terms of genetic and constitutional factors and early experience.

Genetic and Constitutional Factors

Berger and Passingham [2] discuss the proposition that many quantifiable characteristics, behavioral and physiological, are manifest at or shortly after birth, citing studies by Sander [28] Thomas et al. [29], and others. They have little doubt that genetic differences underlie the physiological and behavioral differences between individuals, acting through various structural and metabolic pathways which affect behavior, although little as yet is known of this. They suggest that there is evidence for continuity or a degree of enduring "bias" varying between individuals in the ways in which they interact with the postnatal world, and so determine in some degree the effects of early experience.

Korner [18] has suggested that individual differences at birth when they *do* contain the rudiments of later characteristics may affect development in both the early stages and the long run. She assumes that the differences are possibly neurophysiological in origin and interact with experience to form a persistent style of dealing with and mastering later developmental tasks. Korner suggests that the pattern of impulse control and differing ways of dealing with excitation favor the formation of particular sorts of ego defenses and cognitive characteristics.

Other studies suggest that certain traits, qualities, or characteristics, possibly hereditary in nature, may be predictive of subsequent disorder in early or late childhood. Relatively stable individual patterns of automatic functioning have been described in neonates [25], and identical twins show a greater degree of similarity than do fraternal twins [15]. It has been suggested that there is a relationship between strength of reactivity, conditionability, and later development of neurotic disorders, while automatic lability has been linked with characteristics found in conduct disorders [4, 19], although the latter has not been supported by later studies [31]. The variable of "activity level" regarded by some as genetic or constitutional in origin [12] has been linked to later aggressive behavior. There are marked individual differences in neonates in activity level, which are said to be relatively stable in time. Escalona and Heider [9] have surmised that high activity level in infants is evidence of difficulty in mastering or limiting internal tension. It also elicits a larger variety of responses from people in the environment than does passive behavior. A study by Thomas, Chess, and Birch [34] examines the kind of temperamental characteristics present in children before the onset of behavior disorders.

Chess [6] has discussed the importance of early identification of children with a "high risk" of developing a behavior disorder and the dangers of indiscriminate labeling leading to unnecessary intervention and overprotection. The child's development may be handicapped in that opportunities for learning and constructive mastery are never permitted. Chess regards children with particular characteristics which lead to difficulty in meeting normal demands and expectations as particularly "at risk." A particular category of risk arises from vulnerability due to certain individual traits of temperament or behavioral style. The interaction between such children and family and community environment leads to deviant development and possible behavior disorder. Even if constitutional predispositions do exist either as neurophysiological patterns or as temperamental styles, the subsequent development of emotional disturbances must also depend on individual psychological development and experiences, including social learning.

The Child "At Risk"

The human organism as a self-maintaining organism is inevitably exposed to hazards and dangers from the environment throughout life. These may be of a simple physical kind, the wear and tear of daily existence, or more intense hazards from chemical changes in the atmosphere or extreme fluctuations in temperature as in certain occupations [33]. At this least complex level of risk, continuous cell replacement of various tissues, an aspect of growth in general, maintains a homeostatic balance and acts as a permanent insurance against the risks of damage from the environment [33].

The concept of "risk" under discussion is much more complex and includes hazards of a nonphysical kind such as genetic loading for psychiatric disorder, adverse environmental influences before, during, or after birth, the mechanical hazards of birth itself, and certain types of experience during infancy and early childhood. The notion of infants at risk arose from the findings that in a population of children who had survived the neonatal period there would be a small number requiring special care and treatment for a variety of handicapping conditions, thus meriting special attention by the Health Service in Great Britain. This attention included not only parent counselling and support, both psychological and material, but also protection at certain critical periods in the child's development. The emphasis was originally on disabilities affecting physical and intellectual functioning, but more recently the concept has been widened to include impairment of growth and development in general, including personality development. Handicapping condi-

tions vary widely from phenylketonuria, where the incidence is
known and where preventive measures can be applied to modify or
eliminate the effect of the cogenital enzyme defect, to a variety of
psychiatric disorders in children, where the frequency is more
difficult to estimate and where preventive measures have yet to be
evaluated.

Attempts were made to identify these children at risk *before* signs
of physical handicap became obvious to parents so that medical
help was sought. It was hoped, on the one hand, that early detection
of certain factors would lead to early identification of handicapping
conditions, possibly more effective treatment of the primary handicaps, and mitigation of secondary handicaps. There was also the
implicit hope that early identification of major hazards to growth
and development might lead to some means of eliminating them
entirely or reducing their effects. One example is the benefit derived
from inducing pregnant mothers to give up smoking. Smoking has
been shown to be associated with increased risk of perinatal death
due to the lowered birth weight of babies of mothers who smoke [5].

The earliest efforts at identification were aimed at screening
children with a history of some known cause of impairment or deficit
not visible or detectable until some time after birth, for example,
deafness, visual impairment, cerebral palsy, and mental subnormality,
all incidentally handicaps which are well known for their psychological and psychiatric concomitants. Efforts were later made to
extend the screening methods to cover a larger number of factors,
and the At Risk Register of vulnerable children came into being.
This was criticized on the grounds of difficulty in defining precisely
the factors that put an infant at risk, so that risk categories in
registers become longer and more inclusive. In some cases as many
as 60 percent of all live births were included on the register, thus
negating the advantages of selective screening.

A very recent study in Great Britain, The National Child Development Study (1958 Cohort) [8], has used perinatal and follow-up
data on 14,000 children to select the combination of perinatal
characteristics which offered the "best" prediction of later handicap.
Two groups of handicap were studied, one comprising 14 percent of
the sample included children with deafness, partially sighted children, those with cerebral palsy, severe mental subnormality, and a
small group with multiple handicaps. Good predictions of these

subsequent handicaps were high birth rank (fifth or later birth), an abnormal delivery, and abnormal signs or serious illness in the first week of life. The second group comprised children who because of educational or mental backwardness were receiving or were thought to be in need of special education at 7 years, 2.3 percent of the total sample. Good predictions of these later handicaps were high birth rank (fifth or later birth), illegitimate birth or father an unskilled worker, abnormal delivery, abnormal birth weight (below 2.500 grams or less), or born before 37 weeks or after 43 weeks.

The limitations and difficulties of using at risk factors in selective screening of infants to predict later educational backwardness is shown by the fact that in the second group a "high risk" group of 25 percent of the children on the register as a percentage of all live births would have included just over half of all the children later found to be affected. This shows how difficult it is to reach the goal set by Lindon [2], that a high risk group comprising 20 percent of all children would include a substantial majority of children later found to be handicapped. Davie et al. [8] comment that if suspicion of retarded development in the first year of life had been added to the perinatal factors mentioned above, prediction would have been improved. There was also no information available in the study on family history of defect, which might also have added to prediction.

Data of this kind show the difficulty of predicting later incidence of developmental handicap or psychiatric disorder using our present information on genetic loading, predisposition to different traits of temperament and behavioural response, and adverse early experience such as severe and persistent psychosocial deprivation. There are suggestions, but nothing more, from the Cohort Study of a cumulative effect of certain factors in increasing accuracy of prediction. However, at our present state of knowledge based on prevailing studies, we can say only that certain forms of physical handicap in infancy and early childhood are more predictive than others of later psychiatric disorder, for example, neuroepileptic disorders [27].

Adopted Children

There is a group of children, adopted children, who are worthy of study from the point of view of "high risk" in terms of genetic

and constitutional factors and early experience. In some instances
information about genetic loading is available [26], and a recent
study on illegitimate children [7] has set out the risks to which
mothers and babies are exposed in terms of pregnancy and paranatal
stress. The same study showed that those illegitimate children who
were adopted did better in later life than those who were not,
suggesting that there are factors in family life which reduce risk. On
the other hand, we know that adopted children are overrepresented
in clinical populations attending psychiatric facilities.

Risk-Taking

Anthony [1] has written of personality traits in certain anxious and
obsessional children who operate with wide margins of safety in
their daily activities and so seldom take risks, whereas impulsive,
overactive, and antisocial children enter into situations of danger
and risk more frequently and repeatedly. Studies of children with
excessive susceptibility to accidents have shown that in a small
number the accident seemed to be satisfying emotional needs for
attention or resolving tensions but was more often associated with
bolder and more daring behavior and poor control in competitive
situations with older peers [20].

Fuller [13] found that nursery school children with the greatest
number of accidents showed common features of exceptional physical
strength, daredevil attitudes, emotional instability, and impulsivity
with the highest rate among those who were "insistent and obstinate"
and "rude" [14]. Other studies have shown accident repeaters to be
more aggressive in doll play [17], aggressive and dominating in social
relationships by using their superior gymnastic skills and strength,
and also poor losers [3] and generally more emotionally and socially
maladjusted [23].

Mannheimer and Mellinger [22] have studied personality and
behavioral traits in 453 boys and 231 girls of 4 to 18 years matched
for age and social class with high, intermediate, and low accident
liability. The findings showed that daring, active, exploring, and
extroverted children were more likely to sustain accidental injuries.
The *boys* with more accidents tended to have characteristics that
impaired coping ability, so that with greater accident frequency there
was greater tendency to hostility to parents and peers, competitive-

ness, showing off, anger and impulsiveness when frustrated, careless-
ness and inattentiveness and social maladjustment. The pattern in
girls was less marked but similar, with a stronger association between
accident frequency and need for attention. Their conclusions were
that extreme accident repeaters are a small group showing a large
variety of characteristics and differing in degree and not kind from
less extreme accident repeaters but showing an increased probability
to accidents.

Mastery

The concept of "at risk" includes the notions of vulnerability and
liability, including susceptibility, to particular diseases, injuries, or
psychiatric disorders. This is in marked contrast to the elements of
activity, force, and power and the notion of overcoming which are
embodied in the term *mastery*.

Mastery in everyday use means a state or condition in which
authority, dominion, and sway are exerted to achieve subjection of a
person, complete understanding of facts or propositions, or complete
skill or facility in some motor activity (OED). The notion of
subjection and control of excitation, instinctual drives, painful affects
and ideas, and infantile conflicts is a central feature of formulations
about ego defenses in psychoanalytic psychology [10]. However,
Freud [11] wrote of children repeating in their play the impressions
of everyday life, so abreacting the affects experienced and thereby
mastering the situation, and Wills [32] has discussed how the limitations of capacity for play in blind children holds up their mastery
of their inner and outer world. Murphy [24], in her concept of
"coping mechanisms" whereby children deal with everyday demands
of life, regards this as a broader concept than defense mechanisms
since it includes the direct activities of children in dealing with the
environment, while Anna Freud [10] regarded these activities as
belonging more to the sphere of learning, education, and normal
psychology.

Current psychological research is as much concerned with
exploration, curiosity, spontaneity, manipulation, and activities
depending on external stimulus or arousal as with activities depending on internal drive states. White [30] has used the terms competence
and sense of competence to signify the degree to which a person feels

able to produce effects on his environment, human and nonhuman, to reach important goals, and to elicit desired behavior from others. The motive to perfect or master a skill in order to deal with the environment—effectance motivation—is regarded as important in the child's achievement of motor skills, grasping, reaching, walking, bowel and bladder control, reading, writing, painting and so on. Mastery in this framework includes not only control of impulse and affect but also cognitive and conative aspects in the sense of intellectual command of facts or propositions and facility in using instruments and materials.

Kagan [16] states that the motive for effectance seems to have its own primary foundation based on three related factors. The desire to match behavior to a standard (this requires a representation of some ideal state), the desire to predict and control environmental events, and the desire to define the self. Mastery can be gratified in almost any behavioral context; conversely, one can assume that gratification could be hampered by the limitations imposed by low intelligence, poor neurophysiological integration, and physical handicaps.

Summary

It is tempting to see mastery as one psychological process by which the organism adapts to limitations imposed by genetic and constitutional predispositions to inappropriate development or functioning:

Individual organisms are able to adjust their activities to suit those of the surroundings by processes of "adaptation" or more specifically "phenotypic modification" to distinguish it from adaptation of the genotype as a result of natural selection. . . . The process of phenotypic adaptation by the individual consists in receiving information that modifies the structure or functioning in such a way that it provides a better representation of environmental conditions. [33]

References

1. Anthony, E. J. The behaviour disorders of childhood, in *Carmichael's Manual of Child Psychology*, Vol. 2, P. H. Mussen, Ed. John Wiley & Sons, New York, 1970, pp. 667–704.
2. Berger, M. and Passingham, R. E. Early experience and other environmental

factors: An overview, in *Handbook of Abnormal Psychology*, rev. ed., H. J. Eysenck, Ed. Pitmans, London, 1972.

3. Birnbach, S. Comparative study of accident free and accident repeater pupils. Dissertation. New York School of Education, New York University, 1947.

4. Boyle, R. H., Dykman, R. A., and Ackerman, P. T. Relation of resting autonomic activity motor impulsivity and EEG training in children. *Arch. Gen. Psychiat.*, 12, (1965) 214–323.

5. Butler, N. R. and Alberman, E. *Perinatal Problems*. Livingstone, London, 1969.

6. Chess, S. Temperament and children at risk, in *The Child in His Family*, E. J. Anthony and C. Koupernik, Eds. John Wiley & Sons, New York, 1970.

7. Crellen, E., Kellmer Pringle, M. L., and West, P. *Born Illegitimate: Social and Educational Implications*. N.F.E.R., London, 1971.

8. Davie, R., Butler, N., and Goldstein, H. *From Birth to Seven*. Longmans, London, 1972.

9. Escalona S. and Heider, G. M. *Prediction and Outcome*. Basic Books, New York, 1959.

10. Freud, A. *The Ego and the Mechanisms of Defence*. Hogarth Press, London, 1968.

11. Freud, S. *Beyond the Pleasure Principle*. Hogarth Press, London, 1922, p. 15.

12. Fries, M. and Woolf, P. Some hypotheses on the role of the congenital activity type in personality development, in *The Psychoanalytic Study of the Child*, Vol. 8, R. Eissler et al., Eds. International Universities Press, New York, 1953, pp. 48–62.

13. Fuller, E. M. Injury prone children. *Amer. J. Orthopsychiat.*, 18 (1948), 708.

14. Fuller, E. M. and Baume, H. E. Injury-proneness and adjustment in second grade: A sociometric study. *Sociometry*, 14 (1951), 210.

15. Jost, H. and Sontag, L. W. The genetic factor in autonomic nervous system Function. *Psychosom. Med.*, 6 (1944), 308–310.

16. Kagan, J. Personality development in behavioural science, in *Paediatric Medicine*, N. Talbot, J. Kagan, and L. Eisenberg, Eds. W. B. Saunders, Philadelphia, 1971, pp. 283–349.

17. Krall, V. Personality characteristics of accident repeating children. *J. Abnormal Social Psychol.*, 48 (1953), 99.

18. Korner, A. F. Individual differences at birth. Implications for early experience and later development. *Amer. J. Orthopsychiat.*, 4 (1971), 608–619.

19. Lacey, J. L. and Lacey, B. *The Relationship of Resting Autonomic Activity to Motor Impulsivity in the Brain and Human Behaviour*. Solomon H. Cobb, S. Penfield, and W. Williams, Eds. Williams and Wilkins, Baltimore, 1958, pp. 144–209.

20. Langford, W. S., Gilder, R. J., Jr., Wilking, V. N., Genn, M. M., and Sherill, H. H. Pilot study of childhood accidents—Preliminary report. *Paediatrics*, 11 (1953), 405.

21. Lindon, R. L. Risk Register. *Cerebral Palsy Bull.*, 3 (1961), 481–487.

22. Mannheimer, D. I. and Mellinger, G. D. Personality characteristics of the child accident repeater. *Child Devel.*, 38 (1967), 491.

23. Marcus, I. M., Wilson, W., Kraft, I., Swander, D., Southerland, F., and Schulhofer, E. An interdisciplinary approach to accident patterns in children. *Monog. Res. Child Devel.*, 25, no. 2 (1965).

24. Murphy, L. B., The problem of defence and the concept of coping, in

The Child in His Family, E. J. Anthony and C. Koupernik, Eds. John Wiley & Sons, New York, 1970.

25. Richmond, J. B. and Lustman, S. L. Autonomic function in the neonate: Implications for psychosomatic theory. *Psychosom. Med.,* 17 (1955), 269–275.

26. Rosenthal, D. A programme of research on heredity in schizophrenia. *Behav. Sci.,* 3 (1971), 191–201.

27. Rutter, M., Tizard, J., and Whitmore, K. *Education, Health and Behaviour.* Longmans, London, 1970.

28. Sander, L. W. Regulation and organization in the early infant caretaker system, in *Brain and Early Behaviour,* R. J. Robinson, Ed. Academic Press, London, 1969.

29. Thomas, A., Birch, H. G., Hertzog, M. E., and Kann, S. *Behavioural Individuality in Early Childhood.* New York University Press, New York, 1963.

30. White, R. W. Competence and the growth of personality, in *The Ego,* J. H. Masserman, Ed. *Science and Psychoanalysis,* Vol. XI. Grune & Stratton, New York, 1967, pp. 42–49.

31. Williams, T. A., Schachter, J., and Rowe, R. Spontaneous autonomic activity, anxiety and "hyperkinetic" impulsivity. *Psychosom. Med.,* 27 (1965), 9–18.

32. Wills, D. Problems of play and mastery in the blind child. *Brit. J. Med. Psychol.,* 41 (1968), 213–222.

33. Young, J. Z. *An Introduction to the Study of Man.* Clarendon Press, Oxford, 1971.

34. Thomas, A., Chess, S., and Birch, H. *Temperament and Behavior Disorders in Children.* New York University Press, New York, 1968.

The Study of Competence in Children at Risk for Severe Psychopathology*

Norman Garmezy, Ph.D. (U.S.A.)

Introduction

The purpose of this chapter is to emphasize a particular aspect of the study of children at risk: their manifestations of competence. The study of competence or incompetence may well be the key to the patterning of vulnerability or invulnerability to psychopathology in those children within our society who are thought to have a heightened predisposition (relative to randomly selected children in the population) for the ultimate expression of behavioral disorder or aberration. I have used the twin terms of "vulnerability" and "invulnerability" to sharpen the problem posed by our efforts to predict disorder in children designated as being at risk, despite their variable outcomes—a heterogeneity evident to the joint focus on "risk" and "mastery" at the Bled Conference devoted to such vulnerable youngsters. In recent months the issue of invulnerability or freedom from disorder has been brought home more forcefully to our Minnesota research group following an extensive review generated jointly by Keith Nuechterlein and myself in which we

* Supported by a Research Career Award (MH-K6-14914), a grant from the Supreme Council Thirty-three, A.A. Scottish Rite, Northern Masonic Jurisdiction, and U.S. Public Health Service Contract PH43-68-1313.

focused largely on an unpublished literature devoted to the attributes
of competent disadvantaged children. A growing awareness of the
adaptive efforts of other children who are victims not of sociological
but of genetic disadvantage leads us in a similar direction. Indeed
we are led to the inescapable conclusion, atypical for a psychopathologist, that whatever etiological model for severe mental disorder one
espouses, more children, if followed into adulthood, are likely to
escape our dire predictions than will fall victim to them [9]. What we
are asserting is that our theories of the etiology of mental disorder,
whether rooted in biogenetic, sociological, psychological, or developmental factors, generate prediction errors of considerable magnitude
when applied to long-range forecasting of vulnerability in children.

Unfortunately, such errors pose a significant methodological
problem for investigators engaged in longitudinal-developmental
studies of children at risk who seek to determine, prior to breakdown,
those children who will succumb to, as opposed to others who will
resist, the encroachment of psychopathology. The problem is compounded by another research reality of equally significant dimensions.
In most instances of severe pathology, we are seeking to predict
adaptation or maladaptation not during childhood but rather at some
distant future time in adulthood extending into the middle years of
life. Consider the problem of risk for schizophrenia. More than a
dozen research teams in different parts of the world have taken on
this challenging problem. It is challenging because (1) one is coping
with a disorder of as yet unknown etiology (which poses the problem
of how best to select for risk), (2) with potential dispositional parameters which have not yet been demarcated clearly (introducing the
unresolved issue of what types of variable warrant study in risk
research), (3) accompanied by an anticipated heterogeneity in onset,
prognosis, and course (thus heightening the problem of the prediction
of outcome), and (4) in which the projected age of onset of the
formal disorder itself can extend up to a terminal point somewhere
in the vicinity of age 45. To attempt to predict ultimate outcomes for
a disorder as mysterious and as pervasive as schizophrenia requires
an invulnerable experimental spirit, and an extraordinary amount of
clinical and experimental acumen, together with a conceptual clarity
which the complex nature of the disorder tends to obscure.

Since few investigators possess all of these cardinal qualities, I
would urge that our research goals be of less heroic proportions and

that we develop a more circumscribed working strategy for risk research which, although more contained initially, might in the long run prove to be more productive.

Central to the strategy is the concept of competence—a concept that has proved its predictive power in the many studies of recovery or nonrecovery from schizophrenia which have been conducted over past decades. How shall we define competence? What are the qualities of the "competent" individual? Grinker [10] has attributed to Whitehorn an aphorism that sums up most succinctly a large segment of the literature, notably on the healthy personality, which has great relevance for prognostic factors in schizophrenia:

> Concerning mental health and the absence of a concept of positive mental health, I would like to give you a kind of cookbook definition developed by John Whitehorn, although it is not a complete statement. What I frequently tell my students is that people who are mentally healthy usually work well, play well, love well and expect well. I think that "expect well" is the most important in that there is an anticipation that the future will have something of value to them. (p. 23)

Variations in the degree to which one works, plays, and loves 'well' foretell who will recover from severe mental disorder. The designation of *process* versus *reactive schizophrenia* encompasses in its premorbid description these central aspects of quality of functioning. The Phillips Scale of Premorbid Adjustment in Schizophrenia [17], which has been used with marked effectiveness to delineate patients with either a favorable or an unfavorable outcome, emphasizes the form and quality of the patient's patterns of love and play during the period before the onset of disorder. This emphasis on sexual and social patterns can provide effective predictions of recovery from schizophrenia primarily because the process-type schizophrenic patient typically operates at such a marginal level of premorbid functioning. To broaden the base of prediction to include recovery from less severe forms of psychopathology, or to apply the concept of competence to normal samples, requires that the criteria for effective functioning be extended to include other facets of adaptation: level of intellectual and cognitive functioning; achieved occupational and educational status; consistency of employment; activity in the community; and the constructive use of leisure time. In *Human Adaptation and Its Failures*, Phillips [18] discusses this broadened definition of adaptation:

In our view adaptation implies two divergent yet complementary forms of response to the human environment. The first is to accept and respond effectively to those societal expectations that confront each person according to his sex and age. Included here, for example, are entering school and mastering its subject matter, the forming of friendships, and later, dating, courtship, and marriage. In this first sense, adaptation implies a comformity to society's expectations for behavior. In another sense, however, adaptation means more than a simple acceptance of societal norms. It implies a flexibility and effectiveness in meeting novel and potentially disruptive conditions and of imposing one's own direction on the course of events. In this sense, adaptation implies that the person makes use of opportunities to fulfill internally established goals, values and aspirations. These may include any of a universe of activities, as for example, the choice of a mate, the construction of a house, or the assumption of leadership in an organization. The essential quality common to all such activities is the element of decision-making, of taking the initiative in the determination of what one's future shall include. (p. 2)

To this set of criteria Phillips has added such factors as account-ability, obligation, and reciprocity in personal relationships. By doing so, a nexus has been formed with Whitehorn's emphasis on effective-ness in work, love, and play. Phillips, however, has not mapped the criterion "to expect well," a neglect that I suspect is primarily the result of its essentially derivative nature; to expect well speaks to the quality of self-esteem and a positive self-concept which are formed from skills that reflect economic, social, and sexual adequacy. Such competence qualities not only are effective for predicting the future of the already-disordered but may also have relevance for under-standing those prone to later disorder.

In his paper on the experience of efficacy in schizophrenia, White [28] describes the schizophrenic patient's major liability—his victimi-zation by ineffective actions, and his failure to initiate and to persist in problem-solving—a liability which extends back to a period that long antedates the disorder:

... weak action on the environment has very great generality in schizophrenic behavior. Poor direction of attention and action, poor mastery of cognitive experience, weak assertiveness in interpersonal relations, low feelings of efficacy and competence, a restricted sense of agency in leading one's life—all these crop out in almost every aspect of the schizophrenic disorder.

I should like now to entertain the hypothesis that this ineffectiveness in action is central not only in the picture of the schizophrenic's ultimately disordered behavior but also throughout his whole course of development—that from the start it is the future schizophrenic's major liability. It characterizes his behavior from an early point in life, and it leads to a precarious development in all the spheres I have discussed, including interpersonal competence and self-esteem. (p. 202)

The last paragraph bridges the study of the disturbed adult locked into a network of schizophrenic pathology and the study of children who are at risk for that tragic disorder.

COMPETENCE IN CHILDREN AT RISK

What role can the concept of competence play in the prediction of psychopathology in such children, whether they be defined by biogenetic, familial, sociocultural, or deprivation factors [9]? The methodology of risk studies and some of its limitations make clear the central significance of competence indicators.

The study of risk implies a longitudinal research design and that immediately brings to the fore powerful problems of a logistical and conceptual nature. Such studies seek to predict disorder and deviant outcomes in adulthood from earlier patterns of childhood behavior. The fact that the numbers of children studied in most risk projects are small, as is the anticipated frequency of later deviance, makes the prediction of outcomes difficult. In terms of empirical probabilities, investigators who study the risk of disorder in children born of schizophrenic parentage can project a morbidity risk for their subject of approximately 10 percent (ref. 22, p. 117). Children who are truly at high risk, faced with the unfortunate circumstance of having been born to two parents who have had a schizophrenic disorder, show a morbidity rate that arises to approximately 35 percent (ref. 22, p. 117).

Clearly the proportion of assumed deviance in these children would also rise if the concept of risk were to be broadened to include less severe forms of maladaptation. In either case, variability in outcome must be anticipated and planned for in the design of risk experiments. The projection of variability in outcomes has its advantages. It is equally important to study children at risk who escape disorder as it is to evaluate those who are its victims. But the method for doing so may be better achieved by more circumscribed, short-term, longitudinal-prospective studies in which the emphasis is not on disorder per se but rather on a search for behavioral and biological variables that can effectively discriminate high risk from low risk children, and within the high risk group those children

who show patterns of incompetence and maladjustment from those
who appear to be proceeding toward adulthood along paths of
mastery and adaptation.

The study of competence versus incompetence in childhood
emphasizes the utility of *intermediate outcomes*, and this must be
distinguished from research that aims at the prediction of an
ultimate outcome of mentally disordered status versus normality in
adulthood. But if such studies of intermediate outcomes are to prove
meaningful for risk researchers, they must demonstrate that in a
substantial number of cases there exists a continuity to competence
that extends from childhood into adulthood. Phillips' [18] view of
the issue takes this form:

> The key to the prediction of future effectiveness in society lies in asking:
> "How well has this person met, and how well does he now meet, the expectations
> implicitly set by society for individuals of his age and sex group?" What we need
> to learn is the person's relative potential for coping with the tasks set by society,
> compared to others of his age and sex status. Expected patterns of behavior
> change with the person's age. Presumably relative potential for meeting these
> expectations remains far more stable. Thus to the extent that an individual's
> relative standing in adaptive potential remains constant, we should, in principal,
> be able to predict his future effectiveness in adaptation to society. The pragmatic
> question in need of resolution is the extent to which relative adaptive potential
> does, in fact, remain constant. Only to this extent are we in a position to
> predict the person's future. (p. 3)

The issue, then, is one of probabilities, and these seem to stand
in favor of a continuity of competence. I would therefore suggest
that a tenable first stage in risk research is to explore the correlation
between the behaviors of children presumed to be vulnerable to
psychopathology against a criterion of their qualities of competence.

A FOUR-STAGE STRATEGY FOR RISK RESEARCH

The Minnesota strategy in risk research may be thought of as a
four-stage formulation. The basic research goal is the search for
specific behavioral and biological differentiators that will separate
risk from nonrisk children. But the true power of any parameter in
the study of predisposition must, as I have indicated, meet the even
more stringent criterion of discriminating among levels of competence in the risk group. This research for predictor variables
assumes that there exist external criteria of success or failure in
adaptation that are available to the investigator.

Stage 1: Establishing the Criteria of Competence.   If external criteria are not available, then the first priority of the risk researcher must be to provide age-related indices of competence. That task is not easy, for although listings of the attributes of so-called healthy individuals abound in the literature, a far more stringent screening of such criteria is necessary. The procedure of the Minnesota group is to screen in terms of these qualities characteristics of *stress-resistant* children (whom we have termed the "invulnerables" of our society) on the assumption that these children more closely approximate the competent child at risk. This method will be described in a section to follow.

Stage 2: The Search for Differentiating Variables.   Once developmental measures of competence-incompetence have been identified, the selection of variables that can successfully differentiate between and within risk and control groups becomes the focus of a second stage of research. As a first approximation to these variables, I would look for those which have reliably and significantly demonstrated their predictive power in the study of adult schizophrenia [7]. Examples of such variables that would meet this definitional criterion for a Stage 2 study could include physiological responsiveness, attention deployment, and cognitive effectiveness. Other variables, however, may be derived from developmental studies of normal children on the assumption that developmental lags too may forecast future maladaptation. To add power to a Stage 2 study, a Stage 1 (competence) variable should be incorporated to test the power of the potential (Stage 2) differentiator to segregate subjects who differ in levels of achieved competence.

Stage 3: The Short-Term Prospective Study.   The third stage in risk research would involve the selection of several powerful differentiators for use in short-term prospective studies comparing adaptation in children at risk with appropriate control groups. The use of a convergence technique [2] utilizing cross-sectional groups of children of different ages studied over a sufficient period of time to allow each age group to brook into the next successive age level may allow inferences to be made about the developmental nature of the variables under study. This procedure is now being used in the large-scale risk program being conducted at the University of Rochester under Lyman Wynne's direction.

Stage 4 : Intervention. The final stage in risk research would involve intervention efforts cast into a nontraditional format. The critical element in Stage 4 intervention studies would be the employment of experimental-clinical techniques designed initially to modify performance on a Stage 2 variable with later evaluations aimed at studying the effects of such behavioral changes on (Stage 1) competence indicators.

These four stages should not be viewed as a rigid sequence of steps in research. At some point in a research program an investigator may seek to modify his procedures to test new hypotheses and to introduce and elaborate other variables on the basis of data inputs from ongoing studies.

Studies Illustrating the Four-Stage Sequence

STAGE 1: COMPETENCE INDICES

The investigator of risk can often turn, with gain, to the work of other researchers who have studied age-related indices of competence. An illustrative example can be drawn from White's elaborate research in the pattern of human competence evident in the first six years of a child's life [27]. White's description of his efforts to assess young children illustrates the difficulties in developing competence criteria for any given age period:

Initially, we selected as broad an array of types of preschool children as we could. Our original sample consisted of some 400 three-, four- and five-year-old children living in eastern Massachusetts. We reached the children through 17 preschool institutions (kindergarten and nursery schools). These children varied in at least the following dimensions: (1) residence—from rural to suburban and urban, (2) SES (socio-economic status)—lower-lower to lower-upper class, (3) ethnicity—Irish, Italian, Jewish, English, Portuguese, Chinese and several other types. On the basis of extensive, independent observations by 15 staff members and the teachers of these children, and also on the basis of their performance on objective tests such as the Wechsler and tests of motor and sensory capacities we isolated 51 children. Half were judged to be very high on overall competence, able to cope consistently in superior fashion with anything they met. The other half were judged to be free from gross pathology but generally of very low competence. We then proceeded to observe these children each week for a period of eight months. We gathered some 1,100 protocols on the typical moment-to-moment activities of these children, mostly in the institutions, but also in their homes. At the end of the observation period we selected the 13 most talented and 13 least talented children. Through intensive discussions by our staff of 20 people, we compiled a list of abilities that seemed to distinguish the two groups. (p. 74)

The list is dominated by social and nonsocial abilities with sensory-motor capacities generally being ineffective discriminators. Relevant social abilities reflective of competence include the following: attention-seeking from adults in socially acceptable ways; the ability to express affection and hostility to adults and to use them effectively as resources; the ability to behave similarly with peers, to compete with them, and to assume positions of both leadership and followership; to show pride in accomplishment; and to express a desire to grow up as evidenced, in part, by involvement in "adult-role play behavior."

Nonsocial abilities include linguistic and intellectual competence, attentional ability, and "executive abilities" of the type involved in planning multistep activities and effectively using environmental resources.

The Minnesota Studies of Competence

At Minnesota we have focused on competence indices that are applicable both to the middle years of childhood and to early adolescence—the age span that has the focus of our studies. Initially, the literature of the healthy personality was reviewed and as many indices of adaptive functioning as could be found were catalogued. We then exacted two other requirements to reduce the list and derive our basic criteria: (1) the frequency of occurrence of a given criterion in the literature, and (2) the retention of the criterion against a more stringent and meaningful standard, evidence of the presence of that criterion behavior in competent children who might also be considered to be at risk. Using sociocultural disadvantage as the risk component (a choice made necessary by the lack of a substantive literature available on *able* children exposed to genetic risk, early neglect or familial disorganization), Nuechterlein [16] reviewed a largely unpublished literature contained in the studies and documents to be found in the ERIC (Educational Resources Information Center) file. This provided the source for those competence indicators present in adaptive groups of children exposed to the grinding effects of poverty. We reasoned that children who had mastered environments weighted with disadvantage might share attributes of competence with children resistant to psychopathology. Thus, applying the findings of Nuechterlein's review of the ERIC literature, we selected six indices of competence for use in our risk project, believing these to be the most relevant for adaptation during the period of middle childhood and early adolescence. The six competence criteria are these:

1. Effectiveness in work, play and love; satisfactory educational and occupational progress; peer regard and friendships.
2. Healthy expectancies and the belief that "good outcomes" will follow from the imposition of effort and initiative; an orientation to success rather than the anticipation of failure in performing tasks; a realistic level of aspiration unbeclouded by unrealistically high or low goal-setting behavior.
3. Self-esteem, feelings of personal worthiness, a proper evaluative set toward self and a sense of "fate control," that is, the belief that one can control events in one's environment rather than being a passive victim of them (an internal as opposed to external locus of control).
4. Self-discipline, as revealed by the ability to delay gratification and to maintain a future-orientation.
5. Control and regulation of impulsive drives; the ability to adopt a reflective as opposed to an impulsive style in coping with problem situations.
6. The ability to think abstractly; to approach new situations flexibly and to be able to attempt alternate solutions to a problem.

To reduce these criteria to ratable proportions, our research group subsequently devised a graphic Competence Rating Scale for Teachers.[1] The scale was designed for use by teachers for several reasons: teachers provide a common base for observations of target and control children; the schools have been very cooperative in allowing us access to records and classrooms with informed consent from parents); the school setting is a common arena for observing children's competence qualities. Two items from the scale indicate the format we used. The scale's attributes and its utility with four different groups of vulnerable children and their normal control counterparts have been detailed by Lewis [12].

1. *Relationship of achievement to ability level.* The extent to which the child's performance is consonant with his ability level.

---

[1] Members of Project Competence who have been instrumental in the development of the scale include Beverly Kaemmer, Roger Lazoff, Lee Marcus, Keith Nuechterlein, Paul Sanders, and Susan Phipps Sanger.

The level of performance can be high, moderate, or low; rate only its consistency with ability level.

Utilizes abilities well.
  Typically works close to
  potential

┌ Consistent maximum achievement
  in relation to ability

├ Achievement tends to approximate
  ability level with occasional
  underachievement

Often fails to work up to level
  of ability

└ Markedly underachieving

Descriptive incident:

2. *Control of aggression with peers.* Two factors are involved: the intensity of the child's anger, and the appropriateness of it in terms of external events.

Overly aggressive; at times may
  fight or be verbally abusive
  with little provocation

┌ A bully; often cruel; threatens
  others without provocation

├ Generally even tempered; on
  occasion may overreact with
  aggression but regains control
  quickly

Usually well controlled; can be
  provoked but rarely gets
  angry without cause

└ Rarely antagonistic; anger, when
  shown, is justified

Descriptive incident:

A STAGE 1 STUDY: SOCIAL AND ACADEMIC COMPETENCE OF CHILDREN VULNERABLE TO SCHIZOPHRENIA AND OTHER BEHAVIORAL PATHOLOGIES

Our high valuation of the first criterion of competence, "Effectiveness in work, play and love; satisfactory educational and

occupational progress; peer regard and friendships," is rooted in the
literature of prognosis in schizophrenia, socialization in childhood,
and studies of competence in the face of poverty.

Contained within this first criterion is the important constellation
described earlier—economic (or academic), social, and sexual
competence. This factor became the initial study of our research
program in which Rolf measured the academic and social competence
of six groups of elementary school children [20]. Four of these groups
shared a potential vulnerability to different forms of psychopathology.
One consisted of children whose mothers had had a previous history
of hospitalization for schizophrenia ($N = 31$); the mothers of another
group had prior histories that included hospitalization for depression
($N = 26$); a third group consisted of children who were being treated
in community clinics for externalizing (acting-out) symptoms
($N = 36$), and a fourth group of clinic children presented
internalizing (phobic, withdrawn anxiety) symptoms ($N = 27$). As far
as could be determined by a review of their case histories, these
clinic children did not have mentally ill parents. These four groups
of target children, when located, were attending 37 schools in 113
different classrooms in a city public school system. Within each
classroom, Rolf read all the cumulative records of the pupils to select
two control children who, in the opinion of principal, teacher, or
social worker, were behaving competently. These two children and
the target child comprised a triad consisting of a child at risk, a
competent child matched in terms of his or her comparability to the
target child on such factors as age, sex, grade, social class, occupation
of the family head of household, intactness of the family, school
achievement, and IQ test scores (when available), and a competent,
random control child of the same sex and grade but unmatched on
other demographic variables. Thus the total number of subjects that
comprised Rolf's triads was 360 (targets $N = 120$; matched controls
$N = 120$; random controls $N = 120$).

Measures of social competency were derived from the rating of
peers and teachers. Sociometric ratings built around Bower's "class
play" [3] were based on the judgments of some 3400 children who
participated in the project. (Every child in each of the 113 classrooms
successfully joined in the study.) The typecast assignments given to
the members of the triad by their peers was the basis for determining
peer approval or disapproval. In addition, teachers completed rating

scales designed to measure positive academic behavior, emotional stability and maturity, social agreeableness, and positive social extroversion. Academic competence was also analyzed by a thoroughgoing appraisal of the children's cumulative records and included an application of Watt and his co-worker's method for quantifying dimensional attributes derived from qualitative descriptions of the children written by teachers over successive years [26]. This last analysis is still in progress, while the report of the formal analysis of the content of the cumulative record including such variables as yearly grade reports, health status, standardized achievement and intelligence test scores, notations of absences and tardiness, socioeconomic status of the family, and the frequency of address changes per academic year will soon appear [21].

The study of social competence as adduced from peer and teacher ratings has undergone more extensive analysis and provides partial confirmation of some of the negative social correlates of risk status. Since peer regard is a powerful predictor of adaptation [11, 13, 25], Rolf's findings are of particular interest.

Summarizing the results of his study, Rolf [20] writes:

At the *triad level*, the prediction was generally supported that the groups, in comparison with their respective control groups, obtained lower competence scores. At the *target group level*, the trend of *peer-rated* competence score ranks lowest, followed in order of ascending competence by the children with schizophrenic mothers, the internalizing children, and by the children whose mothers had internalizing symptoms. This order was also obtained for the *teacher-rated* competence scores but only for the girls and not the boys. In the latter case, teachers rated externalizers lowest, and internalizers next lowest, but teachers generally did not discriminate, with certain exceptions, between the two male target groups with mentally ill mothers and their respective control groups. (p. 241)

STAGE 2 STUDIES: PERFORMANCE VARIABLES IN RELATION TO COMPETENCE

The study of attentional factors in children at risk may provide precursor sign for subsequent deficit functioning. Reaction time as a measure of attention and preparatory set has had a lengthy, stable, and productive history in the experimental study of schizophrenic processes. Repeatedly, the RT experiment has provided a reliable method for differentiating schizophrenic patients from control subjects [24]. This suggests that the study of attentional factors in children at risk via the RT procedure reeflcts the sort of dispositional parameter indicative of a Stage 2 variable. Furthermore, the linking of an attentional component to independent indices of competence would satisfy the structure demanded of Stage 2 studies.

A recently completed experiment by Marcus [14] using the basic design of Rolf's study with its four different groups of target children and two groups of matched and random controls exemplifies the strategy. These studies constitute the core of Marcus' dissertation research:

1. Attention and set were studied as a function of varying preparatory intervals presented in a simple reaction time procedure using regular and irregular RT sequences. This study essentially replicates the classical RT study of Rodnick and Shakow [19] and those of Shakow and his associates (e.g., [29, 30]).

2. A second study of attentional mechanisms employed the RT procedure with irregular preparatory intervals but with pretrial information given to reduce temporal uncertainty.

3. The third study also utilized the basic RT task, but it was modified to focus on decision making and choice behavior of the children under conditions of risk-taking in which the probability of positive and negative outcomes was varied by the experimenter. An additional purpose of this study was to provide pilot data regarding behavior relevant to several competence criteria including success versus failure orientation, impulsive versus reflective cognitive styles, and internal versus external locus of control.

The Marcus study provides an example of the Minnesota strategy. Reaction time is essentially a Stage 2 variable; it has demonstrable significance as a measure of attentional deficit in schizophrenia and may provide in similar fashion a measure of the task set of children. But it is necessary that a Stage 1 variable also be incorporated into the study to provide a measure of competence that can be correlated with RT performance. Such a proviso was made in three ways: (1) formal evaluation of the children's cumulative school records; (2) teachers' ratings on the Competence Rating Scale; (3) the creation within the experiment of a risk-taking component to measure level of aspiration, locus of control, and cognitive style.

The results of the study will be reported in detail by Marcus in a future publication. We can, however, summarize his major findings here:

1. Children of schizophrenic mothers and the externalizing group of children show marked attentional deficits. However, the introduction of a powerful motivation condition (the risk-taking procedure) eliminates this deficit in the clinic children but fails to do so in the children who are at risk for schizophrenia.
2. By comparison, children of depressive mothers and internalizing clinic children (whom we have consistently viewed as being at lower risk relative to the other two vulnerable groups) reveal greater attentional focusing. The internalizing children sustain attention under all conditions. By contrast, the children born to depressive mothers initially reveal attentional deficits under the regular and irregular procedure, but the imposition of experimental conditions that provide either for cognitive structuring (the information procedure) or motivational facilitation (the risk-taking condition) quickly accelerates their performance to the level of their respective normal controls.
3. The matched and random controls consistently perform at an equivalent high level on the various performance measures.
4. Simple explanations for these findings based upon extra-task factors such as fatigue, motivational decrements, uninvolvement in the task, are effectively eliminated by an analysis of experimental data that were designed to evaluate such effects.

The question of whether RT performance can be related to competence indicators, however, is not entirely resolved. First, we can note that there is overlap in the pool of subjects used by Rolf and Marcus and that Marcus' findings of greater attentional deficits in externalizers and children at risk for schizophrenia parallel Rolf's data revealing increased negative peer ratings that are accorded these groups of children. Teacher's measures also reveal the low competence status of the externalizing children. Similarly, the children born to schizophrenic and depressed mothers are also rated as significantly less competent than their controls, but so too are the internalizing clinic children—the one group that failed to show any evidence of deficit functioning on the reaction time procedures.

STAGE 3 STUDIES: SHORT-TERM
LONGITUDINAL STUDIES

For a description of a program of risk centering on a relatively short-term prospective design, it is necessary to turn to another research program now under way in the Department of Psychiatry at the University of Rochester Medical School. Under the coordinating leadership of Lyman Wynne more than 20 professional staff members have gathered, drawn from four major universities (Rochester, Cornell, Berkeley, Minnesota) and a diversity of disciplines that includes psychiatry, clinical psychology, developmental psychology, psychophysiology, neurology, experimental psychopathology, epidemiology, sociology, and statistics.

The program focus, rooted in the study of children and family members who are at risk for schizophrenia, is comprised of three subprograms, all interrelated and all central to an understanding of the problem of predisposition. One set of studies focuses on children and siblings born to schizophrenic and depressive mothers as the defining samples at risk; another core is oriented to studies of the families and the parents of these children with an emphasis on family organization, modes of intrafamilial communication, and significant aspects of parenting patterns; a third group of studies is epidemiological in orientation and utilizes an instrument uniquely advantageous to epidemiological research—the Psychiatric Case Register for Monroe County, which is housed in the department's Division of Preventive and Social Psychiatry [1, 15].

The program incorporates both a cross-sectional and a short-term longitudinal-prospective strategy which, in combination, may produce within a span of five years a projected developmental picture of the vulnerable child ranging from early childhood to early adolescence. It is hoped that this can be achieved through the convergence procedure referred to earlier. This strategy involves the use of groups of children at ages 1,[2] 4, 7, and 10 who will be followed initially over a span of 4 years, thus providing for retesting of subgroups of children at least at two converging age points, 7 and 10 years.

---

[2] The 1-year-olds are children who are being seen in an infant risk project under the direction of Professors Arnold Sameroff and Melvin Zax of the University of Rochester, with the collaboration of Professor Harouton Babigian.

The variables to be studied are numerous and embrace such diverse components of adaptation as cognitive and social development employing a Piagetian framework, modes of information processing and sensory integration, psychophysiological studies of children and parents, learning efficiency under censure and praise, quality of school functioning, formal diagnostic assessment of children and parents, modes of parenting, patterns of communication within the family, mother-child play interaction, referential communication between mother and child, styles of conflict resolution, and an analysis of pregnancy and birth factors in risk. Since various components of school-related competencies have been made an integral part of the research program [23], the relevance of adaptation to the range of dependent variables to be studied may indicate whether such a relatively short-term longitudinal-developmental program can suggest the pattern of outcomes in these groups of vulnerable children.

STAGE 4: INTERVENTION

There is little to be said about this final stage of risk research, for few data have been brought to bear on the important problem of intervention within the context of a stage strategy. What can one say about intervention when there exists such restricted information about the etiology of schizophrenia?

However, an approximation to an intervention strategy of the sort suggested by the stage strategy is one whose power has been empirically demonstrated by my Rochester colleague, Professor Michael Chandler. Chandler, a developmental psychopathologist, has been interested in patterns of egocentrism and role playing as significant manifestations of adaptation. The ability to demonstrate perspective or role-taking skills he sees as a dispositional attribute of the maturing organism. Children with tenuous adaptive qualities presumably would show a lessened skill to assay the role of another and to perceive clearly a self-other differentiation. Devising and adapting a variety of assessment procedures for measuring egocentrism, Chandler [5] applied his procedures to the study of 75 normal public school children between the ages of 6 and 13. Other groups consisted of children with long histories of social and interpersonal failures including 50 children in the 8 to 13 year age group who were institutionalized for emotional disturbance and an

additional 50 chronically delinquent boys. The disturbed children
initially showed a significant deficit in role-taking skills. Whereas
most normal children by age 10 can adopt the orientation of another,
Chandler found that many disturbed children had difficulty in doing
so and failed to show a maturing of such skills between the ages of
6 and 10. Indeed the typically disturbed child at 13 proved to be more
egocentric as measured by various test procedures than did the
average 7-year-old normal child. Nevertheless, variability prevailed in
the disturbed group. Nonegocentricity characterized those children
who had been brutalized and were hyperalert to and suspicious of the
motives of others.

Chandler's intervention strategy exemplifies best the Stage 4
principle. In effect, he asked: "What would be the consequenecs of
training these disturbed children in role-taking skills?" His procedure
was to take the 50 chronically delinquent boys between the ages of
11 and 13 and to divide them into three groups on the basis of their
pretraining egocentrism scores. One group remained untreated and
was retested after 10 weeks. The remaining children were seen in
groups of five for a total of 30 hours extending over a 10-week period.
Half of these children became involved in making documentary films
during the treatment period. Chandler's comments on the experiences
he provided for the remaining half of the children warrant repetition:

> Having noted the presence of substantial developmental delays in the role-
> taking abilities of various populations of disturbed children, an effort was made
> to formulate and test a program of remedial training intended as a means of
> testing the modifiability of these observed deficiencies.
>
> There is little information in the research literature that provides useful clues
> as to how a curriculum for improving faulty role-taking skills might be devised.
> What seemed required was some vehicle for transporting the subjects into the
> perspective of others and for encouraging and facilitating their efforts to adopt
> roles other than their own. Efforts to satisfy these task requirements led to the
> development of a storefront video film and actors workshop where delinquent
> adolescents were provided closed-circuit television recording equipment and
> encouraged to make films about their own role taking efforts. They were helped
> to develop skits or short plays about persons their own age and required to
> replay and review these skits until each participant had occupied every role in
> the plot.

What, then, were the consequences of this training effort to get the
children to relinquish their egocentric biases and take on the more
mature social skills commensurate with their age? The documentary

film-making group and the no-treatment group together with the role-playing groups were all administered equivalent forms of the pretest role-taking test. However, only the group trained in role taking showed substantial improvement on the posttests.

A broader question, of course, relates to the daily real-life adaptation of children exposed to such a specific regimen of social skills training. Chandler, in response to my direct inquiry on this important point, wrote to me of a group of delinquent and a group of abandoned and neglected children with whom he and his associates have worked:

In both instances the Ss were selected on the grounds that they were ego-centric beyond their years and were enrolled in a three month long intervention effort which relied on the making of videotape movies of dramatic productions as a training vehicle. With the delinquent sample, behavioral ratings were made both before and after the termination of the treatment effort and the delinquent histories of the group members were examined through a search of police and court records. This record search was carried out at the outset of the program and at 6-, 12- and 18-month intervals after the program's termination. Program participants, in contrast to control Ss, did show some minor reduction in the level of their postprogram delinquent involvement. The population of institutionalized abandoned and neglected children was rated by teachers and custodial staff before and after the intervention project. In addition to changing in more manifest behavioral ways, these observed changes were generally in the direction of increased social competence and comfort in social situations.

Despite my enthusiasm for research of this type, I must confess to a concern regarding this fourth stage of an integrated research strategy. Skills training is a piecemeal treatment procedure. Can such training provide for the development of those higher order skills so necessary for adaptation in our complex society? There is virtue in the search for some form of precise intervention, but there remains the discomforting awareness that the future environmental demands that all children must face, whatever their degree of vulnerability to psychopathology, are so great that a broader program of intervention seems necessary. Skill and competence develop, as Bruner [4] has observed, by small daily accretions of experience from infancy throughout childhood. Such skills lead to new mastery, and this, in turn, encourages the development of other skills that generate a deep competence that may be the necessary inoculant that stays the ravaging effects of disorder. But such skill acquisition requires a broad-gauged view of intervention. Bruner's appraisal of the problem

of intervention applied to disadvantaged children provides a fitting
final statement to the critical problem of reducing the risk potential
of vulnerable children:

> ... Little can be done for a human being with a "one-shot" intervention. One
> has to work at it. Head Start alone does not work, if afterward the child is
> dumped into a punishing school experience. When we build an expectancy, build
> a skill, we incur a responsibility for nurturing it. It may, in some instances, be a
> compounding of evils to open the child's vulnerabilities and then disappoint or
> dump him. If we are to be effective in helping disadvantaged children cope
> better, it is their life cycle that must be dealt with not their preschool or their
> nursery or their street life. That is why we need diverse forms of care and can
> hardly tolerate quarrels about this form vs. that form on ideological grounds
> rather than evidence.... The important thing is to get going. We must surely
> praise the attitude that though the first programs may not happen to be our
> preferred ones, nonetheless, we try to make them as good as possible, knowing
> that we shall surely go on from there. (pp. 115–116)

References

1. Babigian, H. M. Schizophrenia in Monroe County, in *Schizophrenia: Implications of Research Findings for Treatment and Teaching*, M. M. Katz, A. Littlestone, L. Mosher, M. S. Roath, and A. H. Tuma, Eds. In press.
2. Bell, R. Q. Convergence: An accelerated longitudinal approach. *Child Devel.*, 24 (1953) 142–145.
3. Bower, E. M. *Early Identification of Emotionally Handicapped Children in School*, 2nd ed. Charles C. Thomas, Springfield, Ill. 1969.
4. Bruner, J. S. Discussion: Infant education as viewed by a psychologist, in *Education of the Infant and Young Child*, V. H. Denenberg, Ed. Academic Press, New York, 1970, pp. 109–116.
5. Chandler, M. J. Egocentrism in normal and pathological child development. Paper presented at The First Symposium of the International Society for the Study of Behavioral Development. Nijmegen, Holland, 1971.
7. Garmezy, N. Models of etiology for the study of children who are at risk for schizophrenia, in *Life History Research in Psychopathology*, Vol. 11, M. Roff, L. Robins, and M. M. Pollack, Eds. University of Minnesota Press, Minneapolis, 1972, pp. 9–23.
8. Garmezy, N. Research strategies for the study of children who are at risk for schizophrenia, in *Schizophrenia: Implications of Research Findings for Treatment and Teaching*, M. M. Katz, R. Littlestone, L. Mosher, M. S. Roath, and A. H. Tuma, Eds. In press.
9. Garmezy, N. and Nuechterlein, K. H. Vulnerable and invulnerable children: The fact and fiction of competence and disadvantage. *Amer. J. Orthopsychiat.*, 77 (1972) (abstract).
10. Grinker, R. R. Psychiatry and our dangerous world, in *Psychiatric Research in Our Changing World*. Proceedings of an International Symposium, Montreal, 1968. Excerpta Medica International Congress Series. No. 187.

11. Hartup, W. W. Peer interaction and social organization, in *Manual of Child Psychology*, 3rd ed, P. H. Mussen, Ed. John Wiley & Sons, New York, 1970, pp. 361–456.
12. Lewis, J. M. Measuring competence in vulnerable, disturbed and normal children: The development of a competence rating scale for teachers. Unpublished summa cum laude thesis, University of Minnesota, 1973.
13. Lippitt, R. and Gold M. Classroom social structure as a mental health problem. *J. Social Issues*, 15 (1959), 40–49.
14. Marcus, L. Studies of attention in children vulnerable to psychopathology. Unpublished Ph.D. dissertation, University of Minnesota, 1972.
15. Miles, H. C. and Gardner, E. A. A psychiatric case register. *Arch. Gen. Psychiat.*, 14 (1966), 571–580.
16. Nuechterlein, K. H. Competent disadvantaged children: A review of research. Unpublished summa cum laude thesis, University of Minnesota, 1970.
17. Phillips, L. Case history data and prognosis in schizophrenia. *J. Nerv. Ment. Dis.*, 117 (1953), 515–525.
18. Phillips, L. *Human Adaptation and Its Failures*. Academic Press, New York, 1968.
19. Rodnick, E. H. and Shakow, D. Set in the schizophrenic as measured by a composite reaction time index. *Amer. J. Psychiat.*, 97 (1940), 214–225.
20. Rolf, J. E. The social and academic competence of children vulnerable to schizophrenia and other behavior pathologies. *J. Abnorm. Psychol.*, 80 (1972), 225–243.
21. Rolf J. E. and Garmezy, N. The school performance of children vulnerable to behavior pathology, in *Life History Research in Psychopathology*, Vol. III, D. F. Ricks, A. Thomas, and M. Roff, Eds. University of Minnesota Press, Minneapolis, in press.
22. Rosenthal, D. *Genetic Theory and Abnormal Behavior*. McGraw-Hill, New York, 1970.
23. Rubinstein, G. and Fisher, L. A measure of teacher's observations of student behavior. *J. Consult. Clin. Psychol.*, in press.
24. Shakow, D. Psychological deficit in schizophrenia. *Behav. Sci.*, 8 (1963), 275–305.
25. Teele, J. E., Schleifer, M. J., Corman, L., and Larson, K. Teacher ratings, sociometric status, and choice-reciprocity of anti-social and normal boys. *Group Psychother.*, 19 (3-4) (1966), 183–197.
26. Watt, N. F., Stolorow, R. D., Lubensky, A. W., and McClelland, D. C. School adjustment and behavior of children hospitalized for schizophrenia as adults. *Amer. J. Orthopsychiat.*, 40 (1970), 637–657.
27. White, B. L. An analysis of excellent early educational practices: Preliminary report. *Interchange*, 2 (1971), 71–88.
28. White, R. W. The experience of efficacy in schizophrenia. *Psychiatry*, 28 (1965), 199–211.
29. Zahn, T. P., Rosenthal, D., and Shakow, D. Reaction time in schizophrenic and normal subjects in relation to the sequence of series of regular preparatory intervals. *J. Abnorm. Soc. Psychol.*, 63 (1961), 161–168.
30. Zahn, T. P., Rosenthal, D., and Shakow, D. Effects of irregular preparatory intervals on reaction time in schizophrenics. *J. Abnorm. Soc. Psychol.*, 67 (1963), 44–52.

A Risk-Vulnerability Intervention Model for Children of Psychotic Parents*

E. James Anthony, M.D. (U.S.A)

Children at psychiatric risk generally belong to families at psychiatric risk and children who are vulnerable to risk may live in families that are vulnerable to risk. In dealing with the problem of risk and vulnerability, therefore, the individual liabilities have always to be considered in the context of the milieu in which the individual is embedded, an added consideration that further complicates the disentangling of the interrelationships between risk, vulnerability, and disorder.

Families can be put at risk by the disasters of disability, disease, death, desertion, and divorce, and these risks are intensified by an economic and social impoverishment of living conditions. They can be rendered vulnerable to these detrimental circumstances by particular types of malfunctioning such as poor communication and emotional contact between the family members, lack of routine and organization, and absence of any plan for the future [1].

In terms of intervention, families at high risk for psychosis can be broadly divided into two groups. The first is characterized by relative openness to the surrounding social orbit to which it is linked by a helpful network of people and agencies, and a sensitivity to change

* Supported by U.S. Public Health Service grant MH 14052-01.

that is also reflected in a tolerance for differences. The second is relatively closed and alienated from the orbit, highly resistant to change, and intolerant of any deviation from the family's code and culture. Families in the first group are usually receptive to intervention, whereas the more encapsulated the system is, the harder it is to penetrate it or establish any helpful networks with agencies in the surrounding community. The individuals within the family tend to take over these characteristics so that individuals at risk may similarly vary in their susceptibility to influence and change.

The Useful Risk-Vulnerability Paradigm

A disease ecologist, Jacques May, has elaborated a striking analogy depicting the relationship of risk to vulnerability. He asks us to imagine three dolls, one made of glass, one plastic, and one steel, each exposed to an equal blow from a hammer. As a result, the first doll breaks down completely, the second carries a permanent scar, and the third gives out a fine metallic sound. The glass doll is obviously at risk from external forces because of its "constitution." In addition, it might have been badly mishandled after leaving the manufacturers or its owner might have neglected it and thus exposed it to being chipped or cracked. This accumulation of risky experiences may leave the doll in a heightened state of susceptibility, the various components of which could be subsumed in such qualities as cohesiveness, strong tolerance, and shatter-proofness, each of which might be measurable. To carry the analogy a little further, one could imagine a protective coating of some sort being applied to the glass doll producing a revised state of vulnerability. The coating may be short lived or long lived, but only time can tell how effectively it protects the doll from further trauma.

A Risk-Vulnerability Intervention Model

In Figure 1 the doll paradigm has been transposed to a human frame of reference whose basic elements are, once again, cumulative risk, the state of vulnerability and its measurement, acute stressful experiences or acute risks as opposed to chronic risks and stresses, the competence to cope with and master both acute and chronic stresses, corrective interventions systematically employed, changes induced in

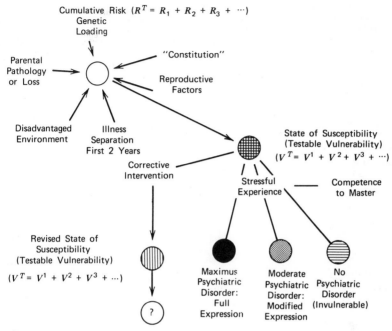

Figure 1 A risk-vulnerability intervention model.

the state of susceptibility, and changes resulting in the occurrence of psychiatric disorder.

We will now deal with the different components of the model in succession.

THE TOTAL RISK ASSESSMENT AND THE RISK PROFILE

Anthony [2] has attempted to classify the commonly encountered risks and chronic stresses under the main headings of genetic, reproductive, "constitutional," developmental, physical, environmental, and traumatic (the R_1, R_2, R_3 . . . in the model). Each subtype of risk is then evaluated separately along seven dimensions of risk relating to that particular subtype with a possible score ranging from 0 to 6. As an example, the assessment of reproductive risk is given in Table 1.[1]

---

[1] A copy of the total risk assessment is available from the author upon request.

Table 1

Reproductive Loading		Check
No apparent reproductive casualty	0	___
Prenatal maternal ill health (vomiting, weight gain, blood pressure rise, albuminuria, swelling, etc.)	1	___
Prenatal fetal ill health (threatened abortion, signs of fetal distress, etc.)	1	___
Paranatal difficulties in the mother (delayed labor, contracted pelvis, instrumental delivery, Caesarean section, placenta praevia, eclampsia, etc.)	1	___
Paranatal difficulties in the child (abnormal presentation, multiple births, prolapsed cord, signs of fetal distress, etc.)	1	___
Postnatal difficulties (anoxia, cyanosis, jaundice, prematurity, low birth weight, excessive molding)	1	___
Neonatal difficulties (evidence of intracranial damage, convulsions, infection, etc.)	1	___
	Total:	___

The other subtypes are treated in the same way: The genetic loading estimates the amount of psychosis in the extended and nuclear family group at the child, parent, grandparent, and great-grandparent levels. "Constitutional" loading is based on the history of activity and sensitivity in infancy, hearing, visual and motor handicaps, body build and temperamental traits. Developmental loading takes into account medical problems at various stages of development from infancy to high school. The physical ill health loading covers acute and chronic illness, allergies, periodic attacks, and central nervous system disorders. Environmental loading relates to experiences in institutions, fostering, frequent residential changes, poor conditions of living, and defect and disorder, both mental and physical, in the parents. The traumatic loading is counted on the history of medical, physical, sexual, and emotional traumata of various kinds. The individual risk scores are then brought together in a common table giving a risk profile and a total risk score (Table 2).

Although the measure is still a crude expression of a complex reaction tendency, it does have the advantage of furnishing a numerical assessment as well as a more analytic approach to a global concept. One obvious defect comes from giving a weight of 1 to each category of risk in all the subtypes, even though the various categories differ both in the amount and nature of the risk involved. This is regarded as a temporary maneuver in an effort to avoid unresearched preconceptions; weightings will be discovered when extensive analyses have been carried out on the correlations of risk with the actual incidents of disorder. The total risk assessment is also a useful tool for demonstrating that different siblings in the same family may

Table 2   The Risk Profile and Total Risk Score

		1 2 3 4 5 6
1. Genetic loading	Low risk	[			|▨|] High risk
2. Reproductive loading		[▨|				]
3. "Constitutional" loading		[	|▨|		]
4. Developmental loading		[		|▨|	]
5. Physical Health loading		[|▨|			]
6. Environmental loading		[	|▨|		]
7. Traumatic loading		[		|▨|	]

Total risk score — High risk (28–42)_____ Moderate risk (14–27)_____ Low risk (0–13)_____

Risk of developing mental disorder during childhood (check one): — High_____ Moderate_____ Low_____

Risk of developing mental disorder during adult life (check one): — High_____ Moderate_____ Low_____ be exposed to very different degrees and kinds of risk, although the children share the same parents and the same familial environment. One of the hunches, still to be tested and proved, is that high scores on the nonenvironmental subtypes genetic, reproductive, "constitutional") would be more likely to be associated with remote effects, that is, the development of disorder in adult life, whereas high scores for environmental subtypes (developmental, physical health, environmental, traumatic) would be more likely to be associated with immediate effects during childhood itself.

THE CONCEPT OF VULNERABILITY AND
MEASURABLE VULNERABILITY

The sampling of different types of behavior in response to psychiatric, psychological, and experimental interfering has suggested a concept of measurable vulnerability pertaining to certain presumptive indices of susceptibility in relation to particular conditions of risk. In the context of the doll analogy, the attribute of fragility is a function of vulnerability in the context of the impact of the hammer; this would not be the case if the risk stemmed from a temperature change. Where the risk for the child has to do with parental psychosis, the presumptive areas of vulnerability would depend on the effects of exposure to psychotic phenomena, and secondly on the method of approach.

In the psychiatric interview the child's vulnerability is gauged on the degree of involvement with the sick parent and his sickness in terms of identification with the sick parent, knowledge of the illness, undue suggestibility and submissiveness, symptomatic behavior similar to that of the sick parent, and test indications as revealed by wishes, artificial dreams, and a doctor's game. Here vulnerability is regarded as a function of involvement. In the psychological interview a standard battery is used comprising the WISC, the Rorschach, the TAT, the Beery, and the DAP, and blind ratings are then carried out, using the test scores, on 13 measures felt to be sensitive to the psychotic influence. Of these, five seemed to have particular relevance to vulnerability from psychotic impact. These were logicality, reality testing, and identity, and, more generally, overall severity and pathology of content (Table 3). The interrater reliabilities for the blind ratings on each variable ranged from 0.867 to 0.985.

Comparing the children of psychotic parents with the children

Table 3   Psychological Evaluation of Vulnerability

Standard battery
  WISC
  Rorschach
  TAT
  Beery (VMI)
  DAP (Draw-a-Person)
  (Sophistication of the Body Test) (Witkin)

Ratings on measures
derived from standard
battery
  Overall severity*
  Logicality*
  Reality testing*
  Identity*
  Pathology of content*
  Concreteness
  Anxiety
  Object Relations
  Internal Control
  Emotionality
  Aggressivity
  Efficacy of Defenses
  Coping Capacity

* Relevant to psychotic vulnerability.
Note: The testing and ratings are done "blindly."

of normal parents in 33 matched pairs (age, sex, ethnic and social class), in the four areas mentioned, the differences between the two groups reached acceptable levels of significance (Table 4).

When the children of white psychotic parents were matched against children of white normals, the differences were even more impressive, indicating that the characteristics of the normal black controls

Table 4   Psychological Evaluation Ratings for Children of Psychotic Parents (Experimentals) versus Children of "Normal" Parents (Controls) ($N = 33$ matched pairs)

	$\overline{X}$	s	$\overline{X}$	s	t Value	Significance Level
Logicality	3.25	1.01	2.61	1.18	2.9263	.005 (E > C)
Reality testing	3.19	0.99	2.64	1.32	2.0897	.05 (E > C)
Identity	3.10	0.58	2.70	0.81	2.6040	.01 (E > C)

approached those of the experimental group as a whole. A simple correlation matrix demonstrated that logicality, reality testing, and identity formation correlated highly not only with one another but also with overall severity of disturbance in the child (Table 5).

In the experimental interview the focus, with respect to vulner-ability, was on self-differentiation, nonself- (object) differentiation, organizational proficiency, reality testing, magical thinking, and puzzlement. The experimental battery for exploring these areas included the "Three Mountains" and "Broken Bridge" tests adapted from Piaget, the Family Relations Test (Bene-Anthony), Witkin's Embedded Figures, and certain subtests of the ITPA.

THE NATURE OF THE STRESSFUL EXPERIENCE

Stress as experienced by the child and stress as estimated by the adult observing the impact of the stress on the child are frequently of very different orders of magnitude, and in our research on high risk children [3] a special emphasis is placed on the "child's eye view" of the psychotic behavior to which he is exposed. It has been found that certain psychoses, in which hallucinations, delusions, seductions, and aggressions actively incorporate the child, are experienced by him as involving, whereas other psychoses, in which the main response of the parent is withdrawal, are experienced by the child as noninvolving. It should be stated, however, that although the child's own involvement in the psychosis of the parent is generally related to the extent to which the parental psychosis involves him, this is by no means always the case, and a small proportion of the children manage to get themselves heavily involved in a noninvolving parental psychosis. There is also no clear-cut indication that the involving psychoses are either geneti-cally or experientially more hazardous for the child than the noninvolving psychoses.

Table 5   Simple Correlation Matrix Ratings on Children
(*N* = 33 matched pairs)

	Overall Severity	Logicality	Reality Testing	Identity
Overall severity	1.000000	0.735269	0.704074	0.653350
Logicality	0.735269	1.000000	0.719528	0.527418
Reality testing	0.704074	0.719528	1.000000	0.482143
Identity	0.653350	0.527418	0.482143	1.000000

In the Family Relations Test (Bene-Anthony) it was found that the children of psychotic parents as a group manifested a decided preference for the "normal" parent[2] and perceived positive attitudes and feelings as coming from the "normal" parent and negative attitudes and feelings as coming from the psychotic parent.

COMPETENCE AND THE MASTERY OF ACUTE AND CHRONIC STRESSES

There has been a recent emphasis in so-called risk research on the notion of competence, and the term is becoming increasingly popular, although its meaning is often diffused beyond usefulness. In its more general use, the level of competence has been judged by performance under challenging conditions such as school achievements, test responses, athletics, and interpersonal relationships. The advantage of "performance competence" is that there

Table 6   Family Relations Test (Bene-Anthony)

Deck of Feelings

POSITIVE   (To and From)   "This is the person I love ..."
                           "This is the person who loves me ..."

NEGATIVE (To and From)   "This is the person I hate ..."
                           "This is the person who hates me ..."

Ambivalence score $(+/-)$ _____
Involvement score _____
Defense score ("Mr. Nobody")_____
Self-preoccupation score ("Me")_____

---

[2] We have no exact figures as yet about the psychiatric status of the "well" spouse, but in other studies clinical disorders have been found in about 10-13 percent of the cases. Our impression is that our figures are even higher.

is a clear executive function to be measured.

In this research we have also been concerned with "representational" competence, which is vaguer and more difficult to assess. This type of competence is based on the skill with which the individual can evaluate, organize, and retain the mass of incoming data and create a coherent and comprehensive frame of reference or schemata, in Piaget's terminology, so that future problems can be analyzed and future performance skillfully directed. There is manifestly a close relationship, therefore, between representational and performance competence.

In our study representational vulnerability is scored on a 4-point scale following a "focal" interview with the child [3] in which the understanding and knowledge of the etiology, diagnosis, the course of illness as observed by him, the treatment, and the prognosis is explored, so that some idea of his total knowledge of the parent's illness is obtained.

THE PSYCHIATRIC DISORDER IN RELATION
TO RISK AND VULNERABILITY

The children of psychotic parents can manifest an array of specific and nonspecific disorders during childhood, adolescence, and adult life. The disorders occurring during childhood may be antecedent types, micropsychoses, or psychoses-in-the-making; parapsychoses, such as *folie à deux*; massive de-differentiations; and reactive disturbances [4]. During adolescence the first psychotic breakdowns begin to appear in the high risk population. The relationship of disorder to risk and vulnerability is discussed elsewhere in this volume [9]. There is no evidence available currently that would support the view that clinical disturbances during childhood facilitate the development of adult psychoses, but there is evidence to suggest a connection with nonpsychotic disorders in the adult. There is also some support for the view that the disturbed group of high risk children would tend to have a higher total risk score as well as a higher vulnerability score.

CORRECTIVE INTERVENTIONS

An ideal intervention program for high risk children, taking into account the current difficulties in finding personnel and funds for such projects, would favor shorter, inexpensive, and technically simple measures preferably using the services of paraprofessionals.

Four types of intervention are being considered in this investigation. *Compensatory interventions* involve various nonspecific procedures aimed at building up ego resources, strengthening self-confidence, and bringing the child into contact with benevolent figures. The opportunities offered include tutoring, camping, "big brother" relationships, outings, recreational and creative opportunities, and a positive alliance with the staff of the research clinic. Most of these activities are being carried out by paraprofessionals who are given only general instructions on the need to bolster the child's morale and maintain a realistic orientation as much as possible at the same time providing acceptable models for mature and autonomous behavior. A log of activities records the amount of intervention time given to any child.

Classical interventions are individual and group psychotherapy. Once again, the amount of intervention time given to each child is carefully recorded as is any work done with the parents and with the rest of the family. The work done with the family is considered as part of the work done with the child and so is included in assessing the amount of intervention.

Cathartic interventions are used during the acute or relapsing phases of the parental illness when defenses tend to be fluid, communications free, and affects highly available. The abreactions may or may not occur during the "focal interviewing" when the impact of the illness on each individual is investigated in detail. Each of the children is asked to report his particular experience of the illness as it develops, envelops, and influences him both inside and outside the family. In the course of this intervention, a whole range of affects, such as fear, shame, guilt, anger, and depression, are abreacted. The wish to drive the psychotic parent out of the house or back into psychosis when he is recovering is often brought up amid a storm of feeling. The family group thus seems to provide a more effective atmosphere for catharsis than does the individual situation. The procedure, however, has proved almost useless outside the acute phase of the illness when defenses are reinstituted.

Corrective interventions are attempts to create specific procedures to reduce vulnerability to the psychotic influences. For example, self-differentiation is furthered by self-orientation and

Table 7   Object Analysis

Qualities: size, shape, color, sound, number considered separately, then summarized as parts of thing.
Functions: tools that cut, measure, fasten, turn
Discovery through senses: smell, taste, hearing, touch
Feelings about things: pleasure, anger, jealousy, sorrow
Numbers of things: cardinal, ordinal, some, all, few, many
Size of things: big, little, long, short, narrow, wide
Things in time and space: yesterday, today, tomorrow, up and down, behind, in front of, here, there, far, near, over, under, right, left

nonself-differentiation exercises, starting from the outside (This is my name; these are my clothes; this is my hair) and proceeding inward (These are my thoughts; my memories; my dreams; etc.). Object differentiation is undertaken through a course of exercises during which the primary and secondary qualities of things are evaluated in terms of the sensations, the function, the feelings, and the ideas that they provoke. The rationale for these two interventions is based on the assumption that complete self-nonself-differentiation requires both a full knowledge of the self and a full knowledge of the nonself, the two delineations proceeding hand-in-hand in the service of differentiation. Furthermore, it also seems that object analysis or nonself-differentiation (Table 7) provides confidence for the more introspective exercise of self-analysis.

The corrective interventions with regard to unrealistic and magical thinking are based on the exploration of the finding of reality solutions to a number of everyday problems. These are constructed as open-ended stories that pose a question with five possible answers ranging from the unrealistic to the realistic (Table 8). In a small normative study, there were indications that the more realistic replies increased with age (Figure 2).

Table 8   Reality Testing

Mary's mother is sick and acts very crabby. Sometimes she yells at Mary for nothing at all. What can Mary do?
1. Talk to somebody about it (5)
2. Stay out of her way (4)
3. Wish for a different mother (1)
4. Don't get upset about it (3)
5. Pray for her to get well (2)

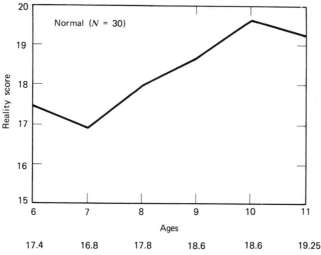

Figure 2   Reality testing.

After the child has made his choice, "reality conversations" are
systematically begun with him covering such topics as his reasons for
choosing his answers, his assessment of what a smaller or older
child might choose, or how his well or sick parent might respond,
and finally what selection the interviewer might make. The interviewer then proceeds to tell the child why he has chosen what
he has chosen, disclosing its basis in realistic thought and action
(Table 9).

The children of psychotic parents, irrespective of age, tended to
be mystified by the incongruities of thought and affect contained in
psychotic phenomena. During the initial sessions with the child,
efforts are made at demystification, furnishing him with not only a
more objective view of mental illness in general but of his parent's
illness in particular. However, the underlying contention is to
increase the representational competence of the child. This might
involve not only decreasing his puzzlement and increasing his
representational competence, but also, at the same time, helping him
to explore self- and object-differentiation, body image, and the
dimensions of reality. It therefore demands a more sophisticated
and professional understanding and approach to the child as
illustrated in the following two cases.

Table 9   Reality Conversations

Interrogation

Have you had any problems like this one?

What did you do about it?

Why did you choose No. _____?

Why did you not choose _____?

Which one would a 3-year-old choose? Why?

Which one would a 15-year-old choose? Why?

Which one would a grown-up choose? Why?

Which one would your mother choose? Your father? Why?

Which one would I (interviewer) choose? Why?

Would you like to know which one I'd choose? I'd choose _____.

Shall I tell you why I would choose _____?

Do you often wish? Do your wishes ever come true?

Do you often pray? Do your prayers ever get answered?

Can you depend on wishes? Why not? What's better?

Shall I tell you what I think? . . . Do you agree? Why not?

CASE 1

A pretty 5-year-old little girl, somehow managing to convey the picture of a leprechaun, followed me into the room, and, for a while, meandered around peering disinterestedly into its different parts. After a while, she came close up to me and asked: "What's your name?" I gave it. She next asked, pointing with her finger, "Is that your head?" I answered seriously that it was adding, with a smile, that I had had it for a long time. She paid no attention to the little joke but continued: "Have you got a mother to go home to?" I said that I did have a mother, but that she lived in another house. She considered this solemnly and then remarked surprisingly, "Why doesn't she love you?" "She doesn't have to stay with me to love me. She loves me even when she doesn't stay with me. Sometimes mothers have to go away from their children, but it doesn't mean that they don't love them." She gazed a little blankly at this and did not appear to have assimilated the message. Suddenly, she commanded: "Smile." I smiled. "Now make your face laugh." I said: "It's difficult to laugh unless you have something to laugh about. However, I'll try for you." I laughed, rather a phoney laugh. She continued: "Are you happy when you laugh?" "You have got it the wrong way around. I laugh when I am happy." "Be cross," she ordered. "That's even a harder thing to do than laughing. You have to be angry with someone to show a cross face and I am not angry." "Are you happy now?" she asked curiously. "Not so happy now, because you don't seem to be so happy. I am a little worried when you are not happy." "Look worried then. Make your face worried. Why don't you cry?" "When something bad happens to me, I feel worried, and because I feel worried my face looks worried, and then if it's bad enough I cry. At present I don't feel so worried that I want to cry." "Are you unhappy when you cry?" "No, you've got it the wrong way around again. I cry when I am unhappy, and I am unhappy when something makes me unhappy." "If I pinched you, would you cry?" "Yes, if you pinched me hard enough, I certainly would cry." She took hold of my cheek and tweaked it, at first gently and then harder and harder, and the harder she tweaked the more painful did my expression become. Eventually she stopped. "Are you unhappy now?" she asked. "Yes, I am unhappy because you pinched hard. I don't want to smile or laugh now because I am unhappy because it was painful." "But you didn't cry," she said almost with a note of disappointment. "That's because it wasn't hard enough. If you had pinched me really hard, then I would feel a lot of pain, and then I would cry." There was a pause during which it seemed to me something was taking place inside her. "It follows," she remarked after a while somewhat surprisingly. She was the child of a severe hebephrenic mother whose affects were utterly incongruous and unpredictable. From this case, we learned something about the process of self-nonself-differentiation in terms of feelings, sensations, and expressions.

CASE 2

In a session with a very frightened little girl, she reported her mother's belief that the food at home was being poisoned and that they were all doomed to die and that her mother had heard people talking in the attic who were busy plotting her death and that they were also attempting to introduce machines into her bed to influence her thinking. The first of many other "demystifying" sessions began, and in the context of illness, she was gently instructed in the ways in which illness could make people imagine a wide variety of phenomena. Every question of the child was answered as realistically as possible and in a matter-of-fact way. The results were so gratifying that it was incorporated as a technique among the corrective interventions.

We have found that organizational competence can be gradually enhanced by exercises that interest and involve the child and stimulate him to order and classify his material, schedule his work efforts, and bring together parts to construct a whole. An important component to the exercises is reversibility, so that the child is encouraged to do and undo, make, unmake, and remake, and go forward and return along his tracks. Models and jigsaws are interesting and challenging tasks for this type of child. An illustration of this approach is given in the next case.

CASE 3

Another equally disorganized and disturbed boy, the child of a psychotic, seemed hopelessly inept in all that he tried to do and was driven further into irreality by his inability to function in any way appropriate to his age and intelligence. He was given, among many other things, some fragments of a model and was helped to put it together with glue into a complete car. His pleasure at having converted a lot of parts into a whole was unbounded. He became intensely preoccupied with model making, and this was encouraged. His high vulnerability score dropped dramatically on retesting. He later reported that he had given one of his early models to a friend and that "It was so well glued together that it would never break up"; his pride was obvious.

Sometimes nature takes a hand unexpectedly in research and helps to illuminate a particular problem. In the following case, a life-threatening event intervened in a way that made the research group realize that although play methods can be effective in bringing about changes in the behavior of children, they cannot hope to match the impact of actual experiences that completely alter the child's way of life.

CASE 4

A 6-year-old boy, son of a chronic paranoid schizophrenic, was severely disorganized, chaotic in his behavior, amorphous in his thinking, and poorly integrated in his personality. His sense of reality was markedly defective, and he was prone to unreal experiences. He remained relatively unchanged for two years under surveillance when he was transferred from the main project to this one. On testing, he scored poorly on self- and nonself-differentiation, on organizational proficiency, on reality testing, on magical thinking, and on logicality of thought. He was frequently very confused. His total score was 28, and we registered him as a seriously disturbed case. At this point, he developed diabetes, and a year later his total score had dropped dramatically to 15. The changes in the family over the same time were minimal. He was doing well at school (when before he could hardly stay in school) and was altogether better differentiated, better organized, and much more realistic and rationally communicative. In the interview, he described his experience with the diabetes. "A diabetic can be quite normal," he informed us. He gave his own shots, tested his own urine, managed his own diet, handled his own hypoglycemic episodes, and charted his own medical progress. It seemed inescapable that the diabetes had acted as an organizing focus in his life. It seemed to us that one type of corrective intervention could take the form of an organizing activity of serious life significance to the individual. It did not have to be an illness.

A Test-Retest Intervention Model

The high risk children of psychotic parents can be presumed as a group to have difficulties around self- and object-differentiation, reality testing, and competent organization of their inner and outer worlds. These may be due to both genetic factors (antecedents of adult psychosis) and environmental factors, (contact disturbances).

By using psychiatric, psychological, and experimental appraisals, a vulnerability score can be elicited. An intervention, classified quantitatively as massive, moderate, minimal, or none and qualitatively as compensatory, classical, cathartic, corrective, or none, can then be made and the vulnerability retested. The changes in measurable vulnerability can then be correlated with the amount and type of intervention carried out, with risk scores, with levels of representational and performance competence, with the presence or absence of disorder, and with changes in the competence of the family as a whole in directing, organizing, planning, and coping with problems of everyday living. This operational model is illustrated in Table 10.

The Risk-Vulnerability Intervention Model in Operation

The children of psychotic parents, when compared with children of nonpsychotic, not only show a greater tendency to become clinically disturbed during the period of childhood and adolescence ($z = 3.89, p = .00005$), but also are more likely to develop adult psychiatric disorders ($z = 2.90, p = .0019$) and adult psychosis ($z = 4.095, p = .00002$). It would seem clear that the amount of cumulative risk to which the individual is exposed does bear a significant relationship with the presence or development of disorder, irrespective of the vulnerability factor, and the same is no doubt true with regard to vulnerability: the degree of vulnerability may determine the presence or development of disorder, irrespective of the risk factor.[3] It may well turn out to be the case, when this investigation is completed, that the upper levels of risk and vulnerability decide the degree of change that is possible regardless of the amount and type of intervention.

There were two other findings in the comparison of the matched samples of high and low risk subjects: first, the global rating of adjustment differentiated them at the .0007 level, giving some indication of the high degree of maladjustment in the high risk group; second, they could be significantly differentiated at the .02

---

[3] For further elucidation of this point, the two-way tables in *The Syndrome of the Psychologically Invulnerable Child* [9] may be consulted.

Table 10   Test-Retest Intervention Model

Area of Expected Change	Corrective Intervention	Test-Retest Change in Vulnerability Score
Self-differentiation	"Who am I?" Self-orientation exercise; self-other exercises	Three Mountains Test (Piaget); Identity Rating (Psychol. Eval.); FRT (Bene-Anthony)
Object-differentiation	"What is it?" Course of exercises in object differentiation	WISC (Vocab., Pict., Concept.); ITPA (Tell me all about . . .); Embedded Figures (Witkin)
Reality testing and magical thinking	"What's real?" Open-ended multiple choice reality questions followed by reality conversations	Retest on multiple choice questions; Broken Bridge Test (Piaget); Logicality and Reality Testing Ratings (Psychol. Eval.)
Puzzlement and representational competence	"What's normal?" Demystification sessions regarding parental mental illness and mental illness in general	Psychiat. Eval. of understanding; attitude questionnaire; disease epistemology
Organizational competence	"How to make things work" Making parts into wholes (models, jigsaws); reversibility ("there-and-back" games)	WISC (object assembly, digits); retest on reversibility game; integrative capacity (Rorschach); coping and defensive skills (Psychol. Eval.)

level by the presence of internalized as opposed to externalized disorder.

Various tentative hypotheses were formulated with respect to the changes that might be expected:

HYPOTHESIS 1

It was expected that the greater the amount of intervention, the greater would be the diminution in the retest vulnerability score.

HYPOTHESIS 2

It was expected, on the basis of a pilot experience, that interventions emphasizing intrapersonal and interpersonal elements (classical) would be more likely to reduce vulnerability scores than those putting stress on ego support, catharsis, and cognitive restructuring. (This hypothesis also reflected the "classical" bias of the investigator!)

HYPOTHESIS 3

It was expected that the families of children showing a greater diminution in the vulnerability score make greater gains in direction, organization, and "planfulness." (In other words, the greater the change in the competence of the family, the greater will be the change in the children in terms of lesser vulnerability and consequently lesser disorder.)

HYPOTHESIS 4

It was expected that the higher the risk score, the greater would be the diminution in the vulnerability score.

HYPOTHESIS 5

It was expected that children manifesting clinical disturbances would tend to show a greater diminution in the vulnerability score than children who were not disturbed, the level of risk being kept constant.

Some Interim Results and Discussion

It should be emphasized that the main purpose for this presentation is to offer a model for investigating the effects of various types of intervention on high risk children with various degrees of vulnerability and to stimulate more work in this area. The research itself is still in interim phase and the data analysis far from complete. Because the *N*s are still small, standard statistical measures have not been employed. The figures given are meant merely to indicate trends.

When massive and moderate interventions were combined and compared with minimal and no interventions, there would seem to be clear support for the first hypothesis indicating that vulnerability, as measured in this investigation, was sensitive to the time factor and that the more time that was spent with the child, the more likely were his specific susceptibilities to be reduced (Table 11).

There was also some support for the second hypothesis suggesting that the classical therapy used in child guidance clinics emphasizing

The Bled Conference

Table 11   Test-Retest Ratings Relating to
Amount of Intervention
(Excluding Corrective Intervention)
(Use of 5-point scale 0-4 with low scores indicating betterment)
($N = 28$)

Amount of Intervention	Test* (mean scores)	Retest (mean scores)	Difference
Massive†	22.47	15.32	7.15
Moderate	18.23	12.74	6.49
Minimal	21.68	22.58	−0.90
None	18.74	16.31	2.43

* The test areas include self-differentiation, nonself-differentiation, organizational proficiency, reality testing, magical thinking, puzzlement.
† Massive = >50 hours; moderate = 10–50 hours; minimal = 1–10 hours.

therapeutic relationships and insight was more effective in reducing vulnerability than the nonclassical interventions (which did not include behavior therapy) (Table 12).

The results from the corrective interventions are at best tentative since the data are still to be fully analyzed, but there is some evidence to show that certain subjects respond with enthusiasm to the exercises for object differentiation, whereas other subjects seem resistant if not actually negativistic. In the reality exercises a few subjects showed changes that were manifest and convincing; although the changes in reality testing remained approximately the same, almost as if there was a resistance to changing the home reality or the intervener's reality, the other subjects showed improvements in the projective aspects of reality as measured on the Rorschach.

In the third hypothesis, the associated reductions in vulner-

Table 12   Test-Retest Ratings Relating to
Type of Intervention
($N = 35$)

Type of Intervention	Test (mean scores)	Retest (mean scores)	Difference
Compensatory (7)	20.34	17.21	3.13
Classical (6)	25.16	11.24	13.92
Cathartic (7)	22.56	21.43	1.12
Corrective (10)	23.62	18.73	4.89
None (5)	18.74	16.31	2.43

Table 13   Concomitant Change in Children and Their Families

Appraisal of Family Change*	Mean Test-Retest Difference in Child	Mean Test-Retest Difference in Family
Small change families	2.78	1.94
Large change families	4.63	38.1

* The extent of change is based on a psychosocial appraisal of direction, organization, and planfulness.

Table 14   Risk and Testable Vulnerability
($N = 20$)

Risk Category	Test Vulnerability (mean score)	Retest Vulnerability (mean score)	Difference
High ($N=7$)	30.29	21.43	8.86
Intermediate ($N=6$)	26.60	25.21	1.39
Low ($N=7$)	22.75	22.60	0.15

Table 15   Disorder and Testable Vulnerability

	Clinical Disorder Present	Clinical Disorder Absent
Mean diminution in vulnerability on retest	43	34
	43	34

ability score with family improvement were of the right order although the differences were small and expectation is that further work will disclose much stronger support for this hypothesis (Table 13).

The support for the fourth hypothesis appeared to be stronger although the *N*s were small (Table 14).

The fifth hypothesis predicting a greater diminution in vulnerability score in the presence of clinical disorder was in the expected direction, but once again the *N*s were small and the difference not too supportive (Table 15).

Conclusion

An attempt has been made to construct a risk profile furnishing a total risk score summarizing a series of inborn and environmental hazards for children with a psychotic parent, and to measure the

vulnerability of these children to the specific risks of psychosis by
evaluating them psychiatrically, psychologically, and experimentally,
focusing on areas that were judged to be sensitive to the psychotic
influence in previous empirical studies. Various types and amounts of
intervention were then applied and compared in terms of the changes
induced in the scores of the measured vulnerability. The durability
of these changes is one of the critical questions underlying the investigation and could only be answered by a short-term follow-up
study.

Although gratifying in bearing out some of the hunches, the
findings were, in certain respects, somewhat disappointing. The
initial expectation had been that the retest would offer much stronger
support for shorter, specific, inexpensive, and technically simple
procedures, but this was not the case. If further research could bring
increased evidence for the efficacy of these simpler and shorter
procedures, an attempt will be made to develop a curriculum for
use by paraprofessionals attached to special units at mental health
centers and mental health hospitals where it is hoped that the families
of the psychotic patients will be screened and helped if necessary,
and where preventive procedures will be available for the more
vulnerable children. We are still far from being finally satisfied with
either our scoring techniques or our intervention procedures, and
further modifications are currently being prepared for use in both
areas.

The figures presented are admittedly too small to draw firm
conclusions and the purpose for giving them is to illustrate the use of
the intervention model.

Our limited experience so far would suggest that not all areas are
equally sensitive to pressures for change. External behavior appears
less resistant than internal behavior, but this could also be due to the
well-known inertia of the internal milieu. Organizational competence
and nonself- or object-differentiation also seemed to make early and
evident gains. The self-concept, sense of identity, and realistic thinking progress more gradually. When the family as a whole changes
with the sick parent remaining well and the well parent realistically
oriented, the changes in vulnerability scores in all areas are dramatic.

We were, of course, concerned with the problem of obtaining
fully matched intervention and nonintervention groups. There
were a number of inherent difficulties, not least of all being the

ethical one of excluding individuals who were both vulnerable and at high risk from the intervention program. Furthermore, those who accepted the invitation for intervention appeared to be more highly motivated, more change-susceptible, and more desirous for change. When dealing with human subjects it is important to acknowledge the inevitability of such scientific limitations and to work as best one can within the situation.

References

All references are by E. James Anthony.

1. The developmental precursors of adult schizophrenia. *J. Psychiat. Res.*, 6 (Suppl. 1) (1968), 293–316.
2. The influence of maternal psychosis on children—folie à deux, in *Parenthood —Its Psychology and Psychopathology*, E. J. Anthony and T. Benedek, Eds. Little, Brown, Boston, 1970, pp. 571–595.
3. A clinical evaluation of children with psychotic parents. *Am. J. Psychiat.*, 126 (1969), 177–184.
4. The behavior disorders of childhood, in *Carmichael's Manual of Child Psychology*, Vol. II, P. Mussen, Ed. John Wiley & Sons, New York, 1970, pp. 667–764.
5. Mourning and psychic loss of the parent, in *The Child in His Family— The Impact of Disease and Death*, E. J. Anthony and C. Koupernik, Eds. John Wiley & Sons, New York, 1973, pp. 255–264.
6. The impact of mental and physical illness on family life. *Am. J. Psychiat.*, 127 (1970), 138–146.
7. The effect of drug treatment on the patient's family. The Role of Drugs in Community Psychiatry. *Mod. Probl. Pharmacopsychiat.*, 6 (1971), 95–109.
8. The contagious subculture of psychosis, in *Progress in Group and Family Therapy*. C. J. Sager and H. S. Kaplan, Eds. Brunner/Mazel, New York, 1972, pp. 636–658.
9. The syndrome of the psychologically invulnerable child. In this volume.

Neurological Findings in Children of Schizophrenic Parents

Joseph Marcus, M.D. (Israel)

The offspring of schizophrenic parents are now considered, on the basis of outcome studies, to be at greater risk for the eventual development of schizophrenia. Rosenthal and Kety [3] have concluded that the transmission of this type of psychosis can be understood on the basis of a diathesis-stress model, according to which the children of such parents begin their lives with a genetically determined vulnerability that is then compounded with the stresses of life in a psychotic family milieu to lay the groundwork for a psychotic breakdown in later life. Although such a genetic diathesis is acknowledged by many, there has been only minimal investigation of the basic characteristics of this diathesis, or of its exact incidence among schizophrenic offspring.

It was in an attempt to identify the incidence and characteristics of such a diathesis or vulnerability that our research group, along with several others [1, 2], undertook a careful study of such children.[1] For the purpose of this conference I wish to report very briefly on only one aspect of a multifaceted, longitudinal project which is still in process. This is the investigation of neurological functioning in these children.

[1] U.S. Public Health Service—National Institute of Mental Health, Project number 06–275–2. Project Officer: David Rosenthal, Ph.D.; Chief Investigator: Schmuel Nagler, Ph.D.

Methodology

A sample of 100 school-age children (ages 7½–14) were examined, 50 children with one schizophrenic parent, and 50 control cases matched for sex, age, school class, and ethnic and social background. Each of these groups was further subdivided into children living in urban nuclear families and those from the kibbutz society. (This was in order to allow an analysis of genetic-environment interaction.) The schizophrenic parents were selected from hospital files with an independent clinician evaluating each case and choosing only those who had undergone a clear-cut schizophrenic psychotic episode according to classical Bleulerian criteria.

In constructing our neurological examination, we attempted to cover all the areas of possible relevance that might reveal the minimal signs of deficiency in neural integration or neurological immaturity. The emphasis was on "soft signs," such as the assessment of fine motor coordination, perception, visual-auditory integration, vestibular functioning, adventitious motor overflow, and primitive postural reflexes. Because of local conditions, we were unable to carry out such specialized investigations as EEG or delayed feedback experiments.

We drew mainly on the work of Paine and Oppé, Prechtl and Stemmer, Cohen, Taft, and Birch, and Stott in constructing the final routine. All examinations were carried out by the same examiner during the second testing session, following the psychophysiological procedure, and the examiner was "blind" to the identity of the children examined. The neurological examination covered the following areas:

General physical state.   Body build, weight, height, head circumference, skin, asymmetries, stigmata.

Motor system: Muscle tone and strength, tendon reflexes, cranial motor nerves, posture, arm rebound, and gait.

Motor coordination: Motor tasks of varying difficulty; walking, hopping, tandem walk, kicking a ball, tiptoe walking, finger-following, finger to nose test, finger opposition, diadochokinesis, match lifting, drawing.

Adventitious motor overflow: Mirror movements, choreiform movements and other involuntary movements, and all forms of associated movements during various tasks, tongue protrusion, hopping, tiptoe and heel walking, diadochokinesis, finger opposition, etc.

Lateral dominance.

Perception and sensory system: Visual acuteness, stereognosis, form perception, and visual motor coordination.

Right-left orientation.

Vestibular function: Directional and optokinetic nystagmus, Romberg sign.

Postural and primitive reflexes: Posture, finger spooning, elbow posture and arm rotations, palmar-mental reflex.

Autonomic nervous system: Triple response.

Language and speech: Phonation, articulation, comprehension, writing.

Audio-visual integration: Birch-Belmont AV Pattern Test.

Whenever this was possible, each item was scored on a scale.

In addition to the scores on individual items, an overall score of nonoptimal neurological functioning was compiled by adding together the total scores from all items in the examination. The examination gives the possibility of assessing gross neurological damage as well as minor developmental deviations, or "soft" signs. Further supporting evidence was obtained from anemnesis, behavioral observation, and psychological tests performed. Although there are no Israeli norms at our disposal which can clearly define the normal age limits for the disappearance of many of these soft signs, various sources seem to indicate that by the age of 7 or 8 years the continued existence of any of the following signs can most likely be considered as indicative of neurological damage, delayed maturation, or faulty integration. The soft signs of MBD include the following:

Motor: Gross awkwardness: hopping, toe-walking, ball-kicking. Fine motor movements: visual-motor, pencil and paper tests, writing. Fine choreoathetosis. Fine tremor. Choreiform movements. Slight ataxia. Awkward tongue movement, dysarthria. Mirror movements, other associated movements or adventitious motor overflow. Mixed or crossed dominance. Muscle asymmetry.

Sensory: Impaired stereognosis and visual integration.

Neuropsychological: Impaired coping of geometrical designs, left-right orientation, and finger-gnosis.

Physical: Body asymmetry and stigmata.

Language: Nonrecognition of words, and lack of understanding of meaning of words.

Deteriorating signs: At least three of the preceding signs on
one side of the body only.

Results

The examinations were carried out under standard conditions,
following the establishment of a good relationship between the
children and the examiner. Though originally provision was made
for adjusting scores for children who showed signs of anxiety,
tiredness, or uncooperativeness, the use of this exigency was found
to be unnecessary. All the children, without exception, were relaxed
and fully cooperative during the examination and showed no
significant anxiety.

A number of items were not included in the final analysis of data
due to two factors: (1) a shift in scores over time was seen, indicating
a gradual and subjective change in the examiner's judgment in
scoring, which made these items invalid; (2) variation was negligible,
that is, the item did not in any way discriminate between subjects.
These items were: head and body posture, the Romberg sign, arm
position, tics, finger to nose test, muscle tonus and power, biceps,
abdominal and palmar-mental reflexes, pattern of rising and
kicking, gait, tongue musculature, nystagmus, stereognosis, letter
recognition, sentence repetition, and skin color.

Overall Score of Nonoptimal Functioning

In line with the thinking of Prechtl, we felt that the best general
measure of neurological deficit or immaturity would be a cumulative assessment of the indications of nonoptimal functioning. Therefore an overall score was constructed from all the remaining items
that were relevant to nonoptimal neurological functioning. There
were 88 possible "points" of nonoptimal functioning, and the actual
scores ranged from 1 to 40. When these scores were plotted against
age in a scattergram, the resulting pattern was clearly a developmental one, with neurological functioning maturing with age
(see Figure 1).

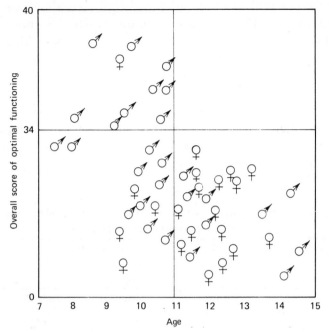

Figure 1   Scattergram.

This scattergram revealed, at the same time, a most interesting finding. If one considers the younger, less mature children under the age of 11, those in whom there is still a moderately wide spread in level of functioning,[2] one finds just *half* of the index cases clustered together in the area representing poor functioning (i,e., with a score of over 24 points of nonoptimal functioning), whereas all the other index cases are evenly scattered among the control cases and show a comparable level of overall neurological functioning and maturity.

This led us to the following line of thought: If the schizophrenic disorder is transmitted through a single dominant gene, as advocated by some, only (approximately) half of the children of one schizophrenic parent should inherit this pathological gene, and if this gene could influence neurological functioning, it would be revealed by a significant degree of nonoptimal neurological performance in the children carrying it.

---

[2] This is both arbitrarily half of our whole sample, and also a logical cutoff point in terms of what we know about the normal curve of such developmental neurological findings.

Therefore we ranked all the subjects according to their overall score and then divided the index group into two halves, those with the highest scores of nonoptimal functioning and those with lower. We then divided the control group similarly, and we compared the high nonoptimal functioning subjects, index versus control, and the low nonoptimal subjects, index versus control. Theoretically, in the first comparison the index subjects should score significantly higher, and in the second comparison there should be no significant difference between the index and control cases. This was born out, as seen in Table 1.

Table 1   Neuropathology Scores of Index and Control Children
(*T* Test for Noncorrelated Means)

$t\,(i-c)=4422$			$t\,(i-c)=-.0741$		
$df=23$			$df=23$		
$p<.01$			N.S.		
Number	Index	Control	Number	Index	Control
1	40	26	1	15	12
2	36	24	2	15	12
3	35	23	3	12	12
4	34	23	4	12	12
5	32	23	5	11	12
6	31	23	6	10	11
7	29	23	7	10	11
8	29	22	8	10	11
9	25	22	9	9	10
10	25	22	10	9	10
11	24	22	11	8	10
12	24	21	12	8	9
13	23	19	13	8	9
14	21	19	14	8	9
15	20	17	15	6	9
16	20	17	16	6	8
17	19	17	17	6	7
18	18	16	18	5	7
19	18	15	19	4	6
20	17	15	20	4	5
21	17	14	21	3	5
22	17	14	22	2	4
23	16	14	23	2	4
24	16	13	24	1	3
25	16	13	25	1	2

If we go back again and limit our comparisons to that half of our sample (50 children) who are under the age of 11, and we compare the high scoring index cases directly with their own matched controls, we find a level of significance of 0.001. Thus this seems to be a clearly differentiated group, representing one-half of the index cases—possibly in line with a single dominant gene theory.

We must emphasize, however, that this is still a small sample. Also, within this particular group of 12 cases there is a preponderance of city males. This might suggest the existence of possible environmental or sex factors as well, which we will discuss later.

Individual Items

Analyses of each individual item were carried out to determine which functions contributed most to the overall score of nonoptimal functioning. Such analyses were carried out on the complete sample ($N = 100$) and on the younger children only ($N = 50$). Also, a direct comparison was made between the 12 index cases with nonoptimal scores over 24 and their controls. The results are seen in Table 2.

These results seem to point to a certain degree of delay in general motor development or possibly some unilateral damage (i.e., asymmetry and unilateral weakness of face muscles). Deficits in certain other circumscribed cerebral functions seem to exist as well (i.e., right-left orientation, perception, and intersensory or (auditory-visual) integration).

Other Analyses of Data

As with all other data in this study, the neurological data were subjected to a quadron analysis (i.e., a t test for matched pairs extended to the case of four matched subjects) for the following comparisons: index versus control (D_1); city versus kibbutz (D_2); interaction (D_3). The results of D_1 were congruent, naturally, with those reported above. The comparison of city versus kibbutz subjects (D_2) showed a greater degree of motor overflow in city children. The only explanation that comes to mind is that the emphasis placed on motor activity and cognitive development in the kibbutz may give these children some advantage in general development, especially

**Table 2   Comparisons of Index and Control Cases on
Individual Items of Neurological Examination
(*T* Test for Matched Pairs: Two-Tailed)**

Items Showing Significant Differences	Total Sample $N=50$ $t=2.02$ $p=.05$ $t=2.69$ $p=.01$		Younger Sample $N=25$ $t=2.07$ $p=.05$ $t=2.81$ $p=.01$		"High Scores" $N=12$ $t=2.23$ $p=.05$ $t=3.17$ $p=.01$	
Asymmetry			.05		.01	
Finger opposition, right					.05	
Finger opposition, left			.05		.01	
Diadochokinesis, right					.05	
Diadochokinesis, left					.05	
Associated movements					.05	
Knee jerk					.05	
Left-right orientation	.50		.01		.05	
Lower face muscles					.05	
Hand coordination, right	.01		.05			
Hand coordination, left	.01		.05			
Perception, item 1	.05		.01		.05	
Perception, item 2					.05	
AV integration	.05		.05		.05	

motor, over their peers in the city. Another possibility (for which we have no hard data) is that the perinatal care given in the city might fall below that given in the kibbutz, so that there may have been more perinatal pathology in the former.

The interaction comparison (D_3) revealed that when contrasting the degree of differences between index and control cases in the city and the kibbutz, the index cases in the city were significantly more pathological as regards the overall score of nonoptimal functioning (right-left orientation, adiadochokinesis, and motor overflow into the left hand during pronation-supination of the right hand).

A sign test of quadrons (of the total number of items) was made to analyze the direction or the general trend toward pathology in the various quadron comparisons (D_1, D_2, D_3). The test showed a significantly stronger trend toward nonoptimal functioning in the index cases (D_1) and in the city cases (D_2). The comparison of differences between index and control in kibbutz as compared to index and control in the city showed a strong, significant trend toward a greater difference between index and control city children, as had been inferred in the previous analyses (see Table 3).

Table 3 Sign Test of Quadrons

D_1				D_2				D_3			
Number Negative	Number Positive	N	S	Number Negative	Number Positive	N	S	Number Negative	Number Positive	N	S
20	36	56	S+	33	18	51	S−	50	9	59	S−

References

1. Anthony, E. J. The developmental precursors of adult schizophrenia, *The Transmission of Schizophrenia*, D. Rosenthal and S. Kety, Eds. Pergamon Press, London, 1968, pp. 293–316.
2. Mednick, S. A. and Schulsinger, F. Some premorbid characteristics related to breakdown in children with schizophrenic mothers, in *The Transmission of Schizophrenia*, D. Rosenthal and S. Kety, Eds. Pergamon Press, London, 1968.
3. Rosenthal, D. and Kety, S. Eds. *The Transmission of Schizophrenia*. Pergamon Press, London, 1968.

A Geneticist's Approach to the Vulnerable Child

Leon E. Rosenberg, M.D. (U.S.A.)

To ask a geneticist to discuss risks of childhood vulnerability with a group of child psychiatrists is a bit like asking an architect to discuss ecology with a group of botanists. In both instances, the speaker and the spoken to are united by intense concern with the subject but may be separated by wide gulfs in professional language, body of facts, and orientation. It is tempting, when faced with these hazards, to retreat into one's own intellectual fortress and discourse on things one knows well, whether or not they promote communication or are truly germane to the topic. I shall try to prevent this Tower of Babel-like result by concentrating on information that both geneticists and psychiatrists need to know if they are to help each other help children.

Biological Perspective

Each human cell contains enough DNA to code for about 7 million proteins. If, as has been suggested, only 10 percent of this DNA is functionally active, this still provides a complement of approximately 700,000 proteins to regulate and modify human growth, development, and homeostasis. Since only about 1 percent of these proteins has been thus far identified chemically or genetically,

the function of the vast bulk of man's genetic machinery remains
to be elucidated.

This genetic material is constantly changing. Based on current
estimates of the rate of human mutation (1×10^{-5} per genetic locus
per generation) and the number of loci coding for proteins (7×10^5),
the total number of mutations expected per gamete is approximately 7. This very large number emphasizes the great potential
that mutational events have in the regulation of all human processes
and provides a numerical base for the appearance of the numerous
inborn errors of metabolism and specific cytogenetic abnormalities
known or yet to be discovered.

We are only beginning to appreciate the magnitude of disease
produced by genetic or congenital abnormalities. Approximately
5 per 1000 newborns in the United States have major chromosomal
abnormalities and 10 per 1000 have inherited metabolic disorders.
Thus in the United States alone more than 20,000 children per
year are born with chromosomal or metabolic disorders. Congenital
disorders rank second only to malignancy as causes for mortality in
children of age 0-5 years and may be responsible for as much as
25 percent of all hospital bed occupancy in the United States. These
figures attest to the important contribution that known genetic
abnormalities play in determining somatic vulnerability in children, and, by analogy, raise the possibility that inherited variation
may also play an important role in emotional illness.

Nature and Nurture

For more than 300 years philosophers, biologists, and politicians
have debated the relative importance of heredity and environment
in determining human intellect and behavior. The English
philosopher John Locke believed that the human mind was blank
at birth (*tabula rasa*) and that all differences between individuals
were environmentally produced. At the opposite extreme are the
views of the French diplomat J. A. Gobineau, who declared that all
differences in man's abilities were entirely innate. Each of these
views has been championed and polemicized, sometimes, as with
Adolf Hitler, to the great detriment of mankind. I contend that
this "nature versus nurture" controversy is artificial and specious.
To say that a human trait is inherited does not imply the absence

of environmental influences but merely the presence of genetic ones. Several examples may help illustrate this very important principle. There can be little doubt that the sex of a fertilized zygote is genetically determined, yet even this fundamental property can be modified dramatically by the intrauterine environment of the embryo. Extirpation of the rudimentary male gonads results in an animal whose cells are genotypically male (XY) but whose external genitalia are typically female. Conversely, administration of masculinizing hormones to a woman carrying a female fetus may produce permanent masculinization in her XX offspring.

Such environmental modifications of inherited characteristics are, of course, not restricted to the prenatal period. An infant born with an inherited deficiency of phenylalanine hydroxylase will become either a helpless retarded ward of society with phenylketonuria or an essentially healthy child, depending on the quantity of phenylalanine ingested during the first 3 to 5 years of life. In like manner, deficiency of glucose-6-phosphate dehydrogenase in black males usually leads to no clinical illness unless the affected individual is given antimalarial drugs or other agents known to precipitate acute hemolytic crises in such patients. I could enumerate many other examples which underscore the principle that the phenotypic expression of single mutant genes of large effect can be modified extensively by nutritional, pharmacologic, and surgical alteration of the individual's environment.

Such nature-nurture interaction is not unidirectional. The concordance rates for tuberculosis and scarlet fever in monozygotic twins are significantly greater than those of dizygotic twins, implying that genetic factors modify susceptibility to infections from Mycobacterium tuberculosis and B-hemolytic streptococci, respectively.

Toward Behavioral Genetics

The importance of hereditary factors in somatic diseases of children and the synergism between such hereditary factors and the environment must be kept in mind as we approach the last and, unfortunately, the least clear topic of this discussion—human behavioral genetics. Just as the developmental geneticist inquires into the nature and location of those genes that control cellular differentiation and determination, so, the behavioral geneticist seeks information about genetic loci which influence normal behavior and searches for mutations which lead to behavioral abnormalities. I see no fundamental difference in these fields since I am as convinced that some genes control personality as I am that other genes determine the color of one's eyes or the length of one's toes. I do not ask whether inheritance plays a role in schizophrenia or manic-depressive psychosis any more than I ask whether genetic factors are etiologically responsible for spina bifida or sickle cell anemia. These convictions are based on a minimum of facts, a modicum of extrapolations, and a maximum of faith.

First let us look at the few facts. Several well-known inherited metabolic diseases may produce severe enough behavioral disturbances to warrant such diagnoses as schizophrenia or autism. I have seen a child with documented homocystinuria whose behavior was bizarre enough to lead expert child psychiatrists to diagnose autism. I have seen young adults with Wilson's disease and acute intermittent porphyria whose initial manifestations were psychiatric aberrations severe enough to be called schizophrenia. These could be chance occurrences, but each has been commented on by other workers as well, suggesting that the phenotypic abnormalities collectively called autism or schizophrenia may be produced by several different mutations which alter apparently unrelated metabolic pathways.

Numerous twin studies have shown higher concordance rates in monozygotic than dizygotic twins for a variety of normal and abnormal personality traits (independence, enthusiasm, guilt, introversion) and for certain psychiatric disorders (schizophrenia, manic-depressive psychosis, psychopathic personality). These studies have been challenged since they have generally not been corrected for the probability that there is greater similarity in the environment of monozygotic than in that of dizygotic twins. In the few studies of twin pairs reared apart, however, the influence of genetic factors on behavioral features and disorders has still been prominent.

Next we should consider the extrapolations. I would like to make brief mention of some studies of behavioral genetics in animals. In rats the ability to run through a maze has been convincingly demonstrated to depend on genetic influences. There is an infectious disease of honey bees which destroys infected colonies. Certain bee strains, however, are resistant to this disease. In such strains worker bees uncap the wax cells and remove the infected larvae from the hive. This behavior is controlled by two recessive genes, one or both genes are resistant to the infection, whereas strains lacking one or both mutations are susceptible.

Perhaps the most exciting work in this field is being done by Benzer and his colleagues with fruit flies (Drosophila). These investigators have isolated large numbers of mutant flies with specific behavioral disorders of many kinds: X-linked mutations leading to loss of the normal ability to move toward a light source (even though the visual apparatus and the locomotor system are intact); X-linked mutations producing distortions of the normal circadian rhythm regulating sleep and wakefulness; different autosomal mutations which lead to sexual aberrations such as homosexuality, lack of courtship success, or (the most pathetic of all) "stuck" in which the mutant male is unable to withdraw his penis after copulation. I hasten to remind you that none of these mutations has yet been documented in the human species, but I believe that Monod was essentially correct when he suggested that "what is true for E. coli is true for the elephant," by which he meant that fundamental genetic concepts such as the genetic code or the mechanisms of protein synthesis which were worked out in bacteria will ultimately be confirmed in mammalian cells, including those of man.

Finally, I resort to faith. I believe that in the years ahead we shall learn that behavior is regulated by biochemical and genetic mechanisms similar or identical to those which modulate the physiology of the liver, kidney, or skeletal muscle. As we learn of these biochemical determinants of behavior, we shall surely find "nature's experiments" in which both the biochemistry and the behavior will be modified by single gene mutations. Such biochemical modifications will lead to diagnostic tests and ultimately to modes of therapy for those many psychiatric disorders which, for lack of more precise definition, we lump today under such headings as autism or schizophrenia. My faith is so deep that I even believe I shall be around to witness these events.

Obstetrical Risk in the Genesis of Vulnerability

A. Minkowski, M.D. and C. Amiel-Tison, M.D. (France)

Today there is general awareness of the risks to the central nervous system encountered by the factors during prenatal life, by the full-term neonate during and after delivery, and by the premature infant. The only question is how to obtain reliable statistics on the incidence of vulnerable offspring in a given population. Thus far the figures and the interpretations based on them that have appeared in the growing literature on risk have tended to be biased by the theoretical orientation of the authors, leading, for example, on one side to the statement that fetal asphyxia has no more effect on the brain than on the heart [6] and on the opposite side to the assertion that the incidence of severe sequelae among prematures is one in three [11].

In actual fact, most of the figures dealing with CNS involvement are simply extrapolations from mortality rates. Nevertheless, the collaborative project of the U.S. National Institute of Health might in this respect provide us with the most reliable data so far available. In this review of the topic, we will consider the following points in turn:

1. Prenatal damage to the CNS.
2. Perinatal damage during delivery.

3. Prematurity and intrauterine growth retardation.
4. Socioeconomic factors.
5. The mother-child relationship.
6. The prevention of CNS involvement in each group.
7. The management of the vulnerable child.

Prenatal Damage to the CNS

We will not deal here with chromosome abnormalities. Whatever their theoretical interest, they are relatively rare. They raise the problem of early amniocentesis and of the possible need for abortion. Our main concern is the chronic fetal distress occurring between the 28th and the 40th week of pregnancy due mainly to *toxemia* of pregnancy. This condition is very frequently ignored or neglected by the pregnant woman. It can be detected by repeated routine measurements of the blood pressure which, in a pregnant woman, should not exceed 130/90. In Sweden every pregnant woman is routinely seen ten times by midwives and four times by obstetricians. If the blood pressure goes beyond this level at two sequential examinations, the woman should be put to bed at absolute rest for one month. Even if she does not feel indisposed, her uterus may be in a state of continuous contractility, which may result in a retardation of intrauterine growth and fetal distress from brain involvement. In some cases it can progress to *cortical necrosis* [2], an extremely serious state of affairs that is either incompatible with life or responsible for acute *status epilepticus*.

This brings up the question of induced premature delivery or (preferably) Caesarean section to prevent brain damage. The timing of this procedure is crucial: it must be early enough to prevent prolonged brain damage yet late enough to avoid prematurity (i.e., before the 34th week). A thorough examination of the mother can also help to control the factor of infection, mainly urinary, often responsible for prematurity and listeriosis, which is a very important cause of CNS involvement and where the only clinical evidence may be the symptom of a chill.

Another condition to bear in mind is diabetes, which can be detected with the help of the glucose tolerance test. Maternal rubella and toxoplasmosis can also be uncovered through routine testing and the same applies to blood group incompatibilities.

Perinatal Brain Lesions at the Time of Labor and Delivery in the Full-Term Infant

Birth trauma, as it is commonly called, is a process that causes severe damage to the central nervous system, leading to death or heavy neurological and psychological sequelae. It is avoidable in at least half the cases by the proper management of labor. *This means that all through the world hundreds of thousands of handicapped children are produced by poor obstetrical procedures.* Though supposedly a developed country, France not only has a shortage of obstetricians, it also fails to make good use of its midwives. Furthermore, pregnant women in France frequently live under deplorable socioeconomic conditions entailing poor housing, an overload of domestic work, and sometimes inadequate or defective nutrition. A great majority of public and private departments of obstetrics are lacking in modern equipment and cannot, for instance, give intensive care to a newborn who requires it. It is quite obvious that transportation to a distant department where this is available is not only the wrong answer to the problem but can sometimes aggravate the situation.

The factor of bad obstetrical management combined with the poor outcome of extreme prematurity should be our main concern in the reduction of risk. At a time when the Western countries have achieved such advances in medical research, problems that could be solved by common sense are being given little attention. Scandinavia, Holland, the United Kingdom, Israel, and some Socialist countries are the only ones that have adopted a prophylactic position and have dealt with the problems of prevention of birth trauma on a large scale in a sensible and appropriate way.

The main syndrome of brain involvement in the full-term infant at birth can be outlined as follows:

Neonatal status epilepticus. According to Monod and Dreyfus-Brisac, [12] the neonatal status epilepticus (NSE) is characterized in the newborn by repeated clinical or electrical spells of convulsions associated with intercrisis neurological or electrical symptoms and an extremely poor prognosis.

In their study of 150 NSE children, Monod and Dreyfus-Brisac found these obstetrical features: prematurity was present in 9 percent, an abnormal gestational history in 49 percent, an abnormal labor and delivery in 36 percent, and cerebral malformations in 9 percent. There are some problems in the recognition of NSE. The epileptic spells often are difficult to identify: only clonic jerks or rapid, clonic spells or abnormal movements or apnea with a special cry may be present. The electrical seizures are referred to as paronystic tracings, which may or may not be associated with *inactive tracings*. In 88 cases with EEG recordings, typical clinical and EEG tracings were found simultaneously in 38 percent, EEG tracings associated with minimal clinical symptoms in 25 percent; and in 15 percent, typical EEG tracings were not accompanied by any convulsion or abnormal symptoms such as intercritical fits. Occasionally the EEG is not characteristic when convulsions are repeated and typical. The intercritical signs and symptoms can include subcoma or coma with simultaneous convulsions present in 51 percent. Absence of wakefulness does not preclude diagnosis.

With regard to prognostic features, the time of onset is not significant but duration is of great importance: less than three days leaves some hope whereas over five days is very serious. Coma carries a bad prognosis. In terms of the intercritical EEG record, two successive paronysytic or inactive tracings in records obtained within the first 24 hours means an almost 100 percent chance of death or extremely serious sequelae. These infants are not incubated or ventilated. Quite inexplicably, 7 percent with normal EEG records are found associated with a serious prognosis.

Etiological factors are mainly vascular and include subdural hematomata, intraventricular hemorrhages [3] (mainly in premature infants), and diffuse cortical necroses; also involved are cerebral malformations and meningitis.

With regard to late prognosis, these were the findings. Of 120 cases, 13 percent were normal, 14 percent had minor sequelae, and 35 percent had encephalopathy; 38 percent were dead before the age of 3, 26 percent before 20 days, and 15 percent before 5 days.

Treatment was mainly symptomatic: 15 to 20 milligrams of phenobarbital per kilogram per 24 hours. Artificial ventilation and intensive care should be restricted to cases with no more than one abnormal EEG tracing, either paronystic or completely inactive.

Continuous electronic fetal monitoring is now recognized as providing an excellent alarm in case of fetal distress during labor. This evaluation is rapidly growing in accuracy and is based on the degree of oxygenation and brain status. The various components of heart rate change have been studied quantitatively in monkeys in order to utilize the exact values of such changes in estimating the actual state of fetal oxygenation [11]. Fetal heart rate has also been correlated with fetal electroencephalogram in the sheep fetus [11]; and cerebral blood flow, oxygen consumption, and glucose utilization has been investigated in fetal lambs *in utero* [11]. Clinical work is also gaining in accuracy by the development of the automatic analysis of fetal heart rate [2] and the correlation of this with EEG [2]. However, the experimental data of Myers and his group [8] on partial fetal asphyxia in monkeys has tied in so well with clinical experience that a few guidelines may already be of interest. Myers reproduced the cerebral lesions found in humans by partially asphyxiating full-term monkey fetuses for a few minutes to a few hours. The changes found in relation to the duration and severity of asphyxia were classified as no apparent pathological changes in the brain, mild to moderate cerebral edema, and acute cerebral necrosis comparable to the lesions of human perinatal injury or cerebral palsy.

A detailed obstetrical history thus is of the utmost importance in making an initial assessment of possible brain lesions in the full-term newborn. Partial fetal asphyxia leads to cerebral edema or necrosis and actual mechanical difficulty (difficult breach delivery, high midforceps delivery) to subdural hemorrhage. Both might ensue, for instance, when a forceps delivery follows on a dynamic dystocia. On one hand, cerebral necrosis is nearly always found in neonates who die following status epilepticus, the most dreadful result from pro-longed and severe asphyxia [8], and, on the other, the Myers' data allow us to assume that cerebral edema is the main lesion in the surviving newborn with marked neurological signs following on moderate fetal asphyxia (without status epilepticus). The main clinical difficulty is to recognize this edema and treat it accordingly as early as possible. In the absence of reliable signs indicating its presence in the newborn, one is faced with the prospect of treating without being able to measure the efficacy of the treatment. With regard to outcome, the lack of precision has to be admitted. There are already some data correlating obstetrical factors and neurological disorders in full-term neonates [2]. Normal EEG tracings and a neonatal course of short duration are the main arguments in favor of a good prognosis; when neurological abnormalities are rapidly

disappearing by the end of the first week, in most instances there
were probably no cellular lesions and the chances are that the child
will develop normally.

To predict accurately the neurological outcome from birth injury
is somewhat difficult. Follow-up studies are rather disappointing;
they have little value since both nosography and care may have
changed in the interim. For full-term neonates, the prognosis is very
poor with cerebral necrosis, equally poor with status epilepticus,
much better with the moderately impaired group, and good to
excellent when neurological symptoms and signs are transitory [2].

Although about 50 percent of obstetrical factors seem to be avoidable, it is nevertheless likely that a fraction of birth injury cases will
remain very difficult to eradicate completely.

Prematurity and Intrauterine Growth Retardation

In the follow-up of vulnerable neonates in this field, a great deal
of data have become available. They can be summarized as follows:

1. Among premature children, that is, children born before
   37 completed weeks, one must expect one-third of them to be
   handicapped with sensory defects, various school problems
   including reading disabilities, convulsions, abnormal EEGs,
   speech problems, and major brain impairment in the category
   of children below 1000 grams of weight and below 30 weeks of
   gestational age. It is important to wait until the beginning of
   school attendance (6 or 7 years) to make a worthwhile assessment [3, 9, 10].
2. It is also important to take into account the socioeconomic
   conditions that might equally interfere with development and
   the amount of early anxiety stemming from the mother's
   approach to child rearing [4].
3. One must take into account the past history of pregnancies.
   A child, for example, whose mother who experienced bleeding
   during pregnancy is likely to have twice as much chance to
   suffer from dyslexia as a child from a control series of mothers
   in whom bleeding has not occurred.
4. The "late syndrome of prematurity" described by Berges and
   Lezine [4] gives the best account of the common type of

deficiency to which the premature child is exposed. In part, their findings are derived from a test of motor imitation. The picture is characterized by evidence of organic impairment, by the presence of neurological signs such as tonic postural abnormalities, by delays in cognitive development (especially with the apperception of space and time), and by disturbances in emotional relationships. With severe intrauterine growth retardation, cerebral sequelae are a likely hazard. Many of these fetuses have been exposed to chemical distress [1, 5, 7] and, after birth, possibly to hypoglycemia. Fitzharding has pointed out that of 96 children with fetal hypohypotrophy that he followed for a minimum of 5 years, 25 percent manifested a minimal cerebral dysfunction, 6 percent convulsions, and 1 percent cerebral palsy.

Socioeconomic Factors

This is one of the major factors to take into account in any follow-up study. Most of the studies have made use of categories of paternal employment (professional, semiskilled, unskilled, others), yearly income (less than $1800, $1800–$2400, $2401–$3000, $3001–$3600, more than $3600), and of parental education (tenth grade or less, eleventh grade, high school graduate, college graduate, university).

Two factors must be emphasized: a mother-child separation should be restricted to what is compulsory in terms of active medical care. But once there is no vital risk, the premature infant must be given his mother. Otherwise, the well-known effects of hospitalism may develop and add their deleterious influence to that of a possible brain damage. Furthermore, the mother herself may be fearful of nursing such a fragile baby and will be inclined to entrust theoretically more skillful hands with its care. And thus a vicious circle may develop and interfere with the establishment of a positive mother-child relationship.

The Mother-Child Relationship

Extensive studies have been carried out showing that the relation is a factor of paramount importance in the fate of the premature infant [4]. The mother's anxiety during the period of hospitalization should be mitigated, for example, by the constant supply of information, by the permission to visit the infant freely, or psychotherapeutic help.

Parents should never be told too soon that the prognosis is gloomy. Well-trained people know that there is no constant relationship between the severity of the initial clinical picture and the degree of sequelae. A more valuable evaluation can be made at the end of the first year, but, finally, it is only at 3 years of age that specific difficulties (mainly in the area of speech and of motor and sensory development) can be diagnosed and adequately dealt with.

This factor has been too frequently overlooked in the past and should be given as much attention as physical intensive care.

Prevention of Brain Impairment on the Larger Scale

It is only by means of energetic preventive measures that the incidence of central nervous system damage will eventually be reduced. Every country should elaborate a prenatal and perinatal policy including such measures as routine examinations of the mother and bed rest if deemed necessary. This latter should be accompanied by a provision to pay the mother if she works or to provide her with domestic help. These measures are currently taken only in Scandinavia, Holland, Bulgaria, Czechoslovakia, China, and North Vietnam etc. and a few other countries.

A Well-Equipped Intensive Care Unit

In some cases the life and future integrity of the child can be served only by a well-equipped intensive care department. The fact should be stressed that at the present time neonatalogists are becoming concerned not only with survival per se but with the survival of good quality.

Only a department of this kind can provide control of biochemical homeostasis, proper supply of calories and nutrients, and artificial ventilation when needed. Obviously, since it is impossible to increase the number of such centers because of limitations of personnel and finance, it might be advisable in countries where the economic situation will allow it to have smaller units widely distributed, as has been accomplished in Sweden. It cannot, however, be emphasized enough that departments of intensive care cannot replace a policy of well-organized and administered prevention.

References

1. Ackerman, B. D., Dyer, G. Y., and Leydorf, M. M. Hyperbilirubinemia and kernicterus in small premature infants. *Pediatrics*, 45 (1970), 918–925.
2. Amiel-Tison, C. Cerebral damage in the newborn. *Biol. Neonat.*, 14 (1969), 224.
3. Amiel-Tison, C. Intraventricular cerebral hemorrhage in the premature infant: Elements of clinical diagnoses. *Biol. Neonat.*, 7 (1964), 57–75.
4. Berges, J., Lezine, I., Harrison, A., and Boisselier, F. Le syndrome de l'ancien prématuré. Recherche sur sa signification. *Rev. Neuropsychiat. Infantile*, 17 (1969), 719–779.
5. Chunga, F. and Lardinois, R. Separation by gel filtration and microdetermination of unbound bilirubin. 1. In vitro albumin and acidosis effects on albumin-bilirubin binding. *Acta Peadiat. Scand.*, 60 (1971), 27–32.
6. Drillien, C. M. *Growth and Development of the Premature Infant.* Livingston, Edinburgh, 1964.
7. Gartner, L. M., Snyder, R. N., Chabon, R. S., and Bernstein, J. Kernicterus: High incidence in premature infants with low serum bilirubin concentrations. *Pediatrics*, 45 (1970), 906–917.
8. James, L. S., Myers, R. E., and Gaull, G. E., Eds. Brain damage in the fetus and newborn from hypoxia of asphyxia. *Report of the Fifty-Seventh Ross Conference on Pediatric Research.* Columbus, O., Ross Laboratories, 1967.
9. Larroche, J. C. Cerebral lesions in the premature infant at birth. *Rev. Neuropsychiat. Infantile*, 12 (1964), 269–275.
10. Larroche, J. C. Hémorragies cérébrales intra-ventriculaires chez le prématuré. 1ère partie: Anatomie et physiopathologie. *Biol. Neonat.*, 7 (1964), 26–56.
11. Minkowski, A., Spears, R., and Swierczewski, E. Foetal oxygenation: Its relation to the central nervous system. Seminar on the occurrence of cerebral lesions before and during birth, Paris, 1961. *Probl. act. Pediat.*, 8 (1963), 129–169. Karger, Bâle, New York.
12. Monod, W. and Dreyfus-Brisac, C. Paroxystic EEG of newborns at term. *EEG C. L. Enur.* 14 (1962), 778.

Mothers at Risk: A Potential Consequence of the Hospital Care of the Premature Infant*

P. Herbert Leiderman, M.D. (U.S.A.)

Introduction

The evidence from numerous pediatric and child psychiatric [1] studies indicates that the premature infant is potentially at risk. Such an infant born prematurely is more likely to show signs of neurological dysfunction, has a greater likelihood of showing behavioral disorders in childhood and adolescence, and performs less well on intelligence tests than a full-term child. Although this statement is generally true, there is evidence to indicate that premature infants born to middle-class parents do not bear the same risk as do premature infants born to lower-class families [2]. Specifically, the physical and psychological retardation for a group of middle-class youngsters born prematurely is less severe than for infants raised in lower-class families. When children with neurological damage are excluded, there appears to be almost no difference between premature and full-term youngsters in the middle-class group.

These observations indicate that while prematurity and the infant's

* This research was supported by grants from the Grant Foundation, New York, and the National Institutes of Health, grant number HD-02636.

subsequent growth and development may be influenced primarily by biological factors, social factors do mitigate some of these biological elements. It may therefore be possible, by examining the social factors in the premature infant's life, to account for some of this decrement in his psychological development.

There are several factors associated with social class that might account for differences between middle-class and lower-class children. Infant malnutrition, maternal attitudes, and maternal behavior vary by membership in specific social class. Therefore, assuming that nutrition is not an important factor in most urban United States environments, it might prove fruitful to explore maternal factors. Of these maternal factors, one of the most intriguing is the relationship a mother establishes with her infant in the early periods of development.

The mother's relationship to her infant, especially in the neonatal period, is influenced by her expectations and attitudes toward the infant, and by the type and amount of social interaction she has with it. For the mother of the premature infant, both expectations and social interaction with the infant differ from the mother of the full-term infant. The mother of a premature has a discrepancy between her expectations and reality due to the early arrival and the small size of the infant; she has very little opportunity, in the typical hospital environment, to be with her infant during the immediate neonatal period since it is cared for by specialists in a separate nursery for periods as long as two to three months.

Accepting the fact that the premature infant is at risk, as stated above, it is the purpose of this essay to look at the possibility of the mother's being at risk, given a situation of early separation from her infant in the modern technologically oriented nursery. The question being addressed is: Does the deprivation of interaction between a mother and her premature infant during the neonatal period have a deleterious effect on subsequent maternal relationships with the infant?

Description of the Study

The research reported here had its genesis in the observation of mothers of premature infants hospitalized in the Stanford University Medical Center nurseries [3–6]. Over a period of 4 years mothers were interviewed and directly observed within the hospital and in the home in order to understand the possible effects of prematurity and maternal separation on subsequent maternal behavior. To accomplish this we arranged that the hospital nursery permit a certain proportion of mothers of prematures to undertake care of their infants while they were still hospitalized in the nursery. Thus we were able to examine the effects of early mother-infant interaction in three population groups: the mothers of prematures who had early contact with their infants; a group of mothers of prematures who underwent the usual procedure of being separated from their infants; and a group of full-term mothers who served as a comparison group for the mothers of prematures.

Studies of infant separation in humans have focused on the consequences of separation for the infant rather than for the mother. This one-sided focus on the infant is particularly unfortunate in light of the many mammalian studies of maternal behavior which emphasize the importance of the young in stimulating this behavior. These studies suggest that the timing and duration of the animal mother's earliest contact with her young are crucial in determining her later behavior toward her infant. If contact with her young is delayed by separating the animal mother from her infant for a period immediately or shortly after birth, she may exhibit maladaptive maternal behavior when contact is once again permitted.

There are no comparable data for the human mother and no data regarding whether or not the neonatal period is a particularly sensitive one for her to undergo separation from her infant. Yarrow, [7], in summarizing the evidence for the human infant, states, "The most sensitive time may be the period in which the infant is in the process of establishing stable, affectional relationships, approximately between six months and two years." Research on animals, on the other hand, has demonstrated that for some species separation in the neonatal period, even for periods as brief as one hour, can produce disturbances in mother-infant relationships observed several months later. Considering the expectancies built up in the human mother, and the physiological changes she has undergone in preparation for parturition, it is reasonable to suppose that the immediate postpartum period may be a time of maximum sensitivity for her. Separation from her infant in the neonatal period may not permit her to develop appropriate attachments to this infant at the time when she is most sensitized to be responsive.

It is extremely difficult to manipulate the human conditions so as to experimentally separate a human mother from her infant in the immediate postpartum period for several days or weeks, then reunite the pair and observe the mother's subsequent behavior. The modern premature nursery is one situation in which this separation is approximated. The usual care for a premature infant requires that the infant be separated from its mother immediately after birth for a period of time ranging from 3 to 12 weeks, depending upon the weight and health of the infant. By rearranging the nursery to permit some mothers to have early contact with their infants, we established the condition whereby we could examine the effects of early contact between the premature infant and mother on maternal attitudes and behavior.

The mothers of prematures and the contrast group of mothers of full-term infants met the following criteria: (1) the mother had no previous history of premature or low birth weight infants; (2) the infant was free from obvious congenital abnormalities; (3) the infant was not of multiple birth; (4) if premature, the infant weighed between 890 and 1899 grams (2.0 to 4.2 pounds at birth); and (5) there was a father present in the home. The mothers of prematures meeting these criteria were randomly assigned to one of two groups. The first group of 20 mothers, the separated group, could view their infants from the nursery window during the 3- to 12-week period the infant was in the nursery, but had no other contact with them during this time, this being the standard practice for premature infants. The 22 mothers in the second group, the contact group, were permitted to enter the intensive care nursery to interact directly with their infants throughout the infant's hospitalization. This caretaking included handling, diapering, and feeding the infant when it was able to suck from a bottle. The 24 mothers in the full-term group experienced the usual nursery procedures, receiving their infants for scheduled feeding during the 3 days of postpartum hospitalization.

When a premature infant reached the weight of 2100 grams (4.6 pounds) it was taken out of the incubator in the intensive care nursery and transferred to a discharge nursery where it remained for 7 to 10 days until its weight reached 2500 grams (5.5 pounds). This also was standard hospital practice. During these 7 to 10 days mothers in both the separated and contact groups were permitted to come in and care for their infants, initially under the supervision of a nurse and later independently. When the infant reached 2500 grams it was discharged to the mother's care at home. The separated and contact phases of the study were alternated in blocks of 3 to 6 months so that at any given time, all mothers in the nursery had the same experiences, either separation or contact.

The contrast group of mothers of full-term infants delivered them without complications, bottle fed them, and experienced full contact with them during the four to five feedings per day while their infants were in the hospital. Insofar as was feasible, the full-term group of mothers matched the prematures with respect to the parity of the mother, the sex of the infant, and the social class of the father.

Participation in the study was voluntary. All families who met the foregoing criteria were told that we were doing a study of families with newborn infants during the first 2 years of life and that we were interested in how parents managed with young infants during this period, and how infants developed until they reached 2 years of age.

The major variables reported in this paper are maternal attitude and maternal behavior. Using a paired comparison questionnaire, maternal attitude was measured by assessing the mother's confidence in her ability to care for her infant. The mother compared herself with five other possible caretakers: father, grandmother, experienced mother, pediatric nurse, and doctor. Comparisons were made for each of six caretaking tasks classified as either social or instrumental. Calming the baby, understanding what the baby wants, and showing affection to the baby were classified as social tasks, whereas diapering, feeding, and bathing were classified as instrumental tasks. The questionnaire was presented to the mother at the time of the infant's discharge from the hospital and again one month following her infant's discharge. Standardized interviews were used to corroborate the questionnaire data.

Maternal behavior was measured by means of observation of selected maternal and infant behaviors during caretaking at two points: one, in the home at 1 week postdischarge, and two, in the pediatric clinic at 1 month postdischarge. During both observations, mothers fed and held their infants. In the home observation at 1 week postdischarge the mother was requested to bathe and change her infant as well as to feed it. Trained observers used a point sampling technique for previously determined behaviors of both mother and infant recorded at 15-second intervals. The frequencies of observed behaviors were converted to percentage scores to equate for varying lengths of observations. Particular behaviors reported in this paper concern distal attachment behavior, which includes looking, talking, laughing, and smiling at the infant. Proximal attachment behavior included percentage of time holding the infant, affectionately touching the infant, and ventral contact with the infant.

The major findings of this study indicate differences in both attitude and behavior between mothers of full-terms and mothers of premature infants. Full-term mothers smiled more at their infants and maintained more ventral contact with them. Both of these behaviors are considered highly specific for the primate group and are indicative of normal mother-infant relationships. The less frequent occurrence of these behaviors in the mothers of prematures suggests an attenuated relationship between the mother and her infant. This attenuation of relationship of mothers of prematures with their infants is consistent with reports in the literature that premature infants are more frequently the victims of battering by their parents and are more likely to have behavioral problems as children.

Within the premature group the effects of separation are consistent with the differences found between the premature and full-term infants, though less strong. Ventral contact between a mother and her infant appears to differentiate the two premature groups, separated and early contact group, even at 1 month postdischarge, with the contact mothers showing greater frequency than the separated mothers, although the difference is not as great as between the mothers of prematures, as a group, and the mothers of full-terms.

The major effect of separation on mothers appears to be an attitudinal one, that is, on maternal self-confidence, which is lower in the separated group. This finding suggests that the immediate postpartum period is a "sensitive" one for the development of appropriate attitudes and behavior for humans. As with animals, if there is a delay in contact such as we found in the separated group, or even a partial delay, as we found in the contact group when compared to full-term mother-infant relations, normal maternal behavior may be attenuated or qualitatively affected.

An additional effect of separation within the premature group is seen in the clinical data. Within the 21-month follow-up period, there were six divorces among the 66 families; five of the divorces occurred in the premature separated group, one in the premature contact group, and none in the full-term group. Within the divorced group there were two mothers, both in the separated group, who gave up their infants to the fathers, a most unusual circumstance in our experience. On the basis of the interview data, it was established that mothers and fathers in both the contact and separated groups had been equally desirous of having a child. Because the distribution into separate and contact groups was not biased, it is a reasonable conclusion that separation of a mother and infant in the immediate postpartum period has a deleterious effect not only on the maternal roles but on more pervasive family dynamics.

Summary

On the basis of the evidence obtained in this study, it appears that the social ecology of the modern American premature nursery forces interactional deprivation for both the mother and infant. This interactional deprivation superimposes on an already fragile infant condition leading to a mother at risk. There is no question that the premature infant is at risk biologically and psychologically as well as socially, as attested to by numerous studies. The findings of this study indicate that the mother of a premature is also at risk, especially those mothers who are deprived of contact with their infants in the immediate postpartum period.

There is sufficient evidence, summarized by Bell [8], to indicate that the human as well as the animal infant does serve as a stimulus for the mother. The barriers set up between mother and infant by the modern technology of the hospital, which provide optimal conditions for the survival of the premature infant, provide decidedly suboptimal, if not deleterious, conditions for the mother of that infant. Thus, given the results of this study, we must consider the possibility that an atrogenically induced condition, "interactional deprivation," is being fostered in our contemporary care of the premature infant. Although we may never have definitive answers on the long-term effects of neonatal mother-infant separation, on the basis of this study, of animal studies, and of experiences derived from traditional cultures, it seems reasonable to reduce or eliminate the barriers between the mother and her infant in the postpartum period so as to decrease the likelihood of mothers at risk.

References

1. Wiener, G. Psychologic correlates of premature birth. "A review." *J. Nerv. Ment. Dis.*, 134 (1962), 129–144.
2. Drillian, C. M. A longitudinal study of growth and development of prematurely born and maturely born children. III. Mental development. *Arch. Dis. Child.*, 34 (1969), 37–45.
3. Barnett, C. R., Leiderman, P. H., Grobstein, R., and Klars, M. Neonatal separation: The maternal side of interactional deprivation. *Pediatrics*, 45 (1970), 197–204.
4. Leifer, A. D., Leiderman, P. H., Barnett, C. R., and Williams, J. A. Effects of mother-infant separation on maternal attachment behavior. *Child Devel.*, 43 (1972), 1203–1218.
5. Seashore, M. J., Leifer, A. D., Barnett, C. R., and Leiderman, P. H. The effects of denial of early mother-infant interaction on maternal self-confidence. *J. Pers. Soc. Psychol.*, 26 (1973), 360–378.
6. Leiderman, P. H., Leifer, A. D., Seashore, M. J., Barnett, C. D., and Grobstein, R. *Ass. Res. Nerv. Ment. Dis.: Early Development,* 51 (1973), 154–173.
7. Yarrow, L. J. Separation from parents during early childhood. In *Review of Child Development Research,* Vol. 1, M. L. Hoffman, and L. W. Hoffman, Eds. Russell Sage Foundation, New York, 1964, p. 122.
8. Bell R. Q. A reinterpretation of the direction of effects in studies of socialization. *Psychol. Rev.,* 75 (1968), 81–98.

Some Relationships between Activity and Vulnerability in The Early Years

Sally Provence, M.D. (U.S.A.)

The child's acting upon his environment is one of the processes through which physical, intellectual, and psychosocial development proceed. In infancy essential elements of healthy adaptation and learning reside, for example, in the role of activity in the development of motor competence, the varieties of active mastery (physical and mental) that are at the heart of what we call coping behavior, the manipulation of objects as a condition for the development of sensorimotor intelligence, the active initiation of interpersonal transactions, the active repetition of the passive experience as a psychic mechanism. Further, it appears a valid assumption that the infant's self-generated activities are basic to at least some aspects of the intrinsic maturational process itself.

The capacity to initiate motor and mental activity is partly determined by biochemical and structural elements of the body, especially of the central nervous system. In addition this capacity is influenced in very important ways by environmental conditions that impinge upon the child, that is, upon what he actually experiences. Thus the interrelationship between innate and experiential factors determines activity as well as other aspects of the developmental process. The assumption is made here that a child who from the beginning of life is enabled to be active (motorically, socially, in play, verbally, and intellectually) will be less vulnerable to stress and trauma than the infant whose activity in one or several of these areas is impaired. A corollary is that disturbances in the capacity to be active are at times indicators of a pathological process and at other times are at the very root of deviant development. Further, if one takes seriously that the infant's self-generated mental, social, and physical activities are essential to development and that they can reduce or alleviate vulnerability, then methods of intervention which include activating the child in various ways are of great importance.

A few familiar observations will illustrate the emergence and role of activity in normal development and in the handling of the ordinary stresses encountered by the child. For example, responsive smiling, which occurs when the adult engages in social interaction with an infant, precedes spontaneous smiling; responsive social vocalization precedes spontaneous social vocalization; the ability to grasp objects handed to him precedes the infant's ability to reach out for them. With the development of the capacity to capture the adult's attention by smiling, vocalizing, or reaching out to the adult or by approaching and grasping *actively*, the infant takes small but significant steps along the path of making his own way.

One sees, not rarely, a well-developing infant whose interest in toys, ability to discriminate among them, and desire to manipulate them has developed far more rapidly than his ability to acquire them through moving toward them. Such a baby may look at the attractive toy beyond his reach straining toward it, breathing heavily with excitement, obviously filled with eagerness and interest. One such infant may settle for what is closest at hand—a nearby toy, his own thumb—or may be content simply to look. For another it appears that the intensity of the wish for the attractive object combined with his inability to change position to reach it results in such a high degree of tension that he dissolves into tears of frustration, disappointment, or anger. His good humor may be restored if the adult puts the desired object within reach or when he becomes able to get it for himself by rolling or creeping.

What one sees in such infants is a temporary imbalance in which the cognitive and emotional interests in the toy have outstripped motoric ability creating for him a situation of stress. Imagine what might happen to him psychologically if his caregivers are unresponsive or if for any reason there is a prolonged period during which he experiences those feelings of frustration and distress. It is important also to recall that the child's active manipulation of toys and other things in his environment, what Piaget calls "hefting" them, is in the Piagetian view an essential component of the development of sensorimotor intelligence.

Another common experience is that of helping an infant or toddler deal with a stressful separation from his mother. We are accustomed to introducing various ways of encouraging the child to be active because they seem to make him less distressed, that is, they "work." Helping an infant or young child wave goodbye to his departing mother or, if he can walk, enabling him to walk away from his parent rather than being walked away from, or, separation having occurred, helping him turn to active play with toys or with a playmate are frequent methods which are far more than distractions. They both lead to and become indicators of successful coping with stress. Something about the child's active participation in the process of leavetaking permits him to feel less helpless and abandoned, more comfortable than he would otherwise be. Similarly, the young child who during the course of a physical examination can participate through having a turn with the stethoscope or reflex hammer is likely to get through his ordeal with less evidence of distress than when such active participation is not offered.

The infant's emotional expressiveness too, as the term expressiveness implies, is an active process. He *expresses* and is responded to more or less appropriately by the people in his environment. The more clearly his mother is able to "read" his expressiveness and respond in accordance with his developmental needs, the more clearly differentiated become his forms of expression and his awareness of his own feelings and those of others. It is difficult to imagine how an infant could come to some appreciation of his own feeling states and what they signify without the kind of interaction just described. We assume that behavioral evidence of progressively differentiated feeling states and moods, of mastery of those things we call "developmental tasks," are concomitant with internal changes.

In focusing upon activity and the value of helping the infant to become active, I do not wish to suggest that other experiences are unimportant. One might argue quite correctly that the infant who has been deprived or traumatized needs to *receive* a great deal. The provision of physical and psychological nurturance, of a variety of stimuli in an emotionally appropriate context, appears to be essential to helping the child move toward self-initiated, well-organized, directed, and differentiated motoric, social, verbal, and intellectual activity.

There is a danger, of course, that the concept of activity is stated so broadly, since one assumes that activity is essential to development and indeed to life itself, that it would lose any value in clinical practice. It is important to focus the discussion by illustrating its usefulness. *The proposition, then, derived from clinical observations in research and practice is that unusual inactivity in infancy, due to biological or experiential factors or to combinations of both, is a frequent characteristic of the psychologically vulnerable child and, further, that therapy which enables the child to be active in his own behalf reduces symptomatic behavior, enhances general developmental competences, increases coping behavior, and leads to decreased vulnerability.*

Of a number of types of psychologically vulnerable infants two general categories are selected for illustration: the normally endowed child who *becomes* vulnerable because of what he experiences and the child with an impaired neuromotor system who is vulnerable from birth. I will not deal here with severe inborn biological defects of the mental equipment nor with that heterogeneous group of primary personality disorders we designate as psychotic, autistic, atypical, and so on.

It is characteristic of the normally endowed infant in a pathogenic environment to react with disturbances in many aspects of development. Distortions of intellectual, social, and emotional growth which characterize the badly nurtured infant have been amply documented. Moreover, because of poor nurturance he may also develop disorders of bodily function that involve any one or several organ systems. Disturbances of physical growth, of motility, of gastrointestinal and respiratory function and skin disorders are commonly encountered as reactions to poor nurturing. The particular set of reactions developed by such a normal infant will depend on many things, among them his biological makeup, the specific nature of the deprivation or trauma, and the phase of development in which adverse experiences occur. His previous developmental progress, which has involved many antecedent interactions between innate and environmental factors, is another determinant of the effect of a stressful situation. If he is born with a defect of the somatic apparatus—sensory defects, motor defects, biochemical aberrations, and so on—vulnerability to interferences in psychological development is increased, and he requires even more consideration and specificity of care to develop in a psychologically healthy manner.

In clinical practice one encounters with considerable frequency infants in whom there are significant innate or acquired somatic problems. One encounters with equally great frequency infants who are experientially deprived or traumatized. For some the nurturance which provides, among other things, the psychological nutriments needed to energize and activate the child is grossly deficient in quantity and/or in quality. Others are seen in whom severe stress, imposed by psychologically traumatic experiences, interferes with the forward progress of self-generated adaptive behavior under ego control and with coping and defensive behavior as well. Noxious combinations of deprivational and traumatic experiences are, however, more common than "pure-culture" deprivational or traumatic experiences.

Case examples of four vulnerable children have been chosen as illustrations.[1]

MATTHEW, A CHILD WITH PSYCHOPHYSIOLOGICAL SYMPTOMS

Matthew, age 10 months, was referred to our hospital for diagnostic study because of rumination of 4 months duration and failure to gain weight for 1 month prior to admission. His parents had been concerned for 2 or 3 months that he had a serious physical illness and his pediatrician had become worried when he failed to gain weight. As a very young infant he had been healthy, but somewhat hypertonic and jittery and given to spitting up a mouthful or two of formula after most feedings. His mother, though repelled by this, had managed to feed him adequately for about the first four months and he had grown normally and seemed healthy. At about this time the mother's patience wore thin, anxiety and anger mounted, and feeding times became fraught with tension on both sides. At the time of admission Matthew was a fair-skinned baby boy with scanty, wispy, blonde hair and large brown eyes with which he continuously scanned his surroundings, looking prolongedly into the faces of the adults who came into his room. Thorough physical evaluation revealed, besides a slightly below average weight, only a mild nutritional anemia. He ate willingly enough

---

[1] The first three cases have been previously reported in S. Provence, Psychoanalysis and The Treatment of Psychological Disorders of Infancy, in *A Handbook of Child Psychoanalysis: Research, Theory and Practice*, B. Wolman, Ed. Van Nostrand-Reinhold Company, New York, 1972.

when the nurses fed him but regurgitated with the classical tongue and mouth movements of a ruminator when they left him. His play with toys was desultory. He sucked his thumb and played with his hands and feet. He sat alone with good trunk control, but made no effort to creep or crawl. Interviews with the mother, besides eliciting the information given above, resulted in the opinion that she was, in many ways, a devoted mother in attitudes and behavior, but the particular symptom chosen by Matthew was one she found especially disturbing. It was decided to give her a few days of relief from feeding and taking care of Matthew, so we encouraged her to visit and to be with him in whatever way seemed comfortable, but not to feel responsible for his care. Matthew obviously recognized his mother, was relieved to see her, though he often whined in a dissatisfied way when she was with him and usually vomited when she left the room. Meanwhile, the nurses and other staff carried Matthew up and down the halls when they could or pushed him in a walker. He obviously enjoyed this, became more active, animated, and more playful. On about the sixth day of his hospitalization, responding to what we knew at that point about his tendency to vomit when people left him, I suggested to the staff that they help Matthew learn to creep, which he seemed close to doing. Their enthusiasm for his efforts and his willingness to tackle a small space between himself and a favored adult culminated in his ability to creep on all fours after another 3 days. Concomitant with his mastery of creeping, the vomiting disappeared. Along with this, most of the unhappy tension between mother and child was replaced by more mutually satisfying experiences. He began to gain weight normally and concern about his physical health vanished. He left the hospital after 2 weeks free of his chief complaint. Obviously, one cannot assume that they lived happily ever after, but a major disturbance had been alleviated and the prospects for a vastly improved situation between mother and child seemed good. The most significant therapeutic elements for the mother were the exclusion of some life threatening or disabling physical disease; the understanding and empathy for her and the period of respite for both of them from the heightened feelings around feedings. For Matthew, the provision of interested nurses, willing to involve themselves personally as substitute caregivers without having to compete with the mother for his favors, the stimulation to play with toys and to engage in untroubled contact with caregiving adults, and the infant's mastery of creeping were obviously therapeutic. I believe that the creeping was both an evidence of general improvement and an indication of a healthier adaptation. It gave him a better way of coping with the threat of the mother's disappearance; he could now control the distance between them, by creeping after her when he wished or experimenting with excursions away from her.

CINDY, A DEPRIVED CHILD

An affluent young couple with two older children conceived a third child as a replacement for a lost parent. The mother, an attractive, intelligent, articulate young woman felt unloved and unlovely during her pregnancy, could hardly wait to get back to her prepregnancy way of life, and could not mobilize interest in her infant daughter. She employed, in succession, three live-in caregivers during the first year, one of whom was around long enough to become emotionally significant to Cindy before she left. Cindy was seen in our clinic at 16 months of age because of delayed speech and motor development of several months duration, resulting in the fear of parents and pediatrician that she might be mentally retarded. Her play was impoverished and constricted. When left alone, moreover, in contrast to most children of her age she rarely made a complaint, nor did she often actively seek to change that situation. She was capable of smiling and otherwise expressing pleasure, but lacked zest. In situations in which a healthier baby of her age would express strong protest, Cindy was only mildly complaintive. She was generally apathetic, quiet, and inactive. The parents, quite interested and involved in the lives of their older children, were shocked at the diagnosis we arrived at of delayed motor, emotional, and intellectual development due to deficits in her experience and expressed the wish to exert every effort to help her. Belatedly, it appeared, they had taken note of her presence in the family. With expert social casework, Mrs. H. was able to work on some of her own problems and to become more involved with Cindy in a way that was more supportive of her development. Cindy's response to her mother's efforts and to the father's participation in her care along with specific suggestions from us were enough to encourage them. Improvement continued and when Cindy was 3 years of age, additional help was arranged through a good nursery school experience. At age 5 years, she did not look retarded and was obviously attached to her parents and siblings, but not in a deep way. She was, to our minds, somewhat pallid rather than robust in her general behavior and we questioned how healthy she really was psychologically. However, there were no overt symptoms of disturbance and her parents were quite satisfied with her. One wonders how much healthier she might now be if the signs of delayed development visible in the first year had been heeded earlier. The experience of repeated loss of the caregiving person could not entirely be overcome, and is unfortunately a very common phenomenon.

ELSA, A CHILD WITH SEVERE ANXIETY

Elsa, age 21 months, and her parents were referred to our clinic for evaluation and counselling by their physician in a city from which they had recently moved. In a series of contacts we learned that Elsa had been a difficult baby to take care of from the beginning. In the newborn nursery her mother had recognized her shrill, piercing cry as distinct from all others and as she recalled the first year, she said it felt as if Elsa had cried almost continuously. While she was free of illness she was difficult to comfort, often irritable, and not at all a satisfying infant to the mother who felt helpless, concerned about herself as a mother, and angry at the infant for inducing these feelings. The crying had lessened appreciably at around a year, but the parents came to us because they were concerned about Elsa's delayed speech and what they called "her shyness." Although she would often play in her room when she and her mother were home alone, she would not leave her mother's side when they visited or were out of doors in the apartment house play yard with other young children and mothers. Her parents shared a picture of Elsa as a child who at times could be a charming, gratifying companion, but was often "whiney," hard to please, and easily frustrated.

When we first saw Elsa, her passivity and anxiety were conspicuous. Over a few play and test sessions it was possible to understand that if one could create conditions of comfort and provide toys, Elsa could be energized to play and to interact without undue anxiety. It was possible to exclude organic factors as contributing to the problem. It seemed to us plausible, from a rather large amount of information gained from Elsa's insightful if troubled mother and from seeing Elsa, to formulate the problem as follows: Elsa, as a neonate and young infant, was a baby who suffered, more than most, from internal distress and heightened organismic tension possibly also from external stimuli. We reasoned that she would not have been easy for any mother. For her own mother, who was far away from relatives that might have been helpful, who was disappointed that this, her first child, was not a boy, who felt inept and unfulfilled as a mother, Elsa was impossible. She developed a pattern of crying episodes alternating with periods of sleep and wide-eyed watchfulness. Self-initiated activity in infancy was sharply diminished over the norm though not entirely absent when conditions of at first physical and later psychological comfort could be created. The story of Elsa has a happy outcome, for both she and the parents were ready for help. We arranged that one of our nursery school teachers would see Elsa individually—a gentle, sensitive young woman able to understand and go slowly with such an anxious, fragile child. The mother at first was in the room with Elsa and her teacher, but after six to eight sessions was able to leave and join the social worker in a nearby office for her own appointments. Although she worked to some extent on her feelings and problems, she did not wish to look closely at them. Further, while she was eager for help for Elsa and wanted the child to change, it was not easy for her to allow the teacher and Elsa to establish a relationship. Gradually, however, as the child became more active, more verbal, less uneasy, more competent, better able to cope with frustration and stress, the experiences of satisfaction and pleasure between parents and child increased. The balance had been shifted in the relationship to a predominance of those that supported Elsa's development. By the time she was 3, Elsa, still appearing as a sensitive, somewhat anxious child, was able to cope with and benefit from a regular nursery school program. Her increasingly apparent high intelligence became both a pleasure to her parents and a source of strength and satisfaction in her own economy. In every way she appeared more robust, more active, much more trusting of her parents and others, increasingly resilient in coping with stress, and possessed of a large repertoire of useful modes of adaptation.

RITA, A CHILD WITH CONGENITAL HYPOTONIA

Rita, age 16 months when first seen, was referred by her pediatrician with a question of mental retardation. Parents, grandparents, and the physician were deeply concerned about the child's failure to walk, delayed speech, her frequent crying, and her general lack of interest in playthings. The younger of two children, her relative inactivity seemed a blessing at first to her busy and somewhat harassed young mother, especially since she was socially responsive and physically attractive. It was only when nearly in the second year she was not walking nor talking that they became worried. I shall omit the details of the diagnostic work-up and simply say that the neurologist arrived at a diagnosis of congenital hypotonia and predicted that her motor deficits could gradually be overcome. Rita, a slender (but not malnourished), inactive baby was visually alert, indeed somewhat hypervigilant. For several months she had had frequent episodes of crying when her mother left her, even to walk into another room at home, which made the mother feel both strongly needed and exasperated. Her play with toys was desultory, though it improved somewhat when her 4-year-old brother played with or alongside her. She enjoyed his toys more than those selected for her. On developmental evaluation, with patient repeated efforts to engage her and some of the sessions being conducted in her home, it became apparent that Rita, when she could be induced to participate, was capable of intelligent insight in the toys and could solve adequately many of the problems that can be presented to a child of her age. However, she had little drive toward self-generated, active use of toys, toward verbal activity, or toward active coping in any way with her feelings of anxiety when she wanted her mother. For example, she could creep in spite of her hypotonia but often did not do so, rather she sat immobile looking distressed or cried woefully until someone came to her.

To shorten a long story, we reasoned that if we could help Rita to be more active in the use of her somewhat delayed locomotor skills, she would feel less helpless in her anxiety about separation from her mother. We also believed that if we could help her to gain more pleasure in the use of toys, her adaptive skills would be broadened and deepened and intellectual development would be enhanced. We believed, too, that we should, in the context of play and social interaction, try to enhance her use of language since it would be of special importance for a child with a motor handicap. The treatment was carried out by the parents and one of the grandmothers under our supervision. The fact that we were able to state that we believed her to be of basically normal intelligence probably made a considerable difference and enabled them to work with Rita with optimism. In all of this the quality of Rita's relationships with her parents and grandmother was of course crucial to her improvement. Because of the hypotonia, gross motor skills such as walking, running, and climbing came along slowly, but Rita was increasingly able to use the motor skills she did possess in the service of learning, of seeking pleasure or comfort, of avoiding danger. Today at age 4 years she is an intelligent, well-functioning, verbal child, a "good player" who is a pleasure to her family and to others. Her style of approaching new situations remains cautious, and there is still a tendency toward immobility in the face of stress. However, she is able to mobilize her resources unless the stress is severe. She would still be considered a somewhat vulnerable child to those who know her well but to the casual observer this would be inapparent.

In conclusion, it appears that the capacity to be active in relation to the external world is an essential component of healthy psychological development in infancy. The assumption is that such activity is both essential to and an indicator of psychic differentiation and of many aspects of early ego development. The assumption also has heuristic value in the development of effective treatment programs for the children we designate as vulnerable.

Epidemiological Strategies and Psychiatric Concepts in Research on the Vulnerable Child

Michael Rutter, M.D., F.R.C.P., F.R.C. Psych.,
D.P.M. (England)

Much of the research on vulnerable children has been concerned
with establishing statistical associations with a variety of risk factors.
Thus delinquency has been associated with broken homes [32, 33],
educational problems with low social class [5–7], and mental retardation with perinatal complications and brain damage [2]. These
findings are important and provide the necessary signposts to areas
worthy of further investigation. However, on their own they do little
to help the practicing clinician, since the presence of an association
does not tell him *why* the association exists or how the risk factors
operate. Moreover, the results can only indicate probabilities. It
is useful to appreciate that the child whose father is an unskilled
laborer has an increased risk of showing difficulties in learning to
read, but many children from such a home will not have reading
difficulties. The clinician needs to know the nature of the mechanisms which underlie the statistical association and, at least as much,
the factors that modify the association or ameliorate the effects of the
risk factor. In short, if he is to help, he must know why some chil-

dren succumb and some escape and what he can do to alter the
balance of probabilities in the child's favor. These are difficult questions to which we have at best only partial and tentative answers. The
purpose of this chapter is to examine some of the research strategies
that may be employed in trying to find answers and to note the way
research findings have forced a modification in some of the psychiatric concepts we employ.

In this connection, attention will be restricted to some of the
strategies which are applicable to an epidemiological approach. This
is by no means the only approach but it is one that has many
strengths and great flexibility, as the chapter will seek to demonstrate.
In essence, epidemiology consists simply of the study of the distribution of disorders in a community together with an examination of
how the distribution varies with particular environmental circumstances. It is sometimes regarded as just a technique to measure
prevalence—a mere counting of heads. But it is far more than that.
Originally epidemiology was used with great success to study the
cause of infectious diseases and other medical conditions [13, 28],
and more recently it has been employed to study possible social
causes of psychiatric disorder [12, 27]. It is as a means of teasing out
possible causal influences that epidemiology will be discussed here.

The basis of the experimental method lies in the manipulation of
circumstances. One variable is waggled to see if it causes another
variable to move. The art of epidemiology lies in seeking out circumstances which differ with respect to the "waggled" variable, thus
constituting a "natural" experiment. To illustrate this theme, five
strategies will be discussed, mainly with respect to investigations in
which the author has been involved.

Populations at High Risk through Background Variables

The first strategy uses a high risk population defined in terms of
background variables, in this case parental mental illness. The
sample consisted of all the families containing a child under the age
of 15 years, living in one London borough, in which one parent had
been referred to a psychiatric clinic for some type of mental disorder.
Since we deliberately chose a sample of consecutive new cases, the
parents showed a very heterogeneous mixture of neurotic, depressive,

psychotic, and personality disorders. The children in these families were compared with a control group matched for age, sex, and school class [20]. As would be expected on the basis of previous research [16], the children in the patients' families showed more behavioral deviance than did the control children. However, in elucidating possible underlying psychological mechanisms, the fact of the children being at increased risk for psychiatric disorder is of less interest than the factors that account for the finding that within this high risk group some children succumb and some escape.

These have been studied with respect to many variables but for present purposes mention will be made of only three: separation experiences, sex, and temperamental attributes. It has often been suggested that separation from parents is a frequent cause of psychiatric disorder in children [3, 4]. We sought to determine whether this was the case, and if it was, what were the psychological mechanisms which mediated the association.

Within the sample of patients' families, we first found that separations from both parents for a period of at least one continuous month were indeed associated with behavioral disturbance in the children [19]. However, this applied only to children in homes where there was marital discord and the association was not found at all in children living in harmonious homes. This was an intriguing finding which suggested that the *reason* for the separation might be the crucial variable. Accordingly, we split separations into those consequent upon family discord or parental mental disorder and those which occurred as a result of the child going on a prolonged holiday away from his family or his going into hospital for a physical illness. It was found that only separations arising from family discord or disorder were associated with behavioral deviance in the children. This result seemed to imply that it was the family discord that did the damage, the separation being incidental or at most contributory. To check on this conclusion, the analysis was repeated with permanent family breakup (as distinct from temporary separations) and the same applied. If the view that it was the discord that caused harm was correct, it should follow that family discord ought to be associated with behavioral disturbance in the children, even if no separation or family disruption had occurred. To check on this situation, the associations between marital discord and deviance in the child were

The Bled Conference

reexamined within the group of children from unseparated, unbroken families. As before, a strong association was found between marital discord and disorder in the child [19].

Throughout these analyses it was striking that the associations were largely restricted to conduct disorders. In spite of diligent search, we found no evidence that family discord was associated with emotional or neurotic disturbance in the children. Since our diagnostic instruments for this age group had been found to be equally satisfactory for neurotic disorders as for conduct disorders [25], we were forced to accept this as a real and meaningful finding.

The study was instructive in showing how an epidemiological approach could be used to examine hypotheses about mechanisms but also it forced a reappraisal of our concepts concerning both parent-child separation [19] and also maternal deprivation more generally [18]. It was concluded that separation as such was not the main factor leading to long-term disorder in the child, but rather that it was the family discord so often associated with separation that did the damage. In view of the demonstrated importance of father-mother and father-child relationships it also seemed that the almost exclusive locus on the mother in earlier writings had been too restricting. Maternal deprivation has often been written about as if it referred to a homogeneous set of circumstances with a single outcome. A review of relevant studies clearly indicated that this was not the case [18]. It is a term which has been useful in the past in bringing to our attention the importance of patterns of upbringing in a child's development. However, it is now evident that the experiences included under "maternal deprivation" are too heterogeneous, the effects too varied, and the psychological mechanisms too diverse for it to continue to have any usefulness. What is now needed is a more precise delineation of the different aspects of "deprivation" together with an analysis of their separate effects and of the reasons why children differ in their responses.

A concern regarding the last point led to a further set of analyses. Although it had been shown that family discord was strongly associated with conduct disorder in the children, the connection was far from invariable. Even in the worst circumstances only some children were affected. So the next issue was to identify possible modifying variables. For the sake of convenience, these may be subdivided into those relating to the family and those relating to the child.

With respect to familial variables the first important modifying factor was the existence of a good relationship with one parent [19]. Among children all of whom were in discordant quarrelsome homes, those who had one good relationship were to some extent protected against the damaging effects of family discord and disharmony. The good relationship did not eliminate the ill-effects but it certainly diminished them. One crucial feature in this connection is that it did not seem to matter which parent had a good relationship with the child. In these circumstances the relationship with the father seemed to serve a similar function to that with the mother (although in other respects, e.g., psychosexual development, the role of the two is obviously different).

The second modifying factor in the family was a change to a happier home situation [19]. This finding is especially important because it points to the modifiability of behavioral patterns even into middle and later childhood. A change to a harmonious family setting did not undo the damage but it considerably ameliorated it. The early years of childhood are certainly influential but they are not "critical" in the sense once supposed [17, 19].

With regard to modifying variables in the child, two sets of factors require mention. First there was a major sex difference in that boys were found to be much more susceptible to the effects of family discord than were girls [20]. This applied to discord in broken and unbroken families, and in another study [31] the same sex difference was found to apply to the stresses associated with short-term admissions into care (often as a result of family discord). However, this greater psychological vulnerability of boys is not seen with all psychological stresses. Thus, for example, other studies have shown that girls are as likely as boys to suffer from the effects of long-term institutional care [30, 34].

The second set of factors concerned temperamental differences. The New York Longitudinal study of "normal" families showed that a child's temperamental features in early childhood were predictive of later behavioral disturbance [22, 29]. Using rather similar measures we found that the same applied to children in families where one parent was a psychiatric patient. Children who were highly irregular in their sleep and eating patterns, whose behavior lacked malleability in that it was difficult to alter, and who were markedly nonfastidious were those most susceptible in this situation [11]. There are probably many reasons why temperamental features are associated with individual differences in susceptibility to stressful family circumstances. Children who lack malleability are likely to find it more dfficult to adapt to the needs of a changing environment. They are thereby more brittle and more prone to be damaged.

The behavioral characteristics may influence the child's threshold for stress but also it may lead to different experiences. The active, outgoing child is going to have a whole range of things happening to him which are outside the experience of the timid, passive, inward-looking child. However, probably one of the key mechanisms is the effect of the child's temperament in terms of the response it elicits in other people. It was possible to examine this possibility in a number of ways. We found that the children with "deviant" temperamental characteristics (i.e., those associated with behavioral disorder) did not differ from other children in terms of family discord, that is, they were no more likely to come from unhappy, quarrelsome homes. But within these families they were more likely to be the target of parental criticism. These irregular, nonmalleable children seemed to act as a focus for parental irritability. When the parents were depressed they tended to "take it out" on these difficult children. In other words, it seemed that the child's characteristics had influenced parental behavior. It would *not* be correct to see the child's temperament as leading directly to psychiatric disorder. Rather it put him at increased risk through its influence on his interactions with his environment.

Populations at High Risk Through Factors in the Child

That naturally leads us on to the second strategy—that which defines a high risk population in terms of factors in the child. There is a wide variety of factors of this kind which could be utilized but we chose to study the effects of organic brain pathology. For this purpose we used a total population sample of children with cerebral palsy and epilepsy and compared their rate of psychiatric disorder with that in the general population of children without overt brain damage [24]. It was found that the children with brain injury had a high rate of psychiatric disorder several times that in the general population, emphasizing the extent to which brain damage increases the risk of child psychiatric disorder. But, just as was the case with the patients' families, some children succumbed and some escaped, and again the interest lay in finding out why this was so and in discovering the mechanisms by which brain damage led to psychiatric disorder.

The results were instructive and clinically relevant. The first finding was that the types of psychiatric disorder associated with cerebral palsy and epilepsy were many and varied. The *form* of the disorder could not be used to diagnose brain damage and the stereotype of the "brain-damaged child" together with concepts of a uniform behavioral response to brain injury had to be abandoned. The truth was more complex but more interesting. By comparing within the neuroepileptic group those children with and those without psychiatric disorder it was possible to identify some of the factors linking brain damage with behavioral disturbance. These fell into three broad groups. First, there was neurological variables; psychiatric disorder was more likely if the brain damage was bilateral. Among epileptic children psychiatric disorder was most frequent in those with psychomotor fits. In short, both the extent and the locus of inquiry seemed to be important. Second, there were cognitive variables; disorder was more likely if the child were of lower intelligence or if he had marked reading difficulties. These associations applied equally to children without brain damage [25]. Third, there were psychosocial variables. Children from broken homes or with emotionally disturbed parents were most at risk, again an association which applied to children without brain damage. It may be concluded that damage to the brain greatly increases the risk of psychiatric disorder, but it does so largely by rendering the child more vulnerable to the same sort of stresses which influence other children.

Studies of the General Population

The third strategy involves studying the general population. The investigation of high risk groups must always carry with it the concern of how far findings are applicable to children at large, that is, how far associations may have been distorted by looking at a minority group. Most children with psychiatric disorder do not have brain damage. To check on possible distortions arising in this way, we studied three general population samples of 10-year-olds [21, 25]

and one of 14-year-olds [10]. In these we used the same type of family
interview methods that we had used in previous studies. The results
showed that in a general population, just as in the high risk samples,
marital discord and parental neurosis were associated with high rates
of psychiatric disorder in the children. In these respects the findings
showed that our choice of samples had not distorted our conclusions,
but the general population sample also added to what had been
found before.

In the patient sample, there were too few families with a marital
relationship characterized by apathy and indifference for us to
differentiate the effects of lack of warmth from those resulting from
the presence of discord. The general population sample was more
suitable for this purpose and it appeared that unloving marriages
were *not* associated with an appreciably raised rate of child disorder
provided that there was no open discord or quarreling. It has yet to
be determined whether this slightly surprising finding is explicable
in terms of more positive compensating factors in the families with
a poor marital relationship but no overt discord or hostility.

One other advantage in the general population studies was the
greater opportunity to examine the validity of the methods used to
diagnose psychiatric disorder. Throughout all the studies using any
of the strategies a particular point had been made of using both
large-scale survey techniques to screen the total population, *and* very
detailed individual clinical assessments to examine the children
selected as having a possible disorder. In this way it was possible to
combine the advantages of large numbers to obtain the general
pattern of findings, and intensive individual study to provide a more
accurate and more detailed psychiatric appraisal. Systematic checks
of many kinds were undertaken to ensure high reliability and validity
of the methods used [23, 25].

Comparative Studies of Two Populations

The fourth strategy involves the comparison of two areas known
to differ in their rates of disorder. Here the question for investigation
is why rates of deviance and disorder are so much higher in some
sections of the community than in others. For this purpose we took
two populations, all the 10-year-olds living in an inner London
borough and all the 10-year-olds living on the Isle of Wight, an area
of small towns and countryside in Southern England. Previous studies

had suggested that psychiatric disorder was much commoner in London children. Accordingly, the first task was to confirm or refute this suggestion. To do this we made an exactly comparable study of the two populations using the same team of investigators and the same research instruments [1, 17, 21, 23, 26]. We confirmed that both psychiatric disorder and specific reading retardation were more than twice as common in London children. The next question was Why? The strategy employed for that purpose was to determine the factors associated with deviance and disorder *within* London and *within* the Isle of Wight, and then to go on to determine if there were differences *between* the two areas with respect to the frequency with which these factors were present in the general population.

The findings were striking and positive. There were four sets of factors found to be associated with psychiatric disorder in both populations, *and* in which the frequency of the factors differed significantly between London and the Isle of Wight. The first set of variables concerned family discord and disruption. Marital disharmony and short-term admissions into care were both associated with child psychiatric disorder. The second set of variables included various forms of parental deviance. Both mental disorder and criminality in the parents were associated with disturbance in the child. The third set of variables involved various kinds of social disadvantage associated with child disorder and the fourth concerned school characteristics. Schools with high rates of teacher turnover and pupil turnover were found to have higher rates of behavioral deviance in the children. In each case, these high risk variables were also more prevalent in London. That is, London families were more often discordant and disrupted, more parents were mentally disturbed or criminal, more families were large and living in overcrowded homes which they did not own, and London schools were more often characterized by a high rate of turnover in staff and pupils. Further analysis showed that these findings were not due to selective in-migration. Rather it seemed that there was something about life in an inner London borough which predisposes to deviance, discord, and disorder. Further studies are required to elucidate just what it is about inner city life which has this effect but the findings are interesting in pointing to a wider range of variables outside the home which have to be taken into account in considering the effects of "deprivation."

This crosspopulation comparison also illustrated how a failure to replicate a finding may throw fresh light on the mechanisms involved. There is an unfortunate tendency in psychosocial research to deal with results like a football score, so that findings are reported in terms of 3 for and 2 against a hypothesis. This is an unnecessarily restricting style of approach. Although not always easy to resolve, one question should always be asked: Why were the findings in the two studies different? The answer may often be highly informative. An example is afforded in the Isle of Wight-London comparison. In London broken homes were associated with behavioral deviance but this was not the case on the Isle of Wight. The issue was explored by examining the circumstances of the children who were subject to breakup of the family, in order to see if "broken homes" meant the same experience in the two populations [26]. It did not, and therein lay the explanation for the apparent nonreplication. First, the reasons for family breakup differed: on the Isle of Wight a higher proportion was due to adoption or parental death (as against parental separation or divorce). Second, in London the parents were less likely to remarry so that more children were living with unsupported mothers. Third, in London among those that did remarry the second marriage was more likely to result in discord and disharmony. In short, the findings again pointed to the conclusion that it is not separation as such which is most crucial, but rather it is the circumstances leading to separation, present during separation, and operating after separation which are most important.

In this cross-population study many factors have been found to be associated with child psychiatric disorder and the next research task is to determine the relative importance of each factor. It is not enough to say that disorders are multifactorially determined and that the result is a bit of everything. Of course, to some extent that is true, but it is also necessary to try to pin down which factors are more important for which outcomes, what types of interactions are present, and what mechanisms are operative. The analyses to these ends are still under way.

Cross-Generational Studies

The last strategy involves an approach which has been very little utilized up to now but which must be included because of its importance and timeliness. That concerns the study of intergenerational transmission and of so-called cycles of deprivation. The question concerns those families in which problems are to be found generation after generation: in grandparents, parents, children, and then grandchildren. What is needed is research that focuses specifically on the factors that lead not to disorder in individuals but rather to the perpetuation of disorder through succeeding generations. How often does this occur? And what is different about the families in which problems persist over several generations as against those in which the problems "die out"? Very little is known on these points but the elegant long-term follow-up studies of Lee Robins [14, 15] show one good way in which the questions may be investigated.

There is one particular issue in this connection that warrants special attention. Intergenerational transmission is most obvious when there is overt disorder in each generation, but is it necessary for overt disorder to be present? For example, we found that girls were much less likely than were boys to develop psychiatric disorder in relation to marital discord. But is it possible that their maladaptive experience in childhood left a mark in other ways? Perhaps the ill-effects lay not in disorder as such but in the impairment of mothering skills which will show itself in the effects on the next generation. This possibility has been very little studied but a recent investigation by Frommer [8, 9] suggests that it might occur. The strategy of cross-generational research has been much underutilized in the past but it offers considerable promise for the future.

Conclusion

The general public sometimes thinks of science as a set of facts or a body of knowledge. But it is not that. Rather, it consists of ways of posing questions and of investigating problems. The process is never complete since one set of answers always raises a new set of questions. In this process lies the excitement of refining the questions to get closer to the mechanisms, biological or psychosocial, which underlie statistical associations. Although sometimes regarded as very different, in fact the research approach has a great deal in common with the clinical approach as applied to the individual patient. The clinician has to ask himself what caused the disorder

in this particular child, why he responded differently to other
children in the same situation, what are the positive factors which
help to ameliorate the difficulties, and what can be done to alter
the situation in the child's favor. In all of this he needs to understand
the psychological processes involved. These questions are closely
related to those considered in the research reported in this chapter.
Research needs to ask not just what factors put a child at an
increased risk for psychiatric disorder, but also why some children
succumb and some escape. There are many research strategies
which may be employed to this end and this chapter has sought only
to outline five that may be used in connection with epidemiological
methods.

References

1. Berger, M., Yule, W., and Rutter, M. Attainment and adjustment in two
   geographical areas. II. The prevalence of specific reading retardation.
   Submitted for publication, 1973.
2. Birch, H. G., and Gussow, J. D. *Disadvantaged Children: Health, Nutrition
   and School Failure*. Grune & Stratton, New York, 1970.
3. Bowlby, J. *Forty-four Juvenile Thieves: Their Characters and Home-life*.
   Balliere, Tindall and Cox, London, 1946.
4. Bowlby, J. *Maternal Care and Mental Health*. W.H.O., Geneva, 1952.
5. Davie, R., Butler, N., and Goldstein, H. *From Birth to Seven*. Longmans,
   London, 1972.
6. Douglas, J. W. B. *The Home and The School*. MacGibbon and Kee, London,
   1964.
7. Eisenberg, L. Reading retardation: I. Psychiatric and sociologic aspects.
   Pediatrics, 37 (1966), 352–365.
9. Frommer, E. A. and O'Shea, G. The importance of childhood experience in
   relation to problems of marriage and family-building. *Brit. J. Psychiat.*, 123
   (1973), 159–160.
8. Frommer, E. A. and O'Shea, G. Antenatal identification of women liable to
   have problems in managing their infants. *Brit. J. Psychiat.*, 123 (1973),
   149–156.
10. Graham, P. and Rutter, M. Psychiatric disorder in the young adolescent:
    A follow-up study. *Proc. Roy. Soc. Med.* (1973), in press.
11. Graham, P., Rutter, M., and George, S. Temperamental Characteristics as
    Predictors of Behavior Disorders in Children. *Amer. J. Orthopsychiat.* 43
    (1973), 328–399.
12. Lin, T. and Standley, C. C. *The Scope of Epidemiology in Psychiatry*.
    WHO, Geneva, 1962.
13. Morris, J. N. *Uses of Epidemiology*. Livingston, Edinburgh, 1957.
14. Robins, L. N. *Deviant Children Grown Up*. Williams and Wilkins, Baltimore,
    1966.

15. Robins, L. N. and Lewis, R. G. The role of the antisocial family in school completion and delinquency: A three-generation study. *Soc. Quarterly*, 7 (1966), 500–514.
16. Rutter, M. Children of sick parents: An environmental and psychiatric study. *Institute of Psychiatry, Maudsley Monographs No. 16.* Oxford University Press, London, 1966.
20. Rutter, M. Sex Differences in children's responses to family stress, in *The Child and His Family*, E. J. Anthony and C. Koupernik, Eds. John Wiley & Sons, New York, 1970.
19. Rutter, M. Parent-child separation: Psychological effects on the children. *J. Child Psychol. Psychiat.*, 12 (1971), 233–260.
18. Rutter, M. *Maternal Deprivation Reassessed.* Penguin Books, Harnondsworth, 1972.
17. Rutter, M. Dimensions of parenthood: Some myths and some suggestions, in *Dimensions of Parenthood.* H.M.S.O., London, 1973.
21. Rutter, M. Why are London children so disturbed? *Proc. Roy. Soc. Med.*, (1973), in press.
22. Rutter, M., Birch, H. G., Thomas, A., and Chess, S. Temperamental characteristics in infancy and the later development of behavioural disorders. *Brit. J. Psychiat.*, 110 (1964), 651–661.
23. Rutter, M., Cox, A., Tupling, C., Berger, M., and Yule, W. Attainment and Adjustment in two geographical areas: I. The prevalence of psychiatric disorder. Submitted for publication, 1973.
24. Rutter, M., Graham, P., and Yule, W. A neuropsychiatric study in childhood. *Clinics in Developmental Medicine 35/36.* Wm. Heinemann/S.I.M.P., London, 1970.
25. Rutter, M., Tizard, J., and Whitmore, K. *Education, Health and Behaviour.* Longmans Green, London, 1970.
26. Rutter, M., Yule, B., Quinton, D., Rowlands, O., Yule, W., and Berger, M. Attainment and adjustment in two geographical areas: III. Some factors accounting for differences. Submitted for publication, 1973.
27. Shepherd, M. and Cooper, B. Epidemiology and mental disorder: A review. *J. Neurol. Neuros. Psychiat.* 27 (1964), 277–290.
28. Terris, M., Ed. *Goldberger on Pellagra.* Louisiana State University Press, Baton Rouge, 1964.
29. Thomas, A., Chess, S., and Birch, H. C. *Temperament and Behaviour Disorders in Children.* University of London Press, London, 1968.
30. Wolkind, S. N. Children in care: A psychiatric study. M.D. Thesis, University of London, 1972.
31. Wolkind, S. and Rutter, M. Children who have been "In Care": An Epidemiological study, 1973.
32. Wootton, B. *Social Science and Social Pathology*, Allen and Unwin, London, 1959.
33. Yarrow, L. J. Separation from parents during early childhood. In *Review of Child Development Research*, Vol. 1, M. C. Hoffman and L. W. Hoffman, Eds. Russell Sage Foundation, New York, 1964.
34. Yule, W. and Raynes, N. V. Behavioural characteristics of children in residential care in relation to indices of separation. *J. Child Psychol. Psychiat.*, 13 (1972), 249–258.

The Risks of the Register: Or the Management of Expectation

Elizabeth E. Irvine, M.A. (England)

It is clear that the child, from the moment of conception, is exposed
to many risks which threaten his development—we all live more
or less dangerously. We can also agree that in many conditions
of handicap or disturbance a number of factors conspire to produce
the problem; etiology is usually multifactorial. Many of these risks
can be predicted, and some can be avoided or counteracted by
appropriate and timely action. It is therefore unquestionable that
research into risk is valuable and should be pursued and that
strategies for counteracting or minimizing risk should be explored.

However, serious questions arise concerning the diffusion of
the knowledge we gain through such research, and the effects of such
diffusion. How far do we have these affects under control, how far
should we try to do so, how far can this be done? The social sciences,
like some branches of natural science, affect what they observe,
in this case largely through the dissemination and popularization
of their findings, or even their hypotheses. Kinsey's report is
published, and widely read, whether in the original or transmuted
and distorted by the media. Sexual behavior is unlikely to be
unaffected by such information. The work of Freud underwent a
similar process. It has been used by some to justify the sexual gratification, and some think the sexual overstimulation, of children;

by others to justify the partial separation of parents and child in the kibbutz. Early traumatic theories of the origins of neurosis and vulgar misunderstanding of the term "repression" were used to justify what most clinicians now consider a harmful degree of over-indulgence, intended to avoid "repressing" the child.

To come to our present topic, the recognition of risk entails anxiety: anxiety for the professionals concerned, anxiety for the parents, the relatives, the social network. We know that anxiety has its uses; it also has its abuses. Anxiety may provide the motive for appropriate action or for more or less inappropriate defensive maneuvers, according to its intensity and according to the ego strength and coping repertoire of those concerned and the environmental support available.

We are not unfamiliar with this at the family level. We know how the anxiety and guilt provoked in parents by handicaps in young children often constitute a serious risk to the child's developmental potential by giving rise to defenses of denial, overindulgence, over-protection, rejection, or simply to despair. We know how these responses may engender risks for other members of the family—neglect of healthy siblings, mutual projection of blame between parents, with consequent threat to the marriage, and so on.

It is relevant here to recall Leiderman's investigation into the unintended interference with the establishment of the mother-child relationship arising from the traditional precautions against infection in the case of premature babies. This work appeared to show the further side-effect of a risk to the parental relationship union. It also suggests the possibility of reducing the double risk of impaired mother-child relationship (and maternal self-confidence) and of a broken home. Similarly, it is common medical practice to postpone contact between mothers (or parents) and babies suffering any obvious physical handicap or deformity, with the good intention of protecting the mother against shock till she is stronger, but with the unintended consequence in many cases of arousing her suspicions (sometimes to the point of horrifying fantasies) and anxieties which can reach traumatic intensity. Here too, the kindly precaution creates a risk both for the mother-child relationship and quite possibly (following Leiderman) for the marriage. It is relevant here that Graham and Rutter [5] found a significant correlation between psychiatric disorder in epileptic children and "nervous breakdown" in the mothers, but not with broken homes. On the other hand, as regards children with cerebral palsy and similar brain disorders, psychiatric disturbance in the child was not significantly associated with maternal breakdown but was correlated with broken homes.

It is hard for a large-scale statistical study to disentangle the various strands of the chicken-egg cycle. Had the mother shown signs of emotional disturbance before the birth of the handicapped child, or should we suppose that she was a vulnerable individual who broke down under this specific stress? How far is the harmony or strength of the marriage related to the vulnerability of either parent? Do vulnerable fathers tend to leave home? Are vulnerable mothers more likely to break down? How often is an apparently satisfactory marriage destroyed either by a psychiatric illness in the mother with which the father cannot cope, or the vulnerability of both parents to the anxiety and guilt aroused by the birth of a handicapped child, and the mutual projection of guilt, with all the subsequent recriminations? Or again, how many fathers are driven away from home by their wives' excessive preoccupation with a handicapped child?

Williams [9] states: "Most authors of studies on handicapped children conclude that parental attitudes to a child and its handicap are of more significance in its personality development than the handicap itself." In particular, he refers to the work of Pond [8] and Drillien [4], who found (in the words of his summary) "that disturbed behavior in children is common where there have been severe complications of pregnancy and/or delivery. When children suffer environmental stress in infancy and early childhood, they are more likely to become disturbed if they suffered complications of pregnancy and birth, and even more predisposed if they were immature. However, *the quality of maternal handling and the early environment of the child is of more significance in personality development and in the causation of behavior disorders than complications of pregnancy, length of gestation or birthweight"* (my italics).

Williams continues:

In examining the contribution of environmental factors to the etiology of behavior disorder, one is struck by the fact that psychiatrists are still predominantly concerned with the gross aspects of child-mother relationships. Such global terms as rejection, over-protection, guilt, withdrawal and denial are used to account for behavior disorder in a child. There is no doubt that these maternal attitudes correlate well with disturbed behavior. But in more cases these maternal attitudes are *secondary phenomena*. This is not to deny that there is a proportion of mothers who are seriously disturbed psychiatrically and who affect their children adversely. But there is a fair proportion of mothers (and fathers for that matter), who have disturbed handicapped children, who have frequently demonstrated their capacity for good parenthood by the normality of their other children. The majority of parents of maladjusted handicapped children are ordinary good, devoted parents. (My italics)

If parental attitudes and behavior are such an important factor in the development *or prevention* of psychiatric disturbance in handicapped children, it behooves us in our deliberations to give very serious attention to the morale of parents—not to say pride of place —*and to the effect on this of our own communications*. It may be legitimate, for scientific purposes, to regard parents simply as adverse environmental factors for their child, even though this seems to fall under the indictment of "treating people as things." Even scientifically, this has its dangers. For obvious reasons, psychiatrists and their colleagues have more opportunity to observe malfunctioning individuals and families than those who master their problems without specialist help. Thus there is a natural tendency to know much more about and to feel much more interest in the pathological than in the normal. Our knowledge of how parents bring up a mentally healthy child, even when there is a serious handicap to contend with, is extremely rudimentary; by and large, we know very much more about "how not to do it." However, this does not matter so much when we talk among ourselves; no doubt we shall achieve a better balance in the long run. But every time we talk in public or publish and mention emotionally disturbed parents as noxious factors in the child's environment without recognition of their existence as suffering people (and I mean people—like us—not "persons") and without recognition of the existence of many parents who do more than any professional can to help their children to contend with their handicaps with psychiatric damage, we are in fact *increasing* the risk of maladjustment among parents, undermining their precious self-confidence, reinforcing those social beliefs and stereotypes which favor parental demoralization and incompetence, and thus increasing the risk for an incalculable number of children.

There was a phase when many child psychiatrists heavily scapegoated the parents. This has now been corrected to a great extent, but the attitudes of many doctors, social workers, public health nurses, and journalists are still affected by this literature and the stereotypes derived from it, while the work of Ronald Laing and his associates has recently poured fresh fuel on the flames. Some enthusiasts among sociologists and others are already proclaiming the death of the family, and there is a real danger that before we get around to serious study of how many families contribute to the normal development of their children, enthusiastic "reformers" will mount a campaign encouraging society to abandon the family in favor of untried substitutes.

Little has been done to redress the balance against the effects of the scapegoating literature. Few "experts" explicitly recognize, with Williams, that some parents of disturbed handicapped children are at least nonfactors in the child's disturbance, while some provide a quality of devoted and intelligent home nursing which few professionals could emulate all round the clock and all round the calendar. The late D. W. Winnicott was, I believe, almost alone in his loving and scrupulous study of "the ordinary devoted mother" and how she lays the foundations of mental health of her children. He also advised social workers to take as a model "therapy of the kind that is always being carried on by parents in correction of relative failures in environmental provision. What do such parents do? They exaggerate some parental function and keep it up for a length of time, in fact until the child has used it up and is ready to be released from special care." This passage could equally well be applied to children suffering from a variety of handicaps rather than from previous failure of "environmental provision."

But apart from Winnicott, who has described the contribution of "the ordinary devoted mother" to the care and education of a vulnerable or damaged child? Virtually the only literature I have found on this has been written by those few parents who are capable not only of providing such care but also of writing about it.

The most notable of these books is *The Siege* by Clara Claiborn Park [7], who comes across as a gifted, sensitive, and remarkably stable woman, mother of three normal children, struggling very effectively to come to terms with the condition of an autistic child, to understand it as far as possible, and to find ways of expanding the child's interest and abilities—methods which called for incredible patience and delicacy of touch, lest the child take fright and withdraw instead of advancing. Beginning without professional help as a lone inventor, Mrs. Park eventually found first-rate professional advice and support, but this was after a long struggle, and she has an eloquent chapter ("The Amateurs") on the potential contribution of parents and the reluctance of many professionals to recognize or encourage this, let alone guide it. Recognizing the dangers of parental overanxiety, oversensitivity, overactivity, or despair, she goes on to say: "But since we parents, in clinical literature, have found few eulogists, it is up to us to put our handicaps into perspective. Since we are conscious of them, we can go a long way towards overcoming even the severest. And we, and others, should realize that they may be counter-balanced by special vantages that even the most gifted psychiatrist cannot watch."

One of the few professional writers to make this point is Margaret Adams [1] of the Eunice Kennedy Shriver Center who writes: "Parents, because they are fully acquainted by hard experience and a very strong emotional investment in the situation that if not taken into account, may sabotage the more carefully laid, objectively sensible plans." Mrs. Park's point is more than this, since the parental expertise and devotion are resources which we can ill afford to waste. As Mrs. Park says: "Perhaps the most important of all the parents' advantages" is "that they know the child's language . . . gesture by gesture, sound by sound, word (at last) by word. . . . They hear the anxiety in the high squeal the outsider cannot distinguish from laughter; they understand that assent is conveyed by running across the room or jumping up and down."

Despite their outstanding ability and stability, the Parks had difficulty in finding professional advisers who were willing to trust them and to accept them as partners (at this point major partners) in the educational/therapeutic exercise. Mrs. Park writes: "Far from denigrating the knowledge of psychotherapists, I only ask that they let parents share it. I learned from my child slowly and painfully, she and I together. But I would have learned faster, and with fewer gaps, if I had been in contact from the beginning with skilled and sympathetic professionals." She reports a first experience of very thorough professional study of the child, combined with a cold, impersonal attitude to the parents, a passive listening to what they had to say, with minimal feedback, a total lack of interest in the records they had kept, an uninformative report, and a total lack of guidance or encouragement.

Later, she reports, with great gratitude and detailed appreciation, an experience of real partnership with the staff of another clinic. The social worker commented, "the words dropped into my mind like balm" on the unusual persistence and energy shown by the parents. "I think," she said, "that we will be able to learn from *you*." "I could scarcely believe I had heard it. They did not think that in my lonely and presumptuous work I had injured my child. They thought I had helped her. Their present recommendation was not that Elly should begin analytic therapy but that I continue to work with her as before with one difference. I would now have professional guidance from an analyst on the staff of the clinic." For some weeks there were regular, frequent sessions, mainly concerned with the mother's emotions; then the focus shifted to the child, and less frequent office interviews were supplemented with an occasional home visit when the mother could observe the therapist's approach to the child and find new ideas for her own approaches, as she also did later when the child was able to enter a good nursery school.

I have written about this book at some length, because of its intrinsic value also because of its scarcity value. It makes my point about the morale of the parents, about their need for encouragement and appreciation, and about how easily and how often this morale is not only neglected but unintentionally undermined. The Parks were certainly outstandingly able, but Williams has emphasized the good performance of many parents of more average ability and the secondary nature of much of the parental emotional disturbance observed and reported. ("Every handicapped child is a risk for the parents," according to Solnit, in this volume.)

Insofar as the disturbance is secondary to the child's handicap, it is worth considering the possibilities of preventing parental disturbance and thus reducing the risk to the child. Caplan's crisis theory is clearly relevant here and has provided the framework for several attempts at early intervention (e.g., refs. 2 and 6). The project described by Nurse arose partly from the observation that the families of retarded children were subjected to multiple and not necessarily coherent visiting by social workers, public health nurses, and officials mainly concerned with regular school attendance; such families are particularly likely to be transferred from one worker or service to another at times of stress or crisis. "This fragmentation of service and lack of continuity is being inflicted on particularly vulnerable people, and a common experience of social workers in this field is to be confronted with families in which disturbed patterns of adjustment and relationship have become firmly rooted over many years."

Two social workers and a senior public health nurse therefore decided to assemble a group of parents within at least two years of learning that their children were retarded, with the aim of helping them to adjust to their predicament. They hoped that by providing "some superficial support to the parents early in the life of the child" the group could obviate the need for long-term regular visiting by social workers later. However, once the lid came off Pandora's box, superficial support was soon forgotten, and the six months' planned duration also proved to be quite inadequate. (It is worth observing here that the crisis, in Caplan's sense, had already been missed, since the children in question were aged at the start of the group.)

The members were deeply and passionately concerned with grief at the handicap, anger at the child's exacting demands, guilt and problems of "Who's to blame?", desperate wishes that the child could have been aborted, with guilt about these, and conflict about wishes to get rid of the child by sending it to an institution (at a time of great public concern about scandalous conditions in a hospital for the retarded). Since "every handicapped child is a risk for the parents" (Solnit, in this volume) and since every parent who succumbs to this risk increases the risk of maladjustment for the child, it behooves us to consider what we can do to minimize this risk—in fact to give this question a high priority. Much of the risk is inherent in the situation; disappointment, grief, resentment, anxiety, and guilt are normal expectable reactions to severe handicap in a child and are liable to give rise to dysfunctional defenses. All parents have to struggle with these responses with various degrees of success and failure. The outcome of this struggle, for parents and child, is partly determined by what the parents bring to the situation from their store of previous good and bad experiences, in terms of confidence in their ability to love, to create, to repair; partly by the degree of support they enjoy among their friends and relations; partly by the attitude and skill of their professional advisers; and partly by the general climate of opinion which affects the attitudes alike of parents, friends and relations and professional advisers.

If we agree that it should be a major objective to preserve parental morale, we have to approach the problem at various levels. On the one hand, all those parents who are not totally incapacitated by severe mental illness should be treated as partners in the preventive enterprise. Their potential or actual strengths should be recognized and encouraged, just as we hope they will in turn encourage those of their children. Many of them will need some help with their own feelings, as described by Mrs. Park and also by Brody [3], and this is likely to be most effective if given at the point when the diagnosis or the information of risk is communicated. But the help they need is likely to be educational as well as therapeutic. The child's potential for development and for mastery of any handicap needs to be fully and carefully explained (though not exaggerated), together with the most appropriate ways in which the parents can help the child. This may need to be explained one step at a time, and perhaps with the simpler parents many times, or a long-term strategy may be grasped in one or two sessions by the more intelligent. Most parents will need opportunities to report progress at intervals to some encouraging "expert" and will also need advice as to the timing of new methods, as well as help in noting and valuing the very small increments of success which occur in many cases. Two considerations are important:

1. If the parents' potential for helping the child to develop his competence and master his handicap is mobilized, they will have more to give the child than any therapist can give—although expert intervention may occasionally be needed to supplement parental care or to remove some obstacle which prevents the child from accepting it.
2. It is vital for the parents' own stability to be given a method for helping the child to overcome his handicap and encouraged to use it and to enjoy some success. This provides a truly functional outlet for their drive toward reparation, together with reassurance that they are indeed capable of reparation. Failing such help, many parents attempt reparation in ways of their own devising, which are often dysfunctional, such as over-

protection and infantilization; or else they are liable to fall back on more primitive defenses against guilt, such as denial or rejection.

On the societal level, we have to give very serious consideration to the effect of our deliberations and our publications on the parents of those children whom we identify as vulnerable. We know that these communications will be filtered to them through the popular press and through the professional press and its impact on their professional advisers, and we know that distortion is inevitable, but at least we can avoid inviting it by the imbalance of our emphasis, and we should make some serious attempt to counteract the harm which has been done by previous publications which have unintentionally, but nonetheless powerfully, undermined many potentially helpful parents and added to the burdens they already carried in caring for a handicapped or disturbed child. Anything we say about the unwilling and unwitting contribution of some parents to the maladjustment of their children should be carefully balanced by recognition of the role of the parents in relation to all those children who are able to adapt to their handicaps without succumbing to the risk to which they are exposed. When therapeutic or preventive interventions in which parents were involved (Provence, in this volume) are reported, the work with the parents and the contribution which they were able to make should be at least as fully reported as other elements in the interventive program.

We must never forget that scientific meetings, publications, and publicity affect the situations we describe in unintended ways, as well as those we intend. Let us remember how often the arrogance of the "experts" has led society, and parents in particular, in directions we have later bitterly regretted. Since we inevitably leave "footsteps on the sands of time," let us be careful which way they will lead those who follow.

References

1. Adams, M. Social aspects of medical care for the mentally retarded. *New England J. Med.*, 1972.
2. Booth, B. L. Residential courses for families with a handicapped child. *Case Conference*, 13 (1966), 2.

3. Brody, S. Preventive intervention in current problems of early childhood, in *Prevention of Mental Disorders in Children*, G. Caplan, Ed. New York: Basic Books, 1961.
4. Drillien, C. M. *The Growth and Development of the Prematurely Born Child.* Livingstone, Edinburgh, 1964.
5. Graham, P. and Rutter, M. Organic brain dysfunction and child psychiatric disorder. *Brit. Med. J.*, 3, (19—), 695.
6. Nurse, J. Retarded infants and their parents: A group for fathers and mothers. *Brit. J. Social Work*, 2 (1972), 2.
7. Park, C. C. *The Siege.* Pelican Books, London, 1967.
8. Pond, D. A. Psychiatric aspects of epileptic and brain-damaged children. *Brit. Med. J.*, 5264, *1961*, 1377–1382.
9. Williams, C. E. Behavior disorders in handicapped children. *Devel. Medi. Child Neurol.*, 10 (1968), 6.
10. Winnicott, D. W. The mentally ill in your caseload, in *Collected Papers.* Tavistock, London; Basic Books, New York, 1958.

The Bled Discussions: A Review

Cyrille Koupernik, M.D. (France)

The Garmezy-Anthony-Rosenberg Presentations

Members of the International Study Group were both intrigued and
perplexed by *Garmezy's* discourse on competence and the usefulness
of this concept for studying children at high risk for the development of schizophrenia in adult life. *Rutter* agreed with this emphasis
upon competence to explain why a very sizable group of children
appear to come through the most appalling circumstances in a
remarkably healthy state. He wondered to what extent competence
was specific to the type of stress and the type of outcome or whether
there was some general personality variable that enabled children
to survive different types of hazard. He also cautioned against
overlooking circumstances in the child's environment that also
contributed to psychological survival. It was surprising how a single
good relationship within an otherwise disorganized family can help
a child to overcome severe difficulties.

The choice of schizophrenia as the risk factor to be studied
seemed anomalous to *Rosenberg*, who felt that it would eventually
turn out to be a ragbag containing different entities in the same way
as gout has turned out to be a generic cover for 15 to 20 different
kinds of metabolic disease. Furthermore, people had such different
views of it: for some it was a genetic illness, for others a way of life,
and there were those who felt that the mere act of labeling someone

193

schizophrenic generates schizophrenia. With these considerations in mind, it might be difficult to find a single factor of competence.

Lourie pointed out that there was evidence to indicate that individuals in the general population reacted differently to stress. About 25 percent became disorganized in thinking and performing, and about an equal number at the other end of the scale improved under stress and became better organized and more effective. In his opinion, there were four factors involved in bringing about these differing responses: (1) the capacity to tolerate anxiety; (2) the ability to construct fantasies as a rehearsal for actual problem solving; (3) the propensity for thinking flexibly; and (4) the potential for relationship. *Marcus* drew attention to the fact that the criteria for assessing competence are the same as the criteria for diagnosing pathology in reverse. He also thought that the factor of constitutional endowment was critical for the development of competence.

The group oscillated between inborn and environmental factors responsible for the emergence of competence but soon the term itself was questioned as being in danger of becoming a shibboleth without being understood. Some saw it as a rehash of terms already in general service such as mastery, autonomous drive, the capacity for foresight and hindsight, and particular ego functions engaged in controlling and regulating drives. Some also questioned *Garmezy's* use of the term invulnerable, preferring "resistance." There was also some concern that *Garmezy* was starting his study chronologically too late and that infancy was the time to begin. *Jensen* questioned whether the competencies at different stages of development are different or interrelated and *Matic* pointed out that stress (or acute risk) was often quite specific to a particular child at a particular stage of development; he could often cope with it at one stage and succumb at another.

Richmond felt that we needed to extend our language with regard to these new concepts of invulnerability, competence, and functional capacity to resist stress or, to put it another way, to develop a nosology of health just as we have developed a nosology of disease. It also seemed clear that in studying children it is essential to consider the time frame when the children are being observed as well as the particular characteristics that a given child carries right through his development.

In replying to the discussion, *Garmezy* addressed himself to some aspects of strategy in risk research. It may well be that specific competencies correlated to specific situations into the prevention of specific disorders, but he considered it more scientifically parsimonious, when starting out in an area, to deal holistically with a concept rather than immediately fragmenting it. As one proceeded empirically and discovered children who survived in some ways and not in others, and in some situations and not in others, one could begin to narrow down the concept and make it more discriminative. With regard to psychopathology, it may well be, if one regards it in hierarchical fashion, that grosser forms will manifest low levels of competence and more advanced forms higher levels of competence. This would not imply specific competencies but weightings of competence at different points in the hierarchy. For example, if one takes the Phillip's Scale of Premorbid Adjustment in Schizophrenia or the Becker Scale, these cannot predict neurotic adaptation because the ceiling is too low and the competency levels much too constrained and narrow. If one examines the range of competencies manifested by children, one can ask how a child with a very low level of competence copes with the hierarchically ordered series of frustrations as compared to a child who functions at a middle level of competence. In the latter instance, would the stresses and strains need to be greater before one begins to observe signs of deterioration in performance? *Garmezy* was aware that he was answering the clinical questions raised by the discussants in experimental terms but felt that he needed to advance on an empirical basis, first measuring generalized competencies but with enough factorial qualities so that a child might rate high on a first factor and not so high on a second, and in this way he hoped it would be possible to develop some composite rating index. One could then take children who vary in their levels of competence and introduce them to a set of tasks that become increasingly complicated where observations can be made of adaptive sufficiency or insufficiency. The idea of general weightings of overall competence is derived from the prognostic literature of schizophrenia, but it might turn out to be inapplicable in this context. Now what if one finds two children equally weighted in competence indicator signs, but when both are given a problem-solving situation with built-in frustration, one child masters it and the other does not? This should not dismay the investigator since it is from the atypical case that one learns where next to go and what next to do.

One might need to go beyond the competence indicators and take a look at the adaptive functions of the children and try to find out if and how these differed in the two cases. The work of Thomas, Chess, and Birch suggests a possible constitutional difference in temperament, or there may be fortuitous circumstances that would also conduce to differences.

The trend in developmental psychopathology is moving toward increasing complexity and to the realization that there is a whole host of ancillary circumstances that add to existent strengths and weaknesses in the children. *Garmezy* would agree with Slater that the most powerful model available at the present time in studying schizophrenia, particularly in its more chronic and process form, is the genetic one, and that the most powerful variable in the etiology of schizophrenia is genetic. This would not mean that a genetic position on this issue negates the work being done on competence because this is largely derived from investigations of prognosis in the chronic schizophrenic patient. The reason why we continue to use the term schizophrenia in spite of its acknowledged heterogeneity is because dropping it at the present time when we have nothing else to replace it would land us in a veritable wilderness. On the whole, therefore, *Garmezy* would advocate the retention of the term and the use of the genetic model, which would lead us to expect that some children would be more likely to develop disorders than others. This could be restated in another way by saying that some children appear to be more adaptive than others. In both instances the child at risk would be defined in terms of the psychiatric status of mother or father.

Anthony's observations have shown that children of reactive psychotics respond differently from children of process psychotics and that children who shunt off the parental psychosis appear to survive better than children who become enveloped by it. A great many investigators, some genetically oriented and some oriented toward family pathology, are able to accept the concept of schizophrenia while disagreeing about almost everything else so that there would seem to be some support for continuing to use the term in risk research.

The first stage in the four-stage strategy in risk research is to develop various indicator signs of competence for specific age levels. The second stage is the important one for the study of risk because it asks whether certain children at risk remain invulnerable and whether this is accompanied by other signs of good adaptive functioning such as "getting along well." The clinician looks at the child and sees certain attributes which are a combination of stage 1 variables (competence criteria) and stage 2 variables (dispositional parameters). The ability to think flexibly and creatively recurs in the literature on competence. Hypersensitivity, on the other hand, is probably a stage 2 variable. The variables of both stages may occur in children already disordered or in children likely to be disordered at some future point. This is why one needs indicators that are age related and which will allow us to pick up children even before they reach the clinician.

In continuing the discussion, *Leiderman* was disquieted by *Garmezy's* use of the concept of competence. It seemed to him to be retrogressing to a trait psychology where competency was being considered as an isomorphic entity that could, in a variety of situations, be teased out and described as characteristic of the individual. *Leiderman* felt it was important to emphasize the kinds of environment that need to be examined just as closely as what looked to him like "an old-fashioned trait variable." Since the time of Binet, numerous educators have attempted to measure competency in terms of school performance without considering environments, and this is currently in the process of being rejected because of its ideological undertones in the United States. *Irvine* wondered whether competence could be taught and learned and whether dealing competently with a particular problem could help to increase competence in general.

In reply *Garmezy* said that he had a factor analytic study under way that might disprove the existence of the six factors that he had mentioned which were only extracted from the literature. With regard to whether competence could be learned, he cited work of Anthony on intervention:[1] in teaching the child to problem solve better you try to inculcate a reality orientation, demystify the mystifying aspects of psychosis, and provide him with tools for coping better with himself and his environment. He hoped that competence could be learned and could see no reason why it could not in the

[1] See A Risk-Vulnerability Intervention Model for Children of Psychotic Parents, in this volume.

same way that cognitive styles can be learned. *Garmezy* mentioned
a study in Minnesota in which an effort was being made to
train impulsive children to be reflective and then examining the
consequences for this kind of training on other aspects of competence indicators in the school system. It seemed to him that *Anthony*
was trying to provide children at risk with tools to cope with the
disordered parent and this certainly seemed to be a critical direction
in which to go. *Garmezy* was not too perturbed by the thought of
competence being a trait, but he did feel that environmental factors
were extremely important and that we should either choose diverse
environments and study competencies within these environments or
choose diverse children and study those factors of the environment
that are associated with competency and noncompetency. Either way
would be a contribution.

Garmezy also defended the use of the term invulnerability.[2] Some
people have insisted that there is no such thing as an invulnerable
child and that every child has a breaking point. Others have
suggested that a better term would be well-adjusted. He felt that this
was a most inadequate term with which to describe a child who had
come through harrowing experiences. For him, a well-adjusted child
was one whose family was intact, who lived in the suburbs, whose
father was a professor and mother a social worker, and who comes
home from school to find the family all there ready to take care of
him. *Garmezy* would use the term invulnerable for those who are
functioning well in spite of being exposed to severe stresses. In
closing, *Garmezy* agreed that there was already an abundant literature
on mastery but unfortunately nothing on specific competence
indicators by age. He did agree, however, that teachers were not all
that one could desire as raters of competence and adjustment. In one
study, for example, using a sociometric device involving some 3000
children in the school system, it was found that the child rated most
negatively by both teachers and peers was the externalizer. He was
equally unpopular both in the inner city and in the suburbs. The
second most negatively ranked child by peers but not by teachers
was the offspring of the schizophrenic parent. Now why was this?
Was there perhaps some subtle aspect indicated in play that teachers
were not in a position to observe?

[2] See The Syndrome of the Psychologically Invulnerable Child, in this volume.

In response to *Anthony's* presentation, *Richmond* felt that the curriculum for reducing vulnerability (or increasing competence) was similar to what he and Caldwell had devised for disadvantaged infants and toddlers. He felt that *Anthony's* study might also help to throw some light on the medical controversy regarding native versus acquired intelligence. He was also especially interested in the fact that the children who made the greatest gain came from families that were also functioning better and that children with the highest scored risk seemed to show the most change. And he wondered whether this was something in the nature of a law of initial values— the lower you start, the higher you have to climb.

Provence remarked on the interweaving of sophisticated clinical and theoretical knowledge and the use of established and newly constructed measures that could be used, at the very least, as indices. She felt that *Anthony*, in a number of different dimensions, had arrived at a way of combining and systematizing observations from many different sources and had brought them together in a way that permitted one to examine and to think about them. She felt that the corrective interventions were much what one would expect to be able to do in developmental terms and were, in fact, central to the approach to the younger psychotic child.

In his comments on *Anthony's* presentation, *Garmezy* felt that if one could relate the total risk score on the one hand to a broad set of competence parameters and on the other to a set of dispositional variables that he believed were precursor stages involved in the development of psychopathology, it would be extremely helpful to the further refinement of risk strategy. What *Anthony* had was an admixture of the two. What was new in the method of intervention was the attempt to alter a dispositional parameter. If this could be done, would the modification have repercussions on competence? What *Anthony* seemed to be trying to do was to stay the course of vulnerability by acting directly on a stage 1 variable. He was trying to build in competence qualities by a variety of interventions using training and analysis to increase cognitive competences. It was the use of skill training as a direct way of teaching a child to cope. About the ethical question of intervention in high risk cases, *Garmezy* stated that at his center there was no question that they would intervene when necessary.

Anthony, in his response to the discussants, suggested that his approach to competence lay somewhere between that of *Garmezy* (which was experimental) and *Lourie* (which was psychodynamic) and was a clinical orientation aimed at specific areas. Except for the "classical" type of intervention, he did not think that there was much chance of bringing about changes in the global, psychodynamic areas. In the intervention program the corrective approach that was made to the child likely to disorganize under stress was designed to enhance the synthetic function of the ego, helping the children not only to tolerate the sick parent better, to understand the sickness better, but also to deal with the problems arising out of the sickness.

Solnit reminded the group that there were calculated risks in uncovering the problems through research of potentially risky situations. On a short-term basis, the intervention was often an effort to minimize the risk of the research itself in the hope that the knowledge that accrues would, in the long run, cut down on the damaging hazards to which the child was exposed in actual life. Uncovering a problem and not being able to help with the problem uncovered was therefore an important iatrogenic risk to be considered. There was some evidence that the risk, for example, of being battered was heightened rather than reduced by the process of being investigated. He felt that another type of iatrogenic risk related to the new "revolving door" policy in mental hospitals because of which pyschotic parents were being rapidly and often prematurely returned to their families and children on a maintenance dose of phenothiazines or other tranquilizers. It would be important to investigate the effects on family life under conditions when the parent was sent home or kept in hospital. The gains from the revolving door policy may be illusionary and the detriments very real. Judging from their experience, *Anthony* felt that it would be difficult to generalize about this problem. Some children became reactively disturbed with each psychotic relapse whereas others appeared to become habituated. This may well be because the child was developmentally more advanced with each subsequent relapse. With the "involving" psychoses, the children may experience and even express relief with the readmission of the parent and anxiety and resentment with his return home, but both responses may also be accompanied by an inordinate amount of guilt.

With regard to *Anthony's* example of the diabetic child who improved psychologically while learning to handle and control his diabetic condition, *Sapir* was reminded of a program, developed by by Hadary, concerned with teaching basic science concepts to emotionally disturbed and blind children utilizing special teaching materials that had been developed. Not only did the children learn these concepts but in the process of doing so became less distractable and disorganized and their attention was focused on a meaningful learning experience. The same illustration made *Garmezy* wonder to what extent a sense of competence, rather than any specific competence, could be transferred and how it related to the feeling of self-esteem when one faces and masters a crisis. How much does it add to the ego strength for the next critical trial? Another important element was the importance of learning with one's body, sensuously, as well as with one's mind, to smell, taste, touch, hear, visualize, and really experience the learning situation.

In response to *Rosenberg's* presentation, *Anthony* pointed out that his comparison group of tuberculosis parents had striking similarities to the experimental group of schizophrenic parents in the types of psychopathology that were generated in the children, in the premorbid histories of the patients, and in the way that the criteria of process and reaction seemed equally applicable with regard to prognosis. For this reason, he had been compelled to add a normal control sample to the design. In a study of pedigrees in his research, he had also found families that were heavily loaded with psychosis through several generations and he wondered what effect this had on the expectancies as compared with pedigrees with very light loadings of psychosis. *Rosenberg* thought that in the heterogeneous group of entities subsumed under the term schizophrenia, some may well turn out to be sex-linked and others may well have a single gene acting in dominant fashion. In the lightly loaded families, a sporadic case could be a new mutation if, in fact, this were a single gene effect, but is more likely to be related to a biochemical disposition or the disorder.

The genetic predisposing factors are important but of equal importance are the environmental factors that play upon them. To underline this, *Rickards* offered an example of a family in which some of the children were retarded and some apparently normal. There seemed to be no doubt that the genetic defect was a necessary condition, but the way in which it manifested itself appeared to be influenced by the environment. The family was not only genetically

at risk but also environmentally at risk because of factors of
migration, maternal personality, and considerable stresses of living
which included rearing two severely handicapped children.
Antonovich mentioned an EEG study of the family where he found
almost identical abnormalities in some of the children as in one of
the parents where parent and children were both discovered, but
in some cases the same abnormality appeared in a healthy sibling.
This might provide still another method for studying genetic
transmission.

Koupernik referred to a neurological disease in animals, very
similar to multiple sclerosis in man, which is both genetically and
environmentally determined, the environmental factor being a
slow-acting virus. The response to the virus is genetically determined.
In the same way, the response to drugs varies from individual to
individual, and one could imagine a psychological event being
differently "metabolized" by different children.

The discussion then focused on genetic risks, on prenatal
investigations of the fetus, and on the usefulness of genetic
counseling. *Solnit* once again pointed to potential risks in both
genetic investigation and counseling. There were problems about
parents who received counseling and then went on to have a child in
spite of the risk involved. Then there was the problem where a
deviant pattern is found on chromosomal analysis but with no
evidence of manifest deviation. It would be important to know how
frequently this occurred. *Rosenberg* predicted that very shortly all
women over the age of 40 would have their pregnancies monitored.
This could lead to a considerable reduction in the incidence of
mongolism if society chose to act on this information.

With regard to variability in the expression of disorder in the
offspring, the environment cannot be held completely responsible
for it. Various genetic combinations can occur, and mutation is
always possible. One can also anticipate situations in which husband
and wife may have different kinds of heterozygocity, and the offspring
may be homozygotic for one particular kind of abnormality and
heterozygotic for another, or where there are two different mutations
in which the biochemical manifestations may be similar, but the
manifestations in terms of the entire organism may be quite different.
In reply to a queston from *Koupernik, Rosenberg* thought there

was no indication that an individual having a long I chromosome would have any reproducible type of behavioral abnormality. It seemed to be a more ethnic phenomenon. The behavior associated with the extra Y chromosome may have been due to sampling bias from chromosomal screening of prison populations containing a large number of psychopathic individuals. What future generations would do about an apparently healthy male with 47 chromosomes with an extra Y chromosome was still a moot question. But *Rosenberg* believes that geneticists, pediatricians, psychologists, and child psychiatrists will be confronted by this as a major problem in the next few decades.

Discussion of Presentations by Minkowski, Leiderman, Provence, and Rutter

Lourie thought that in the face of all the genetic and reproductive risks that had been brought up, there was a need to revise the concept of the womb as the almost perfect environment for the human individual. If these risks were advertised widely, perhaps they might modify the alleged urge to "return to the womb" and even eliminate claustrophobia as a clinical entity! It was clear that "survival of the fittest" no longer held true in civilized countries where advanced techniques allowed babies to be born alive who in the past would have been stillborn, and allowed them to continue to live, when in the past they would have soon died. The figures given by *Rosenberg* for rates of genetic mutation raised frightening prospects for the future. Twenty-five percent of hospital beds in the United States are occupied by handicapped people, and there are 7,000,000 handcapped children who require 300,000 teachers for their special education. What are we building up for generations to come? Currently we are developing methods for involving the handicapped more completely in society and even making them culture heroes. American television, for example, features one series involving a blind detective, another a detective functioning in a wheelchair. We also have to remember that many of these handicapped individuals are also at psychiatric risk.

Provence reported that researchers at the Yale Child Development Clinic had become increasingly aware that if they saw premature

babies as late as 1 year of age, it was impossible to determine, unless
the children had gross handicaps, whether their functioning just
moderately below the expectable level for their ages was the result
of experiential or biological factors. They noticed, for example, that
parental attitudes, both maternal and paternal, were affected by
the fact of prematurity, but fortunately for many infants and their
parents this was only transiently traumatic, and the infants who
overcame it did well in spite of the hospital practice of separating
mother and child, and in spite of the physician's advice or admoni-
tion to the parents that the infant was a sick, fragile, and extremely
tenuous creature and the parent had to be extremely careful in
touching, holding, or handling it.

All this did nothing to help but only aggravated the situation of
prematurity, and there was no doubt that it also interfered with the
mutual adaptation between mother and infant that is so important
to getting children off to a good start in the first year. The sudden
number of cases, the cumulative effect of disturbed parental
attitudes, are not overcome in spite of positive developments in the
child, and these are the cases one sees at the age of 4 or 5 years
at the child guidance clinic. This type of outcome is not peculiar
to premature babies but also for all kinds of infants who are looked
after in ways that do not support their development; prematurity
and other life-threatening disorders in the postnatal period are,
however, the most frequent offenders with respect to this kind of
nonsupportive, nonsatisfying relationship between parent and child.
What happens in the first year of life between a mother and her
baby is something very special, and one cannot substitute just any
caretaker for the mother. It does not have to be the biological
mother, but the relationship has to have a certain quantity and a
certain quality that is not easily obtained with surrogation.

Richmond thought that *Minkowski's* presentation was a good
example of the astute clinical investigator who, while managing
patients, was able not only to look critically at what he does but
also at the social policy implications of what he does. The class
differences in connection with infant mortality and morbidity are
well known and documented, but to reduce the risk for the lower
income groups requires planning on a national basis. *Minkowski*
has pointed to the effective systems in operation in some countries
for reaching the universe of pregnant women; the Scandinavian

countries, in particular, have been successful in distributing their maternal and child care services and inducing people to utilize them. He admitted that several years ago he had thought that the establishment of proper health services themselves would not be preventive unless the multitudinous and severe stresses related to poverty were corrected. However, the success of the Maternal and Infant Care Program produced by the Children's Bureau of the United States in reducing both infant mortality, morbidity, and prematurity rates in the lowest income group has completely negated this notion. We would strongly approve *Minkowski's* plea for greater investment in the preventive approach rather than in expensive and elaborate rehabilitation services, but it is often very difficult to convince even sophisticated professionals to put more resources into prevention when there are children who currently need treatment. There is an ethical problem involved.

Today we are seeing children with learning disorders and subtle neurological problems, and one wonders to what extent prematurity may not have played a role in these developments. Furthermore, careful neurological assessments of delinquents furnish a considerable yield of neurological abnormalities and once again raise the question as to their relation to perinatal traumata. In discussing *Leiderman's* presentation, *Minkowski* mentioned that the work was undertaken at the time when there were still very strong taboos against bringing nonprofessional people into the premature nursery, and it took both courage and persuasion to bring this off. In addition, his research group helped to direct more attention to the maternal side of the mother-infant equation. *Richmond* predicted that future studies would be both developmental and interactional. *Brazelton's* work was a current example of this, whereas *Leiderman* still focused on the infant or the mother, rather than on the infant and the mother.

Leiderman suggested some simulated prenatal, perinatal, and postnatal experiences to prepare mothers more adequately for the maternal response, but *Richmond* had some question about this. Were reproductive holdups nature's way of telling us about biological and ultimately psychosocial limitations? To what extent was infertility a biological communication regarding parental incapacities? *Marcus* recalled that in the national study in England on 11,000 childen there were two factors associated with reproduc-

tion that correlated significantly with later disturbances: low
birthrate and low socioeconomic status. There was a further risk
inherent in prematurity: about 25 percent of battered children are
premature, and it is possible that the hyperactivity and hyperreac-
tivity that were thought to be typical of prematures and possibly
related to some minimal brain dysfunction might act as provocations
to the battering parent. He also speculated as to whether the isolette
experience might not have sensitized the infant, making it even
harder to hold and handle and therefore setting up a vicious circle
for the mother who is already rejecting the child.

   Belmont discussed the circular feedback model of the child's
input interacting with the auxiliary ego-support in terms of the
past presentations. There could be deficiencies on the supportive
side for social and cultural reasons, but there are also factors that
render the support inaccessible to the child or unusable by him.
There may be a barrier operating within the child, perhaps
genetically determined, that prevents his ego from reaching out
competently to take what is offered by the mother. *Leiderman's*
presentation represented the interposition of an artificial barrier in
the use of environmental support. At his center, *Belmont* has
instituted a program for premature babies whereby they are subjected
to artificial motor stimulations by the nurses. What they neglected
to do was to provide some stimulation for the mother, to insure
her involvement, so that the feedback mechanism could operate.
Leiderman pointed out that it was not enough to provide rocking
beds, mobiles, and various kinds of visual, auditory, and tactile
stimulations without insuring that these are continued when the
infant leaves the hospital. This was one reason why at Stanford they
preferred to work through the mothers. They made it her job.

   In response to *Provence's* presentation, *Richmond* asked what the
follow-up on infantile psychophysiological disorders resulting from
degrees of deprivation such as the failure to thrive, spasmophilia,
rumination, nutritional anemias, and disorders of rhythm had
disclosed. He wondered whether the parents continued to manifest
competence in their management of the child. In reply, *Provence*
thought that some of the interventions seemed to help the parents
over a crisis point and to allow them to develop healthier and more
appropriate responses in future situations. For example, mother
may be a much better mother for her toddler than she was for her

infant, since she has been carried past the crisis point of meeting the infant's dependency needs. Although there were mothers who were poor nurturers all along the developmental line and did not succeed in meeting their children's needs at any stage, or in having a satisfying relationship with them, it seemed to her that the severity of the problem diminished with time following several crisis interventions. With ongoing support, many of these parents managed to become good enough, especially if one did not quarrel with them about their management.

Richmond remarked that he had seen many young mothers still in their teens who seemed grossly incompetent in dealing with their infants, but over the years he had seen these same mothers mature and become fairly competent after they had gotten through satisfying their own adolescent needs. *Provence* emphasized that one dealt with the individual case in an individual way based on one's clinical knowledge and experience, and it was not difficult to be helpful. Where the problem arose was when large numbers of people had need of your services and difficulties arose in providing the delivery of services on this scale.

Lourie felt that it was important to look at each case individually because in generalizing one lost a great many that did not fit a generalization. There were problems in meeting the dependency needs in the poverty areas, but he and his colleagues had found that if you met the dependency needs of the mothers, it helped them to meet the dependency needs of the child. The mothers in these poor communities often have experienced deprivation themselves, and this leads to a cycle of dependent, helpless, and passive mothers perpetuating this pattern from generation to generation. One needed an army of helpers to tackle a job of this magnitude. It seemed that clinicians were able to help because they individualized and personalized their helpfulness. If this helpfulness was then projected onto a larger scale, was there some risk of its becoming attenuated and less effective.

Rutter took an opposing point of view. People were different, and each one was different from everyone else, but if this was all, nothing that we learned about one person could be applied to the next. In fact, for the purpose of planning action, we need to know something about the qualities which people share with others, recognizing that these do not involve everyone. He quoted *Garmezy* as asking, "What is the source of this complacent belief that the factors for programming primary prevention efforts are known to us?" *Provence* had stressed the complexity and individuality, but *Rutter* was of the opinion that we also needed to be comparing different modes of intervention to find out about their relative strengths and weaknesses. It was only by doing this that we could come up with answers about the specific needs of individual children.

Disadvantaged individuals needed to be helped, and researchers would not want to interefere with such action. Nevertheless, the action needed to be monitored and evaluated, so that one could learn from one's inevitable mistakes. *Rutter* stressed the importance of monitoring for two reasons: first, we do not always do what we think we are doing, and second, we need to teach parents methods of coping which extend beyond specific issues. He was not suggesting that we knew how to do this but that this should be one of our goals. In parent education, one should not only focus on what is done but also on how it is done and especially on the parent-child and teacher-child interaction. Although these interventions need to be tailored to the individual case, nevertheless, certain principles are involved, and these are transmittable.

Garmezy, in response to a question, touched on some of the difficulties in defining the concept of competence. He felt that any effort to set criteria for competence, particularly for cognitive or nonaffective criteria, was immediately challenged on the grounds that one was transmitting coping skills but middle-class values were being imposed upon lower-class people. He himself preferred to consider that the values were probably present in the population in some form of distribution that was clearly worth investigating. Studies have shown the distribution of growing deficit scores to children who had been exposed to Head Start, and later to school, showed a decline. However, there were also children who did not produce this pattern, and these are worth their weight in gold to a nation in crisis, because they provide us with the sort of attributes that generate resistance.

In the same way, we would focus on those families that appeared to be providing strength to their children in disadvantaged circumstances, studying, in the most intensive anthropological fashion, just what it was the parents in these families were doing about this immunity. Then we would produce programs in which the competent mothers, drawn from the milieu of disadvantage, would become the teachers of less competent mothers living under the same conditions. *Garmezy* felt that the real danger in making discoveries in this field lay in falling into the cliches of the mental health disciplines and that the only way to rupture these cliches was to look to the atypical cases that fail to match the stereotypes that constituted our theories.

Brody referred to what he called a "Holy Grail" syndrome in which everybody was looking in a visionary way for ultimate solutions. At one time it was thought that public housing would solve the problems of venereal disease, delinquency, and everything else that went with them. Later it was one-to-one psychotherapy. Today it was community psychiatry, the clinician forgetting that he was responsible *to* the community and not *for* the community. There had to be choices made by people other than ourselves, regarding the optimum solutions, and there had to be alliances with other agencies and other professionals. *Brody* observed that following successful experiences in the family, the value system and motivations tend to change in that family. He took a public assistance population of about 1000 mothers, most of them functional illiterates, and provided them with additional money so that they could learn to read. At the end of a period of 2 years, a significant number of mothers had completed the equivalent of high school, and, as a result, the quality of family life changed radically. One of the problems with regard to interveners who have been chosen from the same level as the people who are to be helped is that they started to lose their effectiveness in a period of 8 to 9 months, because their identification was no longer with the recipient, beneficiary group but rather with the establishment.

In this same context, it was mentioned that Mednick was attempting to train children at high risk to cope with frustration by a gently graded series of tasks which would not allow the generating of failure, and *Rutter* thought that the children themselves might possibly possess some kind of inborn capacity to teach their parents the job of parenting, and perhaps we ourselves might learn something from the child in this respect. *Solnit* saw the day care center as an important intervention in the case of children at risk in low-income neighborhoods. The crucial question for such a setting was the number of infants and toddlers that a single mother

could care for. Trying to answer it was a way of testing how we
think that mothers ought to be put to work to get the best out of the
situation. He felt that two important principles were involved in
examining the question of risk and vulnerabilty: never to separate
the child from the context and always to remember that what is seen
through the microscope depends on the power of the lens. It may
show nothing, or some scarring, or some severe pathology, and the
fact is that we all tend to use different powers in examining the
field. *Garmezy* agreed with this and felt it was important to keep
the person doing studies of individual differences in close touch
with the epidemiologist and with all other magnifications in between.

Regarding the issue of the peer as the main intervener, *Provence*
thought that it was quite probable that someone in the same social
class from the same neighborhood who has gone through the same
experience would be highly effective as a helping person, but there
was some danger in this generalization, because she had found that
that the people who were most critical of the black families who
were having difficulties were the black paraprofessionals, and it was
a long time before the latter could adopt a more tolerant attitude
toward the former. It would not discount the professional person,
because what one did share was a common humanity, and if that
got across, then you had it made. It did not matter, then, what color
you were or how many degrees you had.

In his presentation *Richmond* reviewed the history of what was
taken for granted today in the field of risk research and intervention.
He began with his own book on the mother-infant interaction,
based on research which he carried out with Caldwell, mentioning
their concern with individual differences and vulnerabilities to
psychomatic disorders. The question that he asked himself had
been referred to by Alexander as the X factor: Why was it that some
individuals under stress seemed to hold up fairly well while others
developed various psychosomatic syndromes? To explore this
problem more basically, he decided to look at the individual at its
earliest time, during the neonatal period. The population studied
was a low-income one, the highest level being about 3000. So what
struck him in observing the performance of the children in these
families was the gradual decline in performance over time. The
circumstances in which these children were brought up left much to
be desired: They were often parked with adolescents or left with

siblings not much older than they were or carted across town to be deposited with various individuals, not necessarily the same, on succeeding days. Of the first 28 children studied, 26 underwent this developmental decline, as measured by the usual developmental tests, but 2 actually progressed and performed extremely well. He and Caldwell then set about devising the curriculum which should not be regarded as highly structured but rather suggestions for the care-taking adults.

Richmond then traced the history of the Head Start Program, which was intended to be a comprehensive child development program, even though people assigned to it focused at times on cognitive development or on medical care. However, it was designed to be comprehensive, to provide medical care and early education, to utilize the social services and economic resources available in the community, to involve the parents, to involve the community who would be essentially responsible for developing and operating the program. It was decided that there would be no fewer than one professional teacher and two teacher aides for every 15 children, making a one-to-five adult-child ratio. A wide variety of efforts was made to evaluate the effects of this kind of intervention. To summarize the results, it was found that the longer the children were in the program, the greater the gains in cognitive tests, though there was often a leveling off effect.

Regardless of ideological commitments in some of the more research-oriented programs, the children seemed to do about the same, whether they used Montessori or traditional nursery school approaches. When examined closely, it seemed that the various ideological groups were not really doing what they said they were doing; moreover, it often seemed that the enthusiasm of the individual intervener was a crucial factor in helping the children to do better. In place of many different curricula, the movement appeared to be moving pragmatically toward multiple minicurricula incorporating additional approaches, sensory stimulation, and affect stimulation. Looked at from one point of view, it seemed very close to what the middle-class child was obtaining in the course of his daily life experience at home. In the earlier stages, the over-enthusiasm generated the hope that the short exposure in the preschool period would somehow immunize the child forever to an unfavorable ecological set, and a great deal of subsequent data negated this. However, some studies have shown sustained gains and others only transient ones. If, however, Head Start has succeeded in improving the quality of early elementary grades in ghetto neighborhoods and in rural poverty areas, then it will have made its most significant impact on the country, and there is some evidence that would lead to the belief that this was in fact happening.

Why some programs had a sustained effect and others not would have been a function of continuity. For example, by sending a teacher who had known the children and the family into the home for as little as half a day a week made a great difference in the children's capacity to sustain their level of performance in the program.

Another gain from the Head Start Program was the way in which citizens began to participate in the lives of their communities in increasing the effective ways. In one investigation it was found that in the Head Start communities, as compared to controls, the programs generally seemed to improve and the involvement of citizens in political action was more vigorous. Another Head Start effect has been in improving the quality of schools as well as the day care for infants and young children. Of 4 million children born each year, not quite 20 percent will be living under unfavorable ecological circumstances associated with poverty. This represented a really significant number of children at risk.

Commenting on this presentation, *Lourie* felt that the Head Start program and programs subsequently stemming from it were reaching down into the earlier age levels and by contact with the children have led us to find the really neglected ones with the alcoholic mothers, mentally ill mothers, pleasure-loving teenage mothers, and hopeless, helpless, and passive mothers. *Marcus* pointed out that the Head Start population of children were at risk in a very wide and undefined way. Among the 20 percent were children with cultural deprivation, brain damage, low birth weight, and so on. It would seem that the next step would be to make an evaluation of the specific kinds of risk, the specific kinds of deficits, and to develop specialized programs for all these different groups of children.

Richmond pointed out that the program was not intended to deal with clinical problems. Furthermore, depending on the theoretical notions of directors, the focus was placed on different remedial techniques. There was some hope that more individualized

developments would begin in the program. In the future one would
also want professional observers involved with the family at an
early time, to pick up developmental deviations. *Krynsky* felt
that if the problem was as great as this in an advanced country such
as the United States, he could only feel very pessimistic about
Brazil, where 50 percent of the inhabitants were illiterate, where
the average family in the north had 16 to 18 children. There was
a big problem with mental retardation; a great deal of money and
a great many teachers were needed. *Krynski* mentioned that the
United States spent about $3 billion a year to take care of its
retarded population but that this was, of course, beyond the means
of poorer countries.

In response to *Rutter's* presentation, *Hersov* wondered about
Rutter's finding in the general population that disturbances in the
child were associated with marital discord but not with unhappy,
unloving marriages without overt discord. This seemed to run
counter to his experience and if it were the case, this was possibly
due to the fact that families in which overt discord was possible were
also families in which affect could be openly expressed and where
there was less need to scapegoat the children. He also wondered at
what point in the cycle of deprivation the impairment of mothering
skills began.

Garmezy felt that in the less discordant marriages there was also
less opportunity for modeling in terms of parental behavior. He
felt that the intergenerational transmission involved in the cycle
of deprivation demanded longitudinal study and, if this were carried
out, it might be possible to observe during play fantasy expressions
of children that are precursors to inadequate mothering later on.
One might even go further and perhaps create microcosm in the
laboratory precursive parenting patterns in children and observe how
they deal with them. The problem of antecedents and consequences
also arose when *Rutter* correlated the stable school system with
nondeviancy in the children and the unstable system with deviancy.
Were we observing here an antecedent to deviant behavior or a
consequent of deviant behavior? Then there is an increase in
deviancy in schools with the greatest teacher turnover, but if this
matter is discussed with the teachers, they point out that it is the
deviancy in the school that leads them to leave school. *Lourie*
thought that *Rutter's* work in the Isle of Wight demonstrated that

when the child psychiatrist left his hospital or clinic, he no longer thought like a clinician but like a behavioral scientist covering a wide range of factors and forces in his thinking.

Rutter also alerted us to the influence of the environment and the possible detrimental effect of city living. Whenever there was an exodus from rural to urban areas, family adjustment appeared to suffer. In St. Louis Pruitt Igoe was an impressive demonstration of some of the destructive effects of the high-rise on child development. There were problems of coping with separation anxiety when you live above the fourth floor, and urine smells in the elevator created problems because children in the process of toilet training would not quite make it home in time. It is possible that we may be asked to participate in planning the cities for the future and we should be prepared to consider the question in the context of child development. Another important issue was how early to start teaching the process of family life. It used to be taught in the high school and it is now being taught in junior high. It may be necessary to teach it much earlier.

Although he acknowledges the multifactorial influences relating to risk, *Rutter* tends to set them aside and deal with one facet at a time. It is hoped that an integration of these will eventually take place because we cannot afford to disregard the complicated processes at work in these children, making some children succumb while others need only crumbs of good experience to land on their feet. *Leiderman* wondered about the functional relationship between *Rutter's* questionnaires and actual behavior and felt that the questionnaires should be subjected to the same careful scrutiny that was used to select samples, otherwise the scope would be too broad and not specific to the issues. *Richmond* felt that *Rutter* had demonstrated his capacity to move from the macroscopic or epidemiological to the microscopic end of observation. This approach reached out beyond the clinical into a wider social sphere and could help in the identification of areas from which there might be a potentially higher yield. It therefore appealed to the social planner more than it did to the clinician. *Richmond* thought that unless we moved in this direction we would spend a great deal of time reinforcing additional biases rather than breaking new ground. It could also help us in our work toward a better environment, a more favorable ecology. He reminded the group that the original work on inter-

generational transmission carried out many years ago had raised
hopes of a new psychopathology with many of its causal connections
clarified, but this did not prove to be the case. The "cycle of
deprivation" might provide a better route for this.

Sapir mentioned a finding in a study by Bergen and Spock
(supported by the Grant Foundation) in which a mother who was
being counseled about the handling of her young child continually
ignored suggestions and persisted in avoiding direct physical
involvement. There seemed to be no doubt about her interest in
and love for the child. It finally became apparent to counselors that
the mother was deliberately avoiding an overinvolvement to protect
her son from her tendency to overwhelm possessively. Her apparent
rejection, in fact, represented a mature protectiveness based on an
awareness of her own shortcomings. This raised the broader
question of what children "mean" to adults and what children "do"
to adults in terms of evoking feelings of rivalry, competitiveness,
and resentment.

Bergen and Spock were also able, in subtle ways, to stage-manage
marital conflicts even though the repercussions might be hurtful.
One of the reasons why girls are at lesser risk than boys could be
that they get less caught up in parental frictions. Some parents might
be inclined to regard them as "less important" and therefore less
threatening members of the family. Clinical insights of this nature
could well provide the researcher with valuable leads in the
systematic exploration of parent-child interactions.

Jensen felt that *Rutter* had provided a corrective to the overuse
and misuse of the term deprivation, although it should not be
forgotten that the earlier work on separation opened up a new world
of understanding some of the disorders of infancy and childhood.
There was a danger, however, of merely exchanging one word for
another; discord could become a ragbag in the same way as deprivation. *Lange* agreed that the word "discord" could be misleading
unless one defined it more carefully. He thought that we should
distinguish between the prolonged and unproductive form, which
was obviously deleterious to the children, and the intermittent,
productive discord that was worked through during critical periods.
Chronic discord, where nothing was expressed or worked through,
was highly conducive to psychosomatic disorder in the family.
Matic made his point in the discussion by telling a little joke about

a man who goes up to another man, calls him a liar, and slaps his face, whereupon the other man starts to laugh. When asked why he laughed, he said, "Well, I am not a liar!" This was an example of how stress could be stressful to one person and not to another. From the point of view of stress, paternal deprivation was due not to stress but to a lack of stress. The outcome was also different. In a research carried out in Yugoslavia a few years ago on the population of a child guidance clinic, the externalizers, as compared to the internalizers, were drawn very definitely from the underprivileged sections.

In his response, *Rutter* insisted that he was a clinician primarily rather than a researcher and that his methods tended to be primarily clinical. He pointed out, however, that in studying large samples one had to rely mainly on questionnaires, but it was always a two-stage procedure in which he moved from questionnaire data on large populations to very intensive interviews and sometimes observational data on small numbers. The interviews usually lasted about three hours and fairly extensive information was obtained. There were some variables in studying families that responded to questionnaires, some to interviews, and some, like patterns of communication and decision making, that could be obtained only through the direct observation of interaction. It was not a question of which was the better method in a hierarchical sense but which was more appropriate to what was being investigated. The differences found between boys and girls were not a function of the measuring instrument since they had looked carefully at this and had found that in the investigation of other areas, it picked out girls as well as boys. This was true, for example, in the investigation of institutional upbringing, cerebral palsy, and epilepsy; the girls came out as disturbed as the boys.

Rutter agreed that the concept of discord was not completely satisfactory and that it needed to be broken down more finely. It was definitely not a single entity nor a single process. He also agreed that the question of what is antecedent and what is consequent was crucial and difficult to disentangle. Did disturbed children produce certain teacher characteristics or did certain teacher characteristics produce disturbed children? In Britain free meals in school was a convenient index of social disadvantage, and *Rutter* had found that schools with a high proportion of children having free meals also had higher rates of disturbance. Was this disturbance the effect of disadvantage or of the educational environment? In the analysis the free meal children were excluded and the association of disturbance with school remained virtually unaltered. It seemed as if in the presence of certain sorts of children, certain sorts of teacher characteristics became influential. This did not imply a single direction and nor did it refute the fact that teachers do move because schools are difficult. However, the very fact of their moving made the children more difficult.

With regard to urban versus rural effects, *Rutter* had compared children born and bred in London with children who had come in later, and he found that the rates of deviance were equally high. London was not being used as a dump for disturbed individuals from all over the country; it was city living that generated disturbance. He felt that he had been much influenced in his own research thinking by the work on maternal overprotection by David Levy, who first disentangled the elements of this particular form of maternal behavior and then traced them to their source in unhappy and sexually maladjusted marriages. This was the sort of reasoning that *Rutter* followed both in clinical work and in research.

The problems of risk, vulnerability, and mastery were then examined in the light of work being carried out in Yugoslavia. *Beck-Dvorzak* discussed her experience, as a psychotherapist, of the risks entailed for children from neurotic personality disorders in parents. The impact of parental neurosis on the developing child was as serious and as far-reaching as psychosis and psychopathy. The obsessional mother or mother substitute could elicit a great deal of symptomatic behavior in the child ranging from stammering to constipation. Currently 30 neurotic parents and their preschool children were being studied longitudinally throughout the period of childhood and adolescence by intensive psychotherapeutic methods that would attempt to correlate defense mechanisms in the child with the personality structure of the parent.

A second invesigation had to do with working mothers and the problem of early separation without adequate substitution. The risks for the children were considerable, and it will be interesting to see to what extent the subsequent disorders compare with those found in similar circumstances in Western Europe and the United States. The third set of risks for children stemmed from migration

from rural to urban areas, from the less developed to the more
developed parts of the country, and from emigration for economic
reasons. The first two tended to be associated more frequently with
adult neurosis whereas the third frequently generated emotional
disorders in the children, especially when both parents went abroad
and left the children with relatives or neighbors. Not all the children
were equally vulnerable to this; a great deal seemed to depend on
the child's emotional state at the time of separation.

Poljak continued the discussion of the emigration risk, which is
a major problem in Yugoslavia since a large body of workers move
to other parts of Europe, especially Germany, as a labor force. He
had studied two groups of 38 children, ages 5 to 17 years, one group
being made up of those who had been separated from their parents
for at least 6 months in the two previous years. The children in both
groups had been exposed to a variety of risks but the factor of
separation distinguished the two groups. Emigration accounted for
36 percent of the separations and divorce for 29 percent. The
separated group differed from the nonseparated group in several
respects: it averaged more than two symptoms per child as compared
with one symptom per child; there was a significantly higher
incidence of enuresis. He agreed with *Rutter* that separation in itself
was not the principal factor in the risk but the circumstances
surrounding it that disturbed the equilibrium of the family. A factor
that added to the risk in emigration was the ambivalence associated
with leaving. There were economic pressures to go and emotional
pressures to stay, or one parent might want to go and the other
to remain. All this unsettled the family and left it even more
vulnerable to the separation.

Vlatković-Prpić dealt with the risks, on the increase in Yugoslavia,
of working mothers and the effects of surrogation, particularly by
grandparents ("granny service" was a familiar colloquialism in the
country). In addition to the problems of separation and substitution,
there was no doubt that the mothers were exposed to the same
overwork and overstrain of the fathers and that their new emanci-
pated attitudes created frictions within the family as well as in the
community. The rivalry between the mother and mother substitute
for the child's affection further aggravated the mother's guilt feelings, adding to her doubts and ambivalence. In an interview survey,
only 8 percent of the women were of the opinion that a working
mother can meet all her family responsibilities, whereas 26 percent

of the men felt that they could. In spite of feeling negatively toward what they were doing, nearly 50 percent of the working women said that they would continue to work even if there were no financial necessity for it because of the satisfactions derived from it.

The tentative investigation of children referred to the clinic suggested that when the mother enjoyed her work and found satisfaction in it, the children seemed less emotionally deprived. The sample was mainly composed of poorer class mothers with poorer educational background engaged in unskilled work. There was also some evidence that multiple mothering acted as a positive force when the different caretakers worked together harmoniously. In the rural areas in Yugoslavia the children often worked or played alongside the mothers in the fields and the family systems were traditional, extended, and supportive with the role of the parents considerably modified.

Kos-Mikus pointed out how different cultural factions in different parts of Yugoslavia had different problems dealing with neuropsychiatric disorders. For example, in Slovenia, which could be said to have a depressive-obsessive culture, the average child was expected to be obedient, self-disciplined, organized, sane, and quiet. As a result, children with minimal brain dysfunction were very serious problems and very poorly tolerated. *Hadiantonović* referred to the village of Milosevac, which has for a long time made fostering its way of life. Several generations of boys have now passed through the village and have come to look upon it as a home and the villagers as relatives. It was possible that this unique situation had prevention built into it, but the matter has not been studied. *Klain* felt there was some danger that a massive research approach would overlook important, essential and simple things, especially the specific reactions of individuals. Everyone was agreed that the "happy family" was a preventive institution but it was difficult to define all the ingredients that went into it. An important factor in helping children to overcome some of the hazards of development was to help the helpers to understand more fully and dynamically what they were doing, otherwise their efforts could become singularly unhelpful as their personal difficulties intruded on the situation. *Klain* saw this dynamic education as a preventive measure and felt that it should be applied to medical practitioners, teachers, and others in the helping professions.

Provence thought that we should find another name for the working mother because most of the mothers of the world would protest strongly that some women were working mothers while others were not. In the United States at earlier times and even currently in some parts of the country, mothers worked very hard both inside and around the home with the children scattered around her but somehow feeling her presence. This was different from the mother going out to work and the child being taken elsewhere or having substitute care. What we need to do today is to reorganize the working day for both men and women so that both parents can continue to nurture and support the family and promote the development of the children without being removed too much from them. A number of working options should be open to women, including shorter work days, satisfying rather than menial jobs, and professional opportunities that again would not interfere too much with home life. Having this satisfaction for themselves would enable them to give more satisfaction to their children. Whether they work or not should be a choice that they themselves make.

Lebovici, toward the end of the discussion, noted some of the problems for international groups thinking and working together. Words like "competence" had such different meanings in different languages and in different cultures. There were also difficulties in bringing together dynamic and descriptive concepts within the same meeting. Different views of development might also alter one's notions of risk and vulnerability. If the average, expectable development included a normal psychotic stage and a normal neurotic stage, how would this affect our understanding of what is hazardous or what is disordered? As far as risk was concerned, *Lebovici* had some difficulty in accepting the enormous importance given to risks of social difficulties; for example, in France poverty would not appear to be such a crucial factor.

In all these matters it seemed important not to underestimate the role of internal factors within the individual and the interactions within the family. When one came down to the individual case, many of the wide generalizations seemed hardly to apply. To illustrate this *Lebovici* gave the case of 8-year-old Dominique. The mother had a substitute father, an uncle, who died of hemophilia after which the mother immigrated to France with the grandmother where she married a cousin. The first son turned out to be a hemophiliac and the second a transsexual for whom the question of castration became a crucial issue. After a great deal of contradictory and confusing advice, the boy was eventually castrated at the age of 5 and suddenly became a girl who was given the name Dominique. For a long time, she was unresponsive, almost stuporous, and completely denied her new sex and confused the sex of others, usually addressing men as women. Her IQ dropped 20 points. In therapy she showed a total incapacity for internalizing or symbolizing and it was some time before the denial of her new sex diminished. Her mother was equally confused, having dreams that she had a penis and believing that Dominique would one day become a mother. The case was presented to show how intricate the problems of risk could be and how ineffectual some standard form of intervention could be without taking into account the curious background of the mother.

Intervention was a complicated task, as complicated as psychotherapy. To intervene on a case of deprivation one needed not only to help the child but to help the mother with how not to deprive the child, in fact, how to make better mothers, and this is a question beyond the psychiatric field. To quote a well-known saying: "Give me better mothers and I will give you a better world." The International Study Group has been addressing itself to the question of how to create a better world in order to have better mothers.

Both *Richmond* and *Norman Lourie* emphasized the importance of political action and the importance of making professionals more active in bringing about needed legislation. It was noted that matters are improving in this respect and we are becoming more effective and articulate in relation to public policy. There undoubtedly is still a great deal of inertia and ambivalence on the part of the public in general, as Rexford demonstrated, but within the last few decades there had been a considerable increase in antipoverty legislation and a greater focus on the adverse conditions in which children were being brought up in certain parts of the country. Communities themselves were becoming imbued with new interests and enthusiasms for action programs. One of the reasons that we were not well understood by the public is because we did not have an ecumenical movement in the field, some kind of human ecology approach that would bring us all together and thereby get us increased recognition.

After thanking the Yugoslav contingent for their helpfulness in arranging the Bled conference, *Lourie* closed the meeting.

THE DAKAR CONFERENCE

The Dakar Conference* on Environmental Factors in Risk

MEETING OF THE INTERNATIONAL STUDY GROUP ON "CHILDREN AT PSYCHIATRIC RISK" AT DAKAR, SENEGAL, AFRICA, JULY 29-AUGUST 4, 1973

PARTICIPANTS

CHAIRMAN: E. James Anthony, M.D., *President*
                          International Association for Child
                          Psychiatry and Allied Professions

CO-CHAIRMAN: Serge Lebovici, M.D., *President*
                          International Association of Psychoanalysis

SESSIONAL CHAIRMEN: Reginald S. Lourie, M.D.
                          Lionel Hersov, M.D.
                          Henri Collomb
                          Reimer Jensen

RAPPORTEUR: Albert Solnit, M.D.

LOCAL ORGANIZER   Henri Collomb, M.D.
IN AFRICA

INVITED SPEAKERS

Colin M. Turnbull, D.Phil.
Tolani Asuni, M.D.
T. Adeoye Lambo, M.D.**
P. Herbert Leiderman, M.D.
Adewale Omololu, M.D.***
James P. Comer, M.D.
Donald J. Cohen, M.D.

OFFICIAL DISCUSSANTS

Joseph Marcus, M.D.
Stanislau Krynski, M.D.
Elizabeth E. Irvine, M.A.
Jon Lange, M.D.
Winston Rickards, M.D.

ORGANIZERS OF THE INTERNATIONAL CONGRESS OF CHILD PSYCHIATRY AND ALLIED PROFESSIONS, 1974

Herman Staples, M.D.
Theodore B. Cohen, M.D.

PARTICIPANTS FROM AFRICA

Dr. Amoussou Alexis	Dr. Moustapha Diallo
Dr. Tolani Asuni	Dr. Babacar Diop
Dr. M. Hazera	M. Assane Diop
Dr. M. Makang	Dr. Maurice Dores
Dr. M. Sangaret	Dr. Tidiane Gueye
Dr. E. F. Thebaud	Mme. Marie Hladik
Dr. R. Ahyi	M. Georges M'Bodje
Mme. M. Boutet	Mme. Marie M'Bodje
M. Rene Collignon	Mme. Seynabou N'Dao
Dr. Henri Collomb	Dr. Abdou Sanokho
Dr. Paul Correa	Dr. Gabriel Senghor
Dr. Vincent Dan	Mme. Conce Stievenard
Dr. Saliou Dia	Mme. Simone Valantin

* Sponsored by the Grant Foundation, the Commonwealth Fund and the World Health Organization.

** Deputy Director of the World Health Organization.

*** Unable to attend the meeting at which his paper was read.

Introduction: The African Condition

Colin M. Turnbull, D.Phil. (U.S.A.)

Change in Relation to Tradition

It is still commonplace to think of tradition, especially that of
so-called primitive societies, as being static. Even among much of
contemporary African leadership (especially among those leaders
educated in colonial schools) there is the thought that African tradition is somehow detrimental to progress, if not to survival. Yet in
Africa tradition has always been a dynamic thing, and far from being
static the small-scale societies of traditional Africa have been constantly changing, and tradition has enabled them to cope with the
changes and maintain strong *senses* of continuity even in the face of
discontinuity. That same tradition has involved a different concept
of time and space from that generally held in the Western world;
consequently a Western concept of progress is inapplicable within
the essentially vital traditional systems, just as is our more static
notion of normality. Within the traditional system "normality" is
just as subject to change as anything else.

Insofar as there is much of Africa's tradition that is still very much
alive, even though most systems resting on the notion of tribe have
been largely destroyed, many of the problems arising from current
changes are likely to be aggravated by, it not due to, the persistence
of traditional notions of personality, identity, and security, all of
which are intimately linked with a previous, preindustrial condition

227

that still persists in the vast rural areas of the continent. The present condition is one of conflict between an ancient and still highly dynamic conceptual world and a dramatically new and different contemporary empirical world that was initially forced upon Africa, and is now eagerly being sought.

Without entering into a discussion of which of the two worlds is the more desirable, merely accepting the situation as it is at the moment, it seems utterly unrealistic to ignore the persistence of traditional concepts, even in urban areas, and to ignore both the dangers and the potential of their juxtaposition with a totally new life style. Many of the social institutions of traditional Africa that helped societies to adapt to sometimes quite marked changes are still operative, fulfilling their vital function, but are threatened by our ignorance and by other changes that we consciously seek to introduce for the benefit of these societies. What follows is a very brief outline of some of the areas that should concern all those involved with change in the contemporary African scene. This involves a level of generalization that is as significant as it is valid, for beneath the many different outer forms of traditional African social organization there is a remarkable degree of unity, especially when we consider the inner content rather than the outer form.

Two Important Generalizations

One such generalization relates to the technological level of traditional, preindustrial Africa—an Africa still very much alive everywhere except in the relatively few cities and larger towns. Throughout Africa man has a very special and intimate and wholly integrated relationship with the environment. He sees himself as a part of the natural world around him and indeed, in many instances, actually functions efficiently as a part of the total ecology. This is particularly true of the hunter/gatherer who does not seek to interfere with the environment even by the domestication of animals, let alone through the cultivation of the soil, but it is also true to a great extent of the cattle herders and even the cultivators who still adapt to the natural world rather than attempt to control and dominate it. This has vast implications in terms of both African society and African personality.

Another such generalization which also relates to technological level is that in all traditional African societies man has *had* to depend on man; true sociality was the *only* road to survival. Due to the nature of the various environments, and the relatively low population level, and due to man's concept of himself as a part of the natural world around him as well as to his technological level, wealth has never been perceived as something that can be amassed individually, and security has never been perceived in terms of individual survival. Both wealth and security are ultimately defined in virtually all traditional African societies as people or often, more specifically, as family.

It is perhaps man's technological inability to fend for himself that draws him to sociality rather than any inherent, biologically determined characteristics. At any event the traditional African societies without exception are marked by numerous and often highly complex institutions that function to avert conflict at exactly those points where it is most likely to occur, thus reinforcing the essential if not fundamental sociability of the human group.

The African Social System

At this point it will be useful to attempt to find a way of characterizing the very basic difference between African social systems and those we know in the Western world today, for the proper understanding of this difference is vital if we are to be able to lend such skills as our own world has developed to help another world without irreparably damaging it. Intending absolutely no value implications, it might be fairly said that African societies are moralistic as against the legalistic nature of our own. This is again certainly not due to any inherent or cultivated virtue on the part of the African, but shows rather a sensitive and sensible response to the needs of his condition. The same might be said of our response, however much we might deplore it. The hard fact is that in our own much larger scale societies social order can be maintained only through the threat and use of physical coercion, whereas in no traditional African societies (as with most other small-scale societies throughout the world) does one find anything even approaching a police force, let alone one as potentially armed as ours.

When some of the great nations developed out of confederacies of powerful tribes (as with the Ashanti of Ghana) certain forms of

police activity became necessary, and something approaching a
legal system began to emerge, but this was only recently and in
response to drastic changes introduced from outside. The reason, I
believe, is simple enough. With population pressure on land at a
minimum, and with a level of technology that demanded close and
systematic cooperation for survival, there was little need for tribes
to form into nations, and almost by definition a tribe was a community of believers. Almost invariably those societies with tribal
structure (and not all have such a structure, as with hunter/gath-
erers) preserve the family model and either consist of members who
are related to one another in some way and can trace (or claim to
trace) such a relationship, or else consist of peoples who have created
and preserved a myth of common ancestry, all of whom, in either
case, share common beliefs and values. It is out of this community
of belief that order proceeds, without law.

There is of course still coercion, but it is moral rather than legal.
Instead of a policeman with a gun to prevent robbery and murder,
there is often the belief in an omnipresent and omniscient god or
spirit, and instead of the threat of being shot or taken to court and
punished by due process of law, there is often the threat of being
debarred from an honorable afterlife.

Since the outer form of each system of belief tends to be different,
often widely so, generalization is difficult beyond affirming that in all
the traditional African societies, at the level of band, tribe, or
nation, there exists some such moral pressure involving not only
belief, which is a rational process, but an act of faith, which is supra-
rational *and therefore unquestionable.* And in that unquestion-
ability lies the great strength of the moralistic society (and we perceive that perhaps it is only "moral" in our terms). And because
indoctrination in the community belief starts at birth with the very
first ritual act that consecrates the infant to the·society—past,
present, and future—and continues throughout childhood with
increasing intensity, and because the belief is manifest in ritual
action every day, in assocation with just about every act of any
importance, by the time the child reaches the age of puberty and is
ready to accept adult status responsibility he has acquired faith as
well as belief, believing that he behaves in a given (moral, or social)
manner because he wants to of his own free will, whereas in fact he
has been conditioned so to behave. He does not act in a prescribed

way out of fear of supernatural retribution; the positive sanctions
are always far more significant than the negative sanctions.

African Thought

Here something must be said about the very different conceptual
world of the traditional African, though again the outer forms vary
widely. However, at the outset I suggested that those of us who are not
African have to try to enter another way of thinking and perceiving
if we are to come anywhere close to understanding the African
condition, and in particular we have to accept that our own
concepts of time and space are not the only ones. The clue is often
found in the language, and in many languages, for instance, the
same word equally denotes before and after, in both time and space;
in other words, contrasting the here and now with anything that is
not here and now (and is therefore of totally different relevance). A
misunderstanding of this fact, coupled with a dismissal of African
religious systems as "primitive superstitution," has led to many a
disaster, of which the infamous Mau Mau tragedy was only one.

The Mau Mau tragedy basically rested on the fact that to the
British the dead are dead and no longer have rights to land, which is
therefore morally alienable with the consent of the owner. Even
when they recognized that the Kikuyu had some rather complex
notions of communal ownership they were unable to perceive that
the land is both here (on the surface) and in some kind of subter-
ranean other world that is coexistent, and that it belongs not only
to the living but to the entire lineage, which includes also what we
would call the dead and the unborn. Therefore it is inalienable.
Further it is sacred in the sense that it was given by God for a specific purpose, farming, to a specific people, and that the greatest
disaster of all, deprivation of afterlife with the rest of one's lineage,
attends any desecration of this trust.

Without going into a functional comparison of land tenure
throughout Africa, it is safe to affirm that everywhere there is something of this joint reverence for the land and for the ancestors,
thought not always so clearly formulated. For instance, among the
Mbuti pygmies, whom perhaps I know best, and who have among
the least formalized and most fluid of social systems, the "here and
now" of their forest world is equally paramount, but carefully con-

ceived in typically flexible manner. As with many hunter/gatherers all the focus of attention is on the present, for each day brings its own assurance of the replenishment of life supplies. A perfect part of the total ecology, the Mbuti in that respect act as one of the two major predators in the forest, and the only one capable of performing the all-important task of cropping the otherwise destructive elephant population. They recognize their being part of a wholly integrated world and see their affinity with other animals, even with the plants and streams and rocks and stones of the forest. They seldom see the sky so the celestial imagery is minimal; they use water rather than the sky to express their thoughts about the nature of life.

Water, for the Mbuti, is the only reflective substance and in their experience where it reflects most clearly it is most dangerous and unpredictable. Rivers and streams also form natural boundaries between hunting bands (and game populations) and therefore this respect for water serves well to prevent indiscriminate crossing of these frontiers. But what *is* that reflection, asks the hunter; it plainly has to do with me, is a part of me, is like me in almost all respects, yet is not me—and what is that whole world around that other me? And what happens when I put a foot in the water and the other foot comes up to meet mine and merges with it? And what happens when I gradually immerse my whole body, until only my two eyes are looking at only two eyes, that is all that is left of our two selves? And if I take that last step and totally submerge myself—how am I to know that my other self has not emerged and taken my place? Or if we are still one, and I emerge on the other side of the river, which one of us emerges and which stays below in that aquatic spirit world?

So the Mbuti, technologically one of the most "primitive" peoples in the whole world, uses a natural element as a foil for his thoughts about his very nature and being. And he believes that there is indeed another coexistent world into which you probably (almost certainly) pass at death, from which you emerge at birth, and where, in a sense, *you already are.* Some believe, and legends attest to this belief, that you can indeed either by accident or design cross over into that other plane of existence by entering water at the right place and the right moment; in fact that is how sometimes animals manage to escape from the hunt, for they of course have the same quality of here-and-now otherness.

Backward and forward in time and space plainly have different

connotations to people so sensitive to problems of identity, so aware
of reflections and shadows that are sometimes here and sometimes
there, but always attached. Frequently the concept of time is cyclic
rather than lineal; it is something that, rather like space, surrounds
one and into and out of which one can move more or less at will.
Thus there is no notion of progress which, again, for us is a lineal
concept, a movement from here to there. It is rather a movement
from one here to another here, from one now to another now.

This does not mean that there is no goal. There is, but it is a
goal that has already been achieved, and must merely be reachieved
or maintained. Frequently it is stated with reference to "the Way
of the Ancestors," for it was the ancestors who showed man how to
survive and when disaster strikes it is because that way has been lost.

Family and Kinship

Of all generalizations that are possible about Africa, such as the
essential egality of traditional economic systems, the essential
democracy of political systems (both because these characteristics are
necessities rather than virtues), perhaps the least debatable is the
central position of the family. And it is the family that concerns all
those dealing with the health and welfare of either the society as a
whole or of the individual. Yet we non-Africans persist in importing
our own fixed notions of family, again as though our own conceptual
framework were the only possible one, or had some independent
existence beyond the context of our own being. In traditional African
societies, the family is not only the beginning, it is also the end,
for it establishes itself as a model for all social relations and is
reflected even at the level of national organization.

The most basic and primal lesson in sociality is first learned,
among those whose technology has not provided them with mechanical alternatives, at the mother's breast. In many African societies it
is urged if not mandatory that mothers breastfeed their children for
three years, which not only helps keep the population down but also
thoroughly teaches that child the notion of *dependence* (as opposed
to the Western emphasis on independence). It teaches reciprocity,
which the child may eventually interpret as affection or love. This
vital first lesson in sociality has already been extended beyond the
initial binary relationship by the time the child is weaned. He has

learned by then that the father who cannot give him food gives him other things, and is another kind of mother in that the same kind of reciprocity exists. He then learns to classify other individuals such as uncles and aunts as other kinds of fathers and mothers according to the local (tribal) terminological system, which may seem indeed to classify an aunt as a mother or a male cousin as a mother (see Table 1, part 2).

Table 1   Two Examples of African "Kinship" Terminology

Nuclear Family	All those in the hunting band at any given moment

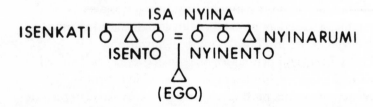

1. **Mbuti Pygmies**. This system in fact classifies age levels rather than kin though the prime model is the nuclear family. The point of reference is "EGO". The terms distinguish four generational levels and only distinguish between the sexes at the parental level.

2. **Nyoro**. Here the system clearly distinguishes paternal kin from maternal kin. The diagram is only partially complete since there are further complications in cousin terminology that still further highlight this prime opposition between the two groups. Whereas the Mbuti system fills a major economic role, clearly designating the vital activities appropriate to each individual according to his age, the Nyoro system is perhaps more political in function, though also with economic implications. The Mbuti are hunters, the Nyoro farmers.

We plainly have to revise our own concepts under these conditions, for the terminology so applied is not a mere conventional
nicety, devised for the amusement of anthropologists, it represents
the family model of reciprocity at a wider level of extension, each
term not denoting or intended to denote any necessary biological
relationship but very definitely representing a real social relationship. In fact some systems, such as that of the Mbuti pygmies, virtually ignore biological kinship and "declassify" kin when they move
out of the hunting band (as they frequently do, to join another band
in another territory) and refer to such absent kin by personal names
until they return. At the same time they classify *everyone* who is a
member of the hunting band at that particular moment as one of
a limited kind of kin. Here in fact the kinship terminology follows
age rather than kinship, separating children, youths, adults, and
elders without regard for sex except at the parental level where, of
course, it is sociologically inescapable. These two very different systems of kinship terminology indicate just how different concepts of
kith and kin can be from one tribe to another; and they also indicate
how very different *all* African kinship systems are from our own,
where our terms merely describe biological relationships which may
or may not correspond to legal or customary social relationships.
This all has a great deal to do with African personality and identity,
which we shall look at shortly.

First, however, mention should be made of the many different
forms of family to be found in Africa, but how again there is an
essential unity underlying them all. Their structure and complexity
invariably match (or are made to match) the needs of that particular
society. Sometimes the form is not unlike our own, though seldom
as restricted in size. But more often there is a great difference in
characteristics other than size. Polygyny is relatively frequent, for
instance, and often children address all their father's wives as
"mother," indicating that they have the same (or similar) affective
and effective relationships with little regard for biology. The lack of
emphasis on the necessity for maintaining the biological bond is
demonstrated by the relative frequency of adoption in some societies,
the important thing being for a woman to have a child, it being
rather less important whether it is hers or not (this naturally varies
with economy and consequent problems of inheritance).

Often the "family," as with the *abusua* of the Ashanti, appears

Table 2   Three Examples of East African
Age-Set Systems Types (simplified)

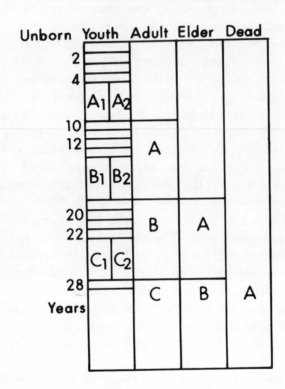

1. Linear. Remembering the very basic generational "kinship"
terminological system of the Mbuti, in these systems we again see
the central importance of age as a structural and conceptual principle.
Many Nilotic pastoralists use a linear system similar to this. The
set goes through grades of, say, nine years in duration. The set being
"born" (marked by mutilation...cutting of forehead, circumcision, etc.)
is open to candidates for four years, then closed. During these four
years each successive year sees its own identity as separate, but nonetheless has succeeded in enlarging the children's social horizons from
the confines of biological "family". For the remaining five years
they see and refer to themselves as a single set, and so pass on, united,
into adulthood as the next set is "born". Each set has its own name,
shared by all members equally.

to be identical with ours—parents and children. But in point of
fact the Ashanti *abusua* adult male and female are not husband
and wife but brother and sister, and the children's father is not
considered a member of the family, because he does not share the
same *mogya* ("blood"), which can only be passed down in the female

Table 3　Three Examples of East African
Age-Set Systems Types (simplified)

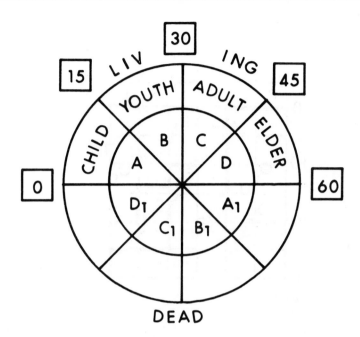

2. <u>Cyclic</u>. Whereas the previous system is non-recurrent, the set names dying as the set dies out, the cyclic system involves a concept of rebirth and significantly is found amongst those people who know of or practice agriculture and whose concepts are more geared to the recurrent life cycle. It provides each individual with a group identity at a lower level than the tribe. At each grade there is a recognized area of activity, responsibility, and authority, and those who live to an old age as the inner wheel turns (every fifteen years here) move into (social) death but have the satisfaction of seeing their set name being reborn, though the children thus born will not be initiated until they are 15.

line since it corresponds to the blood that is shed at birth. The Ashanti, being a much more complex society than many, also recognize paternity, however, but conceive of that as uniting people in a different way, in different families in which *ntoro*, or spirit, is passed down in the male line. Thus one society may recognize two distinct kinds of family, each with its own role or function, each involving every individual in distinct and different loyalties.

In other cases, however, as with the Bushmen hunter/gatherers of southern Africa, the family is considered as a developmental unit

Table 4   Three Examples of East African
Age-Set Systems Types (simplified)

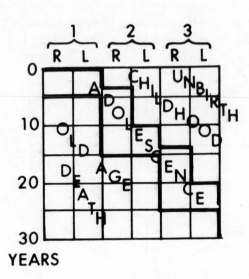

3. Step. This is less common and again corresponds in form to
specific empirical and conceptual needs. The Maasai have a system
similar to this. It separates three age levels, the central one having
a dominant political role, being the protectors of the people and their
cattle. Its internal organization allows for military organization into
regiments, and each set is divided into those of the right hand and
those of the left hand, each with different roles and responsibilities.
However, there is a period of overlapping when the right hand of the
next set is initiated and shares adulthood, briefly, with both halves
of the senior set. In this way continuity is assured, and social
horizons are extended for those of the right hand subsets to both the
set senior to them and the set that is their junior. The initiation of
each new set is accompanied by a formal battle between them and the
senior set they are forcing into retirement.

that passes through four stages, each with its own structure and
identity, each involving different individuals (see Tables 2, 3, and
4). And again the family reveals itself as establishing a model for
social relationships at all levels of social life. For an African chief or
king to be referred to as "father" is no empty thing, and many a
modern African political leader has found, to his cost, just how real
a thing it is to be classified in this way.

Biology is important in African kinship systems merely in that it provides for a natural system (for tracing descent and inheritance), into and out of which system one can be classified, as by adoption. Their concern with incest is consciously at the sociological level, for what is to be gained through inmarriage? Both political and economic considerations are important in marriage, and the need to consolidate intergroup relationships may lead to a system of preferred or prescribed cross-cousin marriage, for instance, whereas if the social context demands the expansion of social horizons, cousin marriage may be proscribed. The same rules that are applied to marriage with such social foresight are applied (more or less equally) to sexual intercourse, with the same kind of social rather than biological consciousness.[1]

When dealing with any African family, then, we have to be prepared to encounter different concepts of family and of kinship, and we have to recognize that the emotions are correspondingly structured, that it is indeed not only possible but likely, if not certain, that a child who calls two people (or twenty) "mother" has the same emotional relationship with both (or all) of them, as well as the same sociological relationship. In fact in all the societies I know personally it is not only difficult to distinguish between biological and sociological kin, it is considered a great impoliteness to do so, involving cumbersome phraseology such as "siblings of the same male sex out of the same stomach" for what we would describe so simply, exactly, and with such little social consequence as "brothers."

The Significance of Name

Not only does the kinship term by which one is addressed or by which one addresses someone else define social role, but so do the

---

[1] In northern Nigeria there is a group where people do not usually know who their mothers are, since it is the custom for men to have successive wives, each leaving her child behind to be brought up by a series of stepmothers as she goes on to give birth to a child to her next husband. The situation is such that it is perfectly conceivable that a man could have sexual intercourse with an older woman without knowing that it is his mother. The men show not the slightest concern about this possibility. They say that normally they do not sleep with older women so it would not normally happen. When pressed they admit that sometimes a young lad will sleep with an older, more experienced woman and brag about it, but when asked if he would have more to brag about if the older woman proved to be his mother, the answer is "only if she were older"; in other words conceptually the prohibited category is age; biological maternity is insignificant.

"personal" names each individual carries, even the nicknames. In fact there is nothing that quite corresponds to our personal names which identify individuals from all other individuals. It is common throughout Africa for people sharing the same name, even a nickname, to believe that in some way they share identity and therefore have a mutual responsibility and can call upon each other in times of need. Family names of course define various group memberships and obligations at the smallest level of family, or at the larger levels of lineage, clan, or tribe. Thus each name defines specific social roles, and so a total name defines a total social personality. It might also be held that individual identity does not exist, only social identity, so functional is the name, and so highly integrative. This brings us back to the matter of security, for in his very names each individual carries an inbuilt social security system which he is expected to, can, and does manipulate to his advantage, just as he himself is manipulated. The security is real, not nominal, as any anthropologist who has been named and classified can verify, for the incorporation into community is real, but it is real only at the technological level where independence is impossible and therefore undesirable.

With the introduction of cash, which is easily stored (unlike food or land or people), individual security becomes a possibility, and modern Western technology makes it possible, especially in the urban context. And of course in the urban and cash economy context it becomes necessary. These factors, together with population increase, in Africa as elsewhere, are in effect necessitating the desocialization of human beings, isolating them into groups that are no longer social. But we have already developed an appropriately individualistic and isolationist system of kinship terminology and inculcate nonsocial, competitive values in our children. For many an urban African the old values still persist and provide a deep-seated area of conflict.

Areas of Possible Conflict and Built-In Mechanisms for Resolution

In the area of conflict and conflict resolution the African is again dramatically different, and it must be emphasized that even in the urban context today many of the old values and even many of the mechanisms still operate, so their proper comprehension is essential.

It may be said as a final generalization that each traditional African society recognizes the fundamental lines along which conflict is most likely to occur. Instead of avowing that such conflict is unnatural, it is accepted as natural and often elaborate institutions develop and make the conflict overt, sometimes by manifesting it in ritualized confrontation, or by ritual role reversal, or by mandatory ridicule. Thus awareness of the danger of conflict is never allowed to drop, the danger lines are constantly kept in mind, and opportunity is given for hostile feelings to be expressed (and thereby expelled) in socially acceptable ways. The major and most general lines so formalized include sex, age, residence (or "territory"), and kinship—*yet these are precisely the major principles of social organization.* They involve elements of the unknown, hence the greater possibility for conflict. A man can never know what it is to be a woman, a child cannot in his childhood know what it is to be old, and an elder in his old age cannot know what it *is* to be a child (only what it *was*); and it is almost universal that peoples living in different places (given the limitations of communications at this technological level) are suspect, as unknowns.

Thus society is divided vertically by kinship and cross-cut by the divisions of age which establish a system of loyalties that have nothing to do with kinship. Both of these are cross-cut by bonds of mutuality or otherwise of sex and residence. Thus each individual has alternatives at every step, and a whole set of different social obligations (and personalities) in and out of which he is constantly moving. This mobility affords him further mechanisms for the avoidance of conflict, by deliberately selecting one of his many roles that removes him from the arena, so to speak. Alternatively he may invoke one or another of these areas of conflict as a principle of social organization and call on his agemates, for instance, to support him in a dispute against kin.

In fact age might be said to constitute another form of "family" and its importance should not be minimized. In Table 5 a few generalized examples of "age families," known more formally as "age-set systems," are given to illustrate the extraordinary weight of importance and complexity surrounding sociality in traditional African societies, one of the very areas in which conflict is most likely to occur being turned to such highly integrative use. Each age level has its own role, thus removing ambivalence, just as the formal initiations or advancement rituals remove all ambivalence as to age status.

Table 5   Two Concepts of "Family" in Africa

---

1.   △ = ○

2.   △ = ○

3.   △ = ○

4.   △ = ○

A. <u>Bushman</u> hunters see the family as having four successive stages,
here illustrated. At stage three the son marries and goes to live with
his wife and hunt with her father's band. The daughter similarly brings
her groom into her band. With the birth of their children the son returns
with his family, and the daughter leaves to permanently join her husband's
band. The grandparents remain in their own territory throughout except
at stage one when, in turn, they would have been in the wife's territory
with her band.

B. <u>Ashanti</u> <u>abusua</u>, a typical matrilineal concept of "family" though
rules of residence vary. Frequently this becomes the residential unit
as the children reach puberty.

Dress and/or other means are used to make one's social status visible
so that again there is little room for ambivalence, and this expressiveness of social personality is a vital constituent of African society.

Conclusion

It is not surprising then that there is little that can be called law (as
supported by physical coercion), for there is little need for it in so

expressive a society where any deviance is not only instantly recognizable but is also so demonstrably dysfunctional. This does not mean that there is no concept of right or wrong, merely that the yardstick used for making such judgments is the social good, for only in sociality can the individual see his own survival. Thus actions are not classified as good or bad, only intent. Anyone may do a wrong thing; that may be unfortunate but not necessarily bad. In an African tribunal, then, the interest focuses not so much on the action, which is seldom in question, but rather on the social personality of the perpetrator of that action, and it is *that* which will determine his fate. Here beliefs such as witchcraft (which we again dismiss with such ignorant facility as superstition) play an important role in providing a means by which a man may be excused for a harmful action, rather like our "extenuating circumstances." For a man may claim that although he stole a chicken, he did not wish to do so, something forced him to do it, maybe witchcraft, or maybe he himself is a witch and does not know it. He is in either case not responsible for his actions and not culpable. But the case does not rest there. Investigation proceeds to see just what the causes of this behavior might be. It may involve a whole series of accusations and counteraccusations, and it may result in nobody or everybody being blamed; the important thing is that in such a proceeding everything is brought out into the open and made public, thus robbing it of much if not all of its potency.

A person who has once claimed the excuse of being a witch may not do so again, for once he admits to having this force within him he is under an obligation to control it by correct ritual behavior, and if he fails to do so he is either socially irresponsible (rather like someone with an infectious disease who continues to walk in public without having it cured) or else he is actively evil, a sorcerer, consciously working against the social good. What is in question is not the action but the personality of the actor, and the measure of judgment is the sociality of that personality.

The degree to which all of this is relevant in the modern urban situation is highly variable, even within any one urban situation, but there is no doubt that it *is* relevant in every African city, and most certainly highly relevant in the much more populous rural areas. It demands of any non-African desirous of participating in and assisting in the development of new African nations that he recognize fundamental differences not only in social organization and structure, but even in personality and in modes of thought and conceptual categories. We may never fully understand the African unless we ourselves become what we are trying to understand, just as one can never truly understand another religion unless one becomes a believer; but we can and must come as close as we can and at least understand the system.

Site Visits in Senegal: Experience of English-Speaking Groups

Elizabeth E. Irvine, M.A. (England) and
Jon Lange, M.D. (Norway)

Prior to the meeting of the International Study Group in Dakar, Professor Henri Collomb made arrangements for the participants to visit areas where they would have an opportunity to observe children in their families and families in their communities coping with some of the problems of living in a developing country. The reporters were asked to keep their practiced clinical eyes as much on the environment as on the people, and to gauge the type of fit between the two.

For the first series of visits the visitors were taken to La Casamance under the guidance of Professor Collomb, whose expertise on the interplay of African culture and African psychopathology is unrivaled. The interpreter was John Gomis, a young philosophy student living in Soukouta.

Witchcraft at Boutjoute

The first visit was to Boutjoute, inhabited by the Manjak people, who offered a stout resistance to the Portuguese in Portuguese Guinea and then immigrated to La Casamance. Here the local witch doctor was holding his clinic in the shelter between several trees.

Along with the witch doctor, who looked remote and at times almost out of touch, was his "manager" and an elderly woman helper. In front of them was an arrangement of sticks carrying drinking horns. On one side was a mound of bones and skulls of animals. In the background a number of women were preparing a cooking pot for the sacrificial pigs, calves, and hens. A great deal of negotiation preceded the actual ceremony, in which libations of wine were poured onto the sticks and passed around in the horns for people to drink.

One client was a young man in European dress with collar and tie who had successfully invoked magical aid to get him to France where he was now living as a house painter, so he had come to give thanks. Another three clients were involved in a business transaction and were hoping for a good omen. The ritual slaughter of the animals was crude beyond the tolerance of the visitors, hardly any of them having the stomach to watch the proceedings. Nevertheless, several young children were close spectators and viewed every event with interest. At no time did any of the young ones watching show any observable apprehension, fear, repulsion, or disgust. One wondered to what extent the urban children from Dakar would have shown the same neutral response.

The Marabout at Soukouta

At Soukouta the visitors were taken to the compound of the local Marabout or religious teacher. The Marabout came in from the fields, changed into smart blue dungarees, and agreed to demonstrate his craft. This was carried out in a special sacred hut in which animal skulls hung from the ceiling. He held a small strip of woven mat which could flap from left to right or right to left, the one meaning yes and the other no. He invoked the genie with prayers and offered to tell fortunes. Through the prayer mat, the genie answered several questions posed to him: Were the visitors all French? No. Were they only French and American? No. Should they continue their work? Yes. Were they all medical doctors? No. The answers were more or less right.

The Marabout then offered to treat any ailments that the visitors had, and it was pointed out that payment for treatment was based entirely on results. After this the Marabout entered an inner chamber where he conversed with the genie, whose replies were an audible series of sounds, somewhat like a crudely played trombone. Here again children were around but seemed more interested in the visitors and their reactions than in what was happening. After the ceremony the Marabout asked if anyone had a Polaroid camera so that he could have a picture of himself immediately.

The Therapeutic Village of Mawa

Mawa was founded 17 years before our visit by the father of the present leaders of the village. The adult males of the leading family were called cultivators and Marabouts, signifying that the village was both religious (Moslem) and agricultural. The founding father traveled widely in Africa studying traditional healing practices and herbal medicine. While traveling in this region, he had a vision telling him to settle here and treat the mentally ill. Every patient came with a relative and with an offering of poultry or animals. The therapy was guided by inspiration given to the therapist in a dream during the first night of the patient's stay in the village. The dream indicated which verse from the Koran was to be given to the patient for meditation. Later dreams were analyzed to find out from where the evil came, and it was thus tracked down to some individual who, in a spirit of anger, had wished the patient ill. In addition to the dream work, herbal medicines were used.

At the beginning most of the patients were very wild or aggressive, and they were restrained by a leg fastened through a hole in a lock. As soon as the patient was well enough not to run away, the restraint was removed, and he began to take part in the ordinary life and work of the village. Some patients settled down permanently in the village, even married into the village. These were said never to relapse. Of those who went back to their homes, some did relapse.

The children in the village appeared to take the psychotics pretty much for granted. Once again they seemed more interested in the visitors and their reactions than in the ravings of the clinical patients or in the crazy ramblings of the schizophrenics. They followed the visitors very trustingly and affectionately into the darkest huts where one or two catatonic patients lay in stupor with elderly women squatting beside them quietly, comfortably, and patiently. The Marabouts and the villagers could hardly understand the questions

posed to them by the visitors about the children. These were questions such as: Were they troubled by what they saw in their contact
with psychosis? Were they frightened by the aggressive or bizarre
behavior ? Did they talk about their encounters with the psychotics
to their parents or other adults? Did they ask questions about the
why and how of psychosis?

As far as the villagers were concerned, the children were just there
in the same way the dogs or goats were there, and it would be just
as stupid to inquire if the dogs or goats reacted to psychosis. On the
face of it this seemed to be true, since none of the visitors observed
any unusual reactions on the part of the children, all of whom
showed an avid curiosity in the visitors, touching them and holding
onto them during the visit. The psychotics were not a strange
phenomenon in the way that the visitors were.

The Village of Enampor

The people at Enampor were Diolas and agricultural. The visitors
were taken into one or two of the houses which were built with three
layers of thatched roof with the central layer sloping inward so that
the rain falling on this part drained and was collected in the middle
of the central room, which was used for living in, cooking in, and
washing in. On the periphery were separate bedrooms for each
family. The rooms were dark and cool in spite of the hot African
sun. The visitors were struck by the sense of physical intimacy, the
closeness of the members of the family to one another, the intermin-
gling of adults and children, and the complete lack of privacy. Even
on superficial observation, it seemed that the children felt safe and
secure in this setting and not at all apprehensive. This factor was
striking throughout the visits—the ease with which we were accepted
by the children and the digit contact that was made. Trivial little
gifts were highly appreciated. There were a few homemade toys
around, but in general the children improvised with the help of
nature in their play.

The next series of visits were planned to demonstrate the differences between traditional village life and the transitional type of
living that was growing on the outskirts of African cities to which
villagers came when emigrating from country to city.

The Center for Social Pediatrics

Pikine is a suburb of Dakar and formed part of a program of slum clearance. However, its population grew faster than the facilities so that very soon the former slum dwellers from Dakar began to turn Pikine into a slum. It was intended for a population of about 10,000, but the present population is somewhere in the region of 300,000. Consequently, all facilities are grossly inadequate. The water supply is from wells, and the sanitary arrangements do not cope with the demand, so that about one-third of the human excreta reaches the public thoroughfare. Unemployment is rife and the main sources of subsistence are begging and food distribution by the government and charitable organizations. The children are vendors, carriers, messengers, baby sitters, and beggars.

The center was sponsored and subsidized by UNICEF and supervised by a public health nurse with special competence in child care and parent education. There were no physicians, the staff being made up of nurses, midwives, and social workers, all of whom work in cooperation with the elders of each district in whose homes part of the training and teaching of mothers takes place. The staff members also make home visits and invite mothers who seem incompetent and unable to cope to the center for additional training in cooking, housekeeping, and infant care. The center also trains teenage girls for future motherhood, and medical students and nurses also receive part of their training here. The infant clinic, with no physicians, sees about 150 patients a day. Studies on kwashiorkor are being initiated to determine differences in intellectual development between an afflicted group and a matched control group. This research kindergarten is not yet open because of staff shortage.

The districts vary in their dedication to child health, but in one district working closely with the center, infant mortality has shown a marked decrease. The family houses were visited and compared with the village houses previously inspected. They seemed grossly overcrowded, with an unemployed father, a paternal grandmother, three wives, and sixteen children, all living in a small three-room house with no water and one squat toilet. The conditions seemed dismal, and there appeared to be very little hope that the children could rise above this sordid and limited existence.

The Fishing Village of Yoff

The visitors were taken next to the Laienne quarter under the
guidance of Dr. Tidiane Gueye. The Laienne is a very strict muslim
sect which forbids smoking, tom-tom playing, dancing, going to the
cinema, and so on. Their population is stable and relatively prosperous and most of the boys reach baccalaureate level. The main
occupation is fishing. The children in this quarter seemed to play
very little, and the sea is regarded as too liquid to bathe in. Very
few toys were in evidence, but ball games involved large numbers of
children.

As usual, African children generally suspend all activities to study
visitors. Drums were elaborated out of bowls and games with pebbles
seemed popular. No dolls were seen, but in their place were baby
siblings, whom little 7- and 8-year-olds carried about on their backs
and hips like their mothers did. Some of the children tried to beg.

Visit to Suburbia

A visit was paid to Sicap, which is a relatively prosperous suburb
that came into being about 1960. The houses had refrigerators, uphol-
stered chairs, pictures and ornaments, and family photographs. There
seemed to be a world of difference between the dark, unfurnished
village huts and these good-looking residences. The children were no
longer wandering around aimlessly engaging in any activity that
seemed to come their way. Here they appeared to have things to do
and a place to be.

As elsewhere in the world, the lives of these African children
roughly reflect the lives of parents and adults around them. The
most unsettled parents were in Pikine and there also we saw the most
unsettled children, and our guess would be that an appreciable
number of children in this slum society carried risk and would
contribute to the not too serious delinquency problem in this region.

Discussion

The site visits had the great advantage of introducing visitors to
Africa in all its variety. There was no other way in which one could

have obtained a feeling of the essential Africa than by going out into the bush and visiting the villages and settlements.

The group discussed the evidence of rivalries and hostilities in polygamous families such as they had observed in Pikine. But *Asuni* felt that this would be expected only in the towns where the families had less territory and wives were not able to have separate huts. If tensions were to occur in the villages, they were probably better regulated and minimized. From what we know about polygamous families elsewhere, tensions are probably never totally absent. *Lambo* said that polygamy was not as common as the visitors might have supposed and that multiple mothering did not depend on polygamy but on close links with aunts and grandmothers in the extended family.

The most intriguing question remained a relative mystery: What was the African child's conception of the world in which he lived? To what extent did he assimilate all the different elements and integrate them into a world picture? It was clear that the Africans we talked to were mystified by the questions we put to them. Clearly we had in mind the subtle and sophisticated internal psyche of the Western child with its high degree of self-consciousness. The African child, in contrast, was not regarded in individual terms as someone who was taking in a world of experience and transposing it into his own diosyncratic frame of reference. As a consequence, there seemed to be very little empathic activity going on between adult and child, the adult trying to view the child's experiences through the child's eyes. The visitors, many of whom were accustomed to working closely and therapeutically with children, found it difficult to feel their way to these children or to get any appreciation of the child's thoughts and feelings from the adults we encountered.

Site Visits in Senegal: Experience of French-Speaking Groups

Cyrille Koupernik, M.D. (France)

The French-speaking group shared with their English-speaking colleagues the same uncertainty as to the meaning of the different phenomena to which they were exposed. Part of the difficulty related to language, which diminished the amount of contact and communication with those who spoke a local language only. This meant that we were restricted to behavioristic observation without even knowing the meaning of the behavioral items that we were attempting to record and interpret. For example, we observed children making what seemed to us threatening gestures, but we were unable to say whether it represented aggressiveness or compliance to a culturally stereotyped mode of bargaining. Almost any type of inference seemed possible. For example, like the other group, we had witnessed the highly complicated transaction conducted by the witch doctor under the sacred tree. On one side were the clients who were seeking to prevent spirits from acting against their best business interests, and on the other side were the witch doctor and a "negotiator." We expected him to be deferential to the witch doctor, but on several occasions he actually seemed to insult him. The "negotiator" used some very cheap red wine, presumably to create the right atmosphere for the proceedings. At one time he tried to establish contact with the visitors by offering them some of this in a horn. All the visitors, medically alert to the presence of parasites, refused, and consequently limited their participation in the ceremony. We remained awkward and alienated, wondering how anthropologists overcame these civilized reactions for the purpose of blending with the natives.

There was possibly another estranging factor at work which was part of history. Some three centuries previously, our ancestors had enslaved theirs under brutal and degrading circumstances, and we were still carrying a burden of guilt related to this. After slavery came colonialism with its authoritarianism and paternalism. With this implicit background, it was almost impossible to establish a comfortable equalitarian relationship that would help to overcome the barriers of language and culture.

What is being said here is that we could not become anthropologists and Africanists in 48 hours. As psychiatrists, we were only able to interpret unusual behavior in terms of our diagnostic classifications without being able to look at it open-mindedly or freshly.

In the therapeutic village that we also visited a "diagnosis" was made based on the patient's dreams, which revealed whether one of his ancestors was dissatisfied with him in some way that would be apparent to the Marabout, who would then seek to negotiate an agreement between the two. This appeared to be a very important part of the general conception of mental illness in this part of Africa.

During the visit we were struck by the way in which the children of all ages confidently and trustfully held onto our fingers as if they simply wanted the contact. A number of questions arose out of these visits: What might be the consequences for a child immersed from his very early years in a world where concepts of magic were prevalent, especially since a 4- to 7-year old child is particularly prone, according to Piaget, to accept magic-phenoministic explanations of the world. With so much reinforcement of a developmental disposition, was it possible that the child would be "fixated" at this level and fail to develop logical thinking? Next, what could be the effect on the child's sense of individuality when he is made to feel a link horizontally in an extended family group and vertically in a long ancestral line that remains active. Then, to what extent can children be habituated to scenes of ritual cruelty and brutality without becoming insensitive to the same events in ordinary life? And, finally, would one expect the children in daily contact with serious mental disorder, as in the therapeutic village, and with surrounding adults rendered helpless by psychosis, to be affected by the process? In answer to the last two questions, it appeared as if the children accepted the unusual with the same amount of unconcern as they accepted the usual. For them, unlike the adult visitors, it was all part of the commonplace realities of their world.

Two different setups of rural maternal services were observed. The first was staffed by a registered nurse, a midwife, and a hygienist with two years of training; the second was run by women in the community who had born children themselves and helped in the childbirth of others. These lay practitioners are given a short course in asepsis and take part in uncomplicated deliveries. As always in Africa, the patient is rarely neglected by the family and usually has a relative staying and caring for her nonmedical needs. The pregnant mothers were brought to the center in carts, often from distant areas. Tetanus of the newborns was rampant under the more or less primitive conditions, and the authorities had not the means for vaccination or immunization. The local group initiated their own preventive measures by building segregated compounds with clean huts and beds above the level of the ground, and, as a result, there has been no tetanus in the past year. The women prefer to be delivered by the midwife and seem embarassed by the idea of male obstetricians.

Risk is a chain event in Africa. As infant mortality is reduced and preventive pediatrics conserves the child population, starvation, which is always in the offing, will become a hideous reality, and inevitably the oldest generation will be allowed to die.

Discussion

In the discussion of the site visits, *Collomb* called attention to the intermediaries in the group, whom he termed "African-Europeanists," and described them from the African standpoint as rather "queer birds" who both blended and yet stood out from the local culture, whether they spoke the native language or not. They were part of the local scene and belonged to it, and they tried to practice their art within a local frame of reference as far as possible.

The International Study Group had behaved as all Euro-Americans did; they brought their knowledge, their training, their Western sophistication and inevitably made the African an object of observation. They had looked from the outside, being unable to feel the situation from the inside, and as far as their very clever eyes and minds could take them, they had made valid observations to be taken away with them; these were export ideas rather than something that could be applied locally. *Sanokho* said that he too had listened carefully to the narration of the brief African odyssey. He thought that the refusal of the wine by the visitors at the witch doctor's ceremony may have represented more than the fear of contamination. There was probably some deep reluctance to being drawn into the darker side of the African continent. To the African, on the other hand, the visitors were travelers and guests, and it was traditional to extend such hospitality and share with these tired, hot, and uncomfortable strangers. It was an attempt to understand something different by stressing the common human need.

From the beginning of the long history of the relationship, the white man has not known how to address the African, since he was not quite human and not quite animal. We are now arriving slowly at the end of this period. Today the Euro-American realizes that he cannot speak in the same old harsh, paternalistic manner, and so he softens his tone, but the message is still the same. We may now belong to the same family, but the African is the child. This means that even for visitors as for weekend anthropologists, there was a risk in the relation, and some Africans would be more vulnerable to its nuances than others. *Sanokho* added that the urbanized and Europeanized African often experienced the same difficulty when dealing with the traditional and rural African, and it had been his experience that the young from both Western and African cultures dealt more naturally with the situation since their young eyes were open to the African reality.

Stievenarb agreed that there were these differences of attitude. In the unusual situations to which the visitors had been exposed, she could detect on the part of the Africans a fear of intrusion. One complex problem is that the Africans were brought up to deal with aggressiveness in quite a different way from the non-Africans. *Moussou* also warned against drawing conclusions from a two-day visit. The culture of African children was obviously different from the culture of African adults, and the culture of the literate African from the culture of the illiterate African. These conditions existed in the United States, and it was therefore unwise to generalize because of them. He tended to believe that there is such a thing as the

"African mind," which is radically different from the European and American mind, but it is difficult to define in its essence.

Thebaugh emphasized that in a rapidly changing society both parents and children are at risk, and, in fact, the family as a whole is. It was not feasible to look for solutions on an individual level, since the risks were global—the whole developing society was at risk. He also disagreed with the visitors who repeatedly drew attention to the absence of toys. It was a mistake to think that because the children had no toys, they did not play. There were very few toys on the continent, but the children did play and did invent their own play material and play items in training for their future roles, as did children elsewhere. *Thebaugh* hoped the visitors would appreciate that this somewhat massive intrusion of foreigners into a traditional milieu inevitably created disturbances which, in turn, modified the behavior of the group. This further limited the conclusions one could draw.

The Vulnerable African Child

T. Adeoye Lambo, M.D. (Nigeria)

Total Environmental Influence on the Development of the African Child

For the purpose of identifying the vulnerable child and the total influences that impinge on development, I shall focus attention on the mother-child relationship and other object relationships in major cultures of Africa. In doing so, I will be drawing on the findings of our work in Nigeria and other parts of Africa dealing with the following areas:

"Viability" of mother-child relation in terms of mutual tempos, needs, resources, gratification, and so on.

Balance of autonomy and support offered by mother from birth.

Mother's handling of basic infancy needs for contact, stimuli, protection, feeding, cleaning, activity.

Pleasure in mother-child relation.

Communication at nonverbal and verbal levels.

Mother's resources.

Impact on the mother-child relation of changes within the mother at different stages, and of changes in drives and ego-development of the child, especially the following: increasing overt aggression and activity with the development of motor skills and drives; loss of intimacy and libidinal gratification from the child with

latency and departure to school; hostility and rivalry emerging
with the birth of new siblings.
Impact on mother and other members of the family of changes in
the child.
Selective and changing patterns of identification in the child.
Interaction of each of the tendencies of the infant suggested
under constitution and equipment (above) with mother's
capacities, needs, limits, goods, problems.

The areas of study encompass such factors as protection from, and
strength of, stimulation and opportunity for sensory, motor, and
integrative experience in the environment. Consistency of relationships and communication with others, empathy, identification with
adults, aspects of child-rearing which are related to emotional security
and optimal mental development, expression of drives, and other
aspects of intimate relationships have also been examined.

It should be realized that even the most careful description of the
data of observation and the most refined method of collecting,
classifying, and correlating these data cannot identify and circumscribe the feeling of the mother. The feeling has to be inferred from
behavior differences toward the child.

In most African cultures the polygamous family, which is patri-
archal and authoritarian, is traditionally a very strong social institution, and to this day there are still a number of positive indications of
its vitality and social value. This powerful cultural institution at
successive stages of the development of the child stimulates his
empathic response, organizes his focus of attention, directing him to
persons, operations, myths, and resources, and regulates his share of
the available values according to the way he responds.

It should be mentioned at the outset that there is a wide diversity
between African cultures and therefore it is untenable to categorize
African personalities into one common mold. The child-rearing
practices vary considerably and if they were to occur consistently in
most African cultures, many factors within these cultures might well
differentially modify the effects. In spite of the basic differences
between major African cultures, there are important areas of
similarity, such as the structure and function of the extended family,
the whole pattern of emotional relations and attitudes toward the

child (breast feeding, toilet training, display of affection, sexual behavior, etc.) and his socialization and role expectation.

Economic and social life of most of the African societies are changing most rapidly and Lambo [1] in his "Concept and Practice of Mental Health in African Cultures" wrote: "In Africa today, scarcely a year passes in which the social conditions of life, the mode of conduct, the very habits and amusements, are not subtly and yet surely altered. . . . We stand bewildered at the shattering of what we had considered the most firmly established assumptions concerning the African family structure." In many urban centers and towns undergoing rapid socioeconomic change, the pattern of mother-child relationships is neither traditional nor Western and cannot be clearly identified; it is, in fact, transitional. This flux may constitute one potential area of vulnerability. In spite of these demonstrable changes the remnants of traditional behavior are manifestly involved in shaping the pattern and social life of the child.

Social Attitudes toward the Child

In most African cultures a child brings the parents and child into a kind of interaction that will itself develop emotionally charged and effective living. It is our observation that the dynamics of growth and normal interactions with the social environment are particularly stimulated in infancy. The most significant observation at this stage is that experiences of frustration are cut down to a minimum and consequently a deep sense of security is inculcated in the infant.

It should be mentioned that our studies covered the influence of the mother's health and attitudes during pregnancy upon her subsequent relationship with the child, in order to investigate the gene-environmental interaction model, especially the "early-neglect" model [2]. We have discovered a relationship between the intensity of her feelings during pregnancy, due to adequate psychological methods of preparation of mothers in these cultures, and her behavior and general maternal feelings subsequently. The subsequent character of the mother's relationship with the child is significantly influenced in these cultures by her attitudes during pregnancy, attitudes which in turn are influenced by the social values and attitudes of the society.

The newborn infant, whose every need is anticipated and fulfilled by a confident mother before he is aware of needing anything, experiences an unbroken state of satisfaction without effort, such as doubtless exists in intrauterine life. He is born into a warm, affectionate, and welcoming culture. During the first few weeks of life the degree of motor activity, the kind of perceptive functions, and the postural capacity of the neonate are optimal and become much more enhanced in subsequent months as human objects impinge certain influences on the child. In the early months he is inseparable from his mother, who feeds him at the slightest whimper, and he enjoys all the emotional security of an extended family, including grandmothers who are notorious coddlers of children.

The child enjoys varying degrees of comfort and security of reinforcing pressure. All these attentions are obligatory, which ensures their continuity and dependability. There is considerable maternal feeling, and in many situations in which many non-African mothers would give evidence of annoyance, impatience, or frustration, those of the African culture manifest supreme control of negatively charged feelings. The mother's sensitivity with regard to the needs of her child, her consistent pattern of behavior and feelings toward the child, and her freedom from anxiety are the direct results of the social and psychological attitudes toward having a child within this culture and the fact that she is usually surrounded and supported by the extended family.

The variation of patterns of maternal behavior under comparable conditions is consistently negligible; maternal behavior patterns are arranged along an ascending line of positive feelings: words (songs), smiles, laughter, cuddling, patting, and stroking. When all the patterns of maternal response to the infant are critically analyzed, it will be found that the effect of this feeling is to sustain the work involved in the care of the infant, intensify the relational behavior in terms of interest and affection, and inhibit any potentially harmful impulse. For example, the work involved in breast feeding can be measured in terms of persistency or continuity, which is also a measure of devotion to the task.

Indigenous custom prescribes breast feeding for an almost indefinite period of time. The mother's supreme interest in the infant is evidence of her relatedness: she is constantly aware of him

regardless of distractions that may arise from boredom, states of
fatigue, or painful or pleasurable body sensations. The infant sleeps
with his mother until about the age of 3 years when he is transferred
to the grandparents or his elder brothers and sisters. This satisfies
the feeling of communion with others and enhances his relatedness
need.

Toilet training is lax and flexible. Lambo [3] commenting on the
child-rearing pattern of the Yoruba tribe of Nigeria observes: "In
fact there is no training at all. The child can evacuate his bowels
under any conditions and this act is usually met by an expression of
delight by the mother or the person caring for him." But the child
generally has acquired effective control by the time he can walk
steadily.

The culture has a built-in system of regard for carrying out this
culturally prescribed sense of devotion and obligation. Kenyatta [4]
says: "When a woman reaches the stage of motherhood she is highly
respected, not only by her children, but by all members of the
community. Her name becomes sacred and she is addressed by her
neighbors and their children as 'mother of so-and-so.' This certainly is
a worthy reward for her reliable presence and positive response."

The function of feeling of maternal behavior thus may be regarded
as a powerful reinforcing agent, strengthening and intensifying
every component in the mother-infant relationship in a positive way.
The direct participation of the grandmothers, aunts, and older
children tends to increase those maternal activities which ensure that
the validity of the child has the highest priority. Thus maternal,
social, and emotional responses within the home are oriented toward
the child. The infant enjoys the warmth of the mother's body and
the closeness of her presence. He is in physical contact all the time—
day and night—with either the mother or the grandmother.

Emotional privation is a clinical term which describes in a specific
sense a lack, or impairment, of the affectional phase, of emotional
warmth, in the mother-child relationship. In clinical work in Africa,
this condition has not been recognized under normal circumstances.
On the other hand, we have found that early childhood experiences
are more easily reactivated in Nigerians than in Europeans. There
is also an overvaluation of childhood memories. This may be due to
the fact that most African children undergo a more prolonged

infancy period of nutritive and emotional dependency. In this respect I find that in many African cultures children are neither actively encouraged to grow up nor discouraged from it. This passive attitude toward the child may also be examined as a potential source of "vulnerability."

Knapen [5] writing on the child-rearing practices among the Bacongo society quoted one of her informants: "We do not insist that a child should grow up; we wait until, according to the order of nature itself, the child arrives at conduct normal for its age." However, in Nigeria and in other African societies a great deal of encouragement is given to get the child to walk and to dance.

Many observers outside the culture have thought that these factors largely contribute to a form of "delayed maturity" of the African child. Maturation, however, has been said not to be the attainment of final state, but rather a process of meeting life's demands and utilizing the available opportunities. In fact, at a comparatively early age in later childhood, African children show profound social insight, confidence, and a remarkable ability to play complicated social roles. Carothers [6] observes: "Childhood, in African theory, is a period of complete irresponsibility; and offenses committed by them at this age are commuted by the parents. Yet, by European standards, African children are highly responsible. Indeed they may often be seen, by the age of 10 years or so, sitting with their elders and even taking part in the conversation with confidence and effect."

Early Childhood

Biesheuvel [7] observed in his study of cultural influences on personality development among the Southern Bantu group: "The African infant lives in a state of virtual symbiosis with its mother during the first eighteen months of life, a state of blissful security when all its needs are completely and promptly met. *There is, however, a sharp discontinuity or contrast between infancy and early childhood experiences. On weaning, there is a marked change in maternal attitude,* the child begins to associate more with his elder siblings and grandparents. There is no feeling of rejection, following on a period of apparent indulgence, because by now the child has learnt to accept *substitutes* early. Indeed overt rejection is minimized by the voluntary attentions of the maternal grandmother or a mother's sister." Does the concept and practice of "substitution" lead to difficulties? This question remains to be answered. Does it have a temporary or lasting effect on the perceptual—affective—cognitive apparatus? Does it simply provoke anxiety?

Identity

At this point I should like to describe the process of identity development in many African cultures. Identification is a process which involves the adoption of values and attitudes that "significantly influence how the individual thinks of himself and how he wants to be seen by others." It is an anchorage of the self in the social matrix. The child-parent identification has been studied extensively and we know that the growing child passes through a number of phases. A useful and positive comment can be taken from the work of Kluckhorn and Murray that every individual, concurrently, is like all other men, some other men, and no other man.

Kenyatta [8] writing on the Gikuyu child observes: "First and foremost he is several people's relative and several people's contemporary." This makes illegitimacy almost an unknown social condition in Africa, and children who are born out of marriage still have social recognition. Laubscher [9] observes that they belong "to some male, either the man who procreated them or the mother's father."

The infant and toddler exist in a phase of differentiating themselves from the environment, but with increasing maturation of systems of perception and of emotional development, a phase of psychological identification with parents tends to appear. In societies with nuclear families and with "one-to-one" confrontation, the process is less complicated. In most African cultures, with their extended families, the concepts of "multiple confrontation" and "selective identification" apply.

The traditional polygamous family is a very large one, consisting of a husband, several wives, children, the grandparents, the uncles, aunts, and many cousins who may or may not live together. Invariably they live close to one another and the paternal grandfather is the sole authority in the home. If he lives away from the other families it is the "social duty" of the father to send the children to live with the grandparents for almost an indefinite period of life, but this in fact does not happen since in most cases the entire extended family lives together.

As a result of the extended family structure and function, the child has many fathers (i.e., grandfather and uncles) who have greater authority and influence over him in every way than his biological father has. In this social context, the psychological process of identification becomes diffuse, less rigid and more flexible, and this may be responsible for the less rigid personality (and behavior) structure of the African with greater flexibility in his social and interpersonal relations. The establishment of these social ties tends to enhance the sense of consciousness of self. Again one may raise a pertinent question here: Can the ego become vulnerable when presented with multiple object relationships at the same time and a wide variation and diversification of the external world?

As growth proceeds, the process of identification will become increasingly abstract and will pertain more to the system of values and style of life of the family and the society than to the parents, and this sociopsychological process will also serve to define more sharply the sociocultural contents of the personality of the individual.

Since the family values are a microcosm of the kinship system value, the development of identification, abstraction of social values, and modification of behavior along community lines become much easier, thus facilitating the development of group membership and group loyalties very early. Thus a child at an early age is able to enter the closed value system.

Possibly due to the importance of maintaining satisfactory social relationship and communication, African children as a whole learn quickly to speak their various complicated languages with fluency and accuracy. I have observed that in Nigerian children verbal ability is found to develop early, and to be markedly profound with ideational and conceptual precision. Also, the dreams of African children show signs of well-defined positive adaptation in relation to their culture at a very early age. As a child grows older in some of these cultures, he develops a true awareness of the intrinsic value of his true emotional need—that of attachment to other human beings.

Through his peers—many of whom are his cousins and relatives in the extended family and kinship system—the child comes in contact with various attitudes toward himself and to many things that are to be valued or rejected. The home, that is, the mother and/or the grandmother, continues to be the major source of emotional satisfaction, for love and affection.

The process of "sharing" her responsibility to care for the child with her mother, aunt, and immediate female relatives enables the young mother to accept the separation or lack of dependence which ensues later as the child moves into a bigger social orbit. There is therefore no feeling of loss on her part and she does not in any way encourage a continuation of dependent relationship. It must also be mentioned that the participation of the maternal grandmother in the mother-child relationship may encourage excessive permissiveness and protectiveness.

It should be mentioned in passing that the value of a male child is rated higher than that of a female child in many of the African cultures which are patrilineal. Since the end-result of all marriage in traditional African culture is procreation, the perpetuation of the kinship is the sole motive. According to Jomo Kenyatta [8]: "If a man dies without a male child, his family group comes to an end. This is one thing that the Gikuyu people fear dreadfully, and it can be said to be one of the factors behind the polygamous system of marriage."

Physical Contact in the Mother-Child Relationship as Prescribed by the Culture (Psychosensory and Psychomotor Development)

I have already mentioned the consistently patterned physical contact in the mother-child relationship in many African cultures. In the early months, and sometimes up to the age of 15 months, the child is inseparable from his mother, who carries him on her back and feeds him at the slightest whimper. Occasionally he is put gently down to sleep but more often he sleeps on his mother's, grandmother's, or older sister's back. From time to time he is held by some other member of the family. The child becomes easily accustomed to these sorties into strange arms with varying degrees of "contact-comfort," security, and reinforcing pressure.

Because most adults love children of any description, they like to hold them, caress them, fondle, rock, and talk to them and generally play with them, and consequently as the infant grows older he is given to more adults and older children for longer periods of time to be fondled and enjoyed. Apart from meeting the physical needs of the child all the expressions of tender feelings—fondling, caressing, singing, and so on—have a deep significance. They convey the feeling that a child is valued, approved of, and wanted, and that he is the object of love, and these feelings are communicated to the very young.

Harlow's studies [10] on the infant-maternal relationship have produced evidence that the physical contact of the infant with a mother whose "skin" is comforting to him adds to "the effects of postural support and nursing in contributing to the significance mother assumes for the child." Harlow writes:

> We were not surprised to discover that contact-comfort was an important basic affectional or love variable, but we did not expect it to overshadow so completely the variable of nursing: indeed, the disparity is so great as to suggest that the primary function of nursing as an affectional variable is that of insuring frequent and intimate body contact of the infant with the mother.

Ribble [11] points out that much of the cohesiveness of a child's personality depends on emotional attachment to the mother and that three types of sensory experience—tactile, kinesthetic, and auditory—contribute primarily to its formation.

Carothers [6] observes that in respect to emotional satisfaction, sensory stimulation, and stable mother-child relationship, therefore, "the African infant's experience seems to be ideal. His needs are better catered for than usually obtained in Western Europe, and it would seem that there is much to be said for adopting African practice in dealing with babies for the 'first few months' of life."

Thus the child in many African cultures comes to recognize love as close and intimate bodily contact, and he derives security from his contact. In addition, all these activities may be correlated with normal maturation changes in the central nervous system. In many gatherings in the villages and towns children are often seen sitting or standing between the legs of a kinswoman or kinsman. In many African children's hospitals, the most remarkable, or one of the most striking features, is the obvious anticipation of these children to touch or hold hands with strangers or visitors. They stand up in the cots, if they can, and show "anticipatory reaching out" by stretching out their hands and initiating response. This may show that the child is not merely a recipient but has become an "active solicitor of affection and active avoider of those who cause unpleasantness."

It is relevant to quote the findings of a controlled study which was conducted in the late 1950s by the Medical Research Council in Uganda, Africa. The study was on the state of development of newborn African children. In the earlier study, Dr. Marcelle Geber [12] examined 107 newborn African children who were considered to be normal at birth by the technique evolved by André Thomas in European children. She concluded as follows:

There seemed to be no doubt that these African children had been born at a more advanced stage of development, judged by the method used, than the normal European child. The results of the examination were so consistent, and the degree of advance was so great, that there was little room for uncertainty. Much of the activity corresponded to an age of 4-6 weeks. Some were even more precocious: for example, the raising of the chin and the scratching of the fingers on the table, when the children were placed on their bellies, might be expected at 6-8 weeks, and so might the maintenance of the head in the mid-position when they were on their backs.

We do not intend at this stage to advance theories or facts in attempted explanation, but it is clear to us that the state of birth is consistent with some clinical observations: that the African child sucks vigorously at the breast almost from the first hour, and that he passes the milestones of development at a very early age. It is consistent also with the findings of psychomotor precocity in the earliest years to which we have already alluded. As we have said elsewhere (Geber, 1956) an extensive investigation of all facets of the development of the African child is planned, and will include twins, children born by Caesarean section, others whose birth has been associated with trauma, and others born before term. The last-named should be especially interesting; it is well recognized that African children whose weight at birth would by ordinary standards cause them to be classed as "premature" are often sturdy and active and can be reared without the special care that has to be lavished on European children of the same weight.

In her second study [13], also of psychomotor development of the African child, Geber examined the psychomotor development of 131 African children aged from 6 months to 6 years, measured by Gesell tests. She observed:

The children came from families of various social levels, from several different tribes. There were four groups: children from Kampala and its suburbs who had come to Mulago hospital for the treatment of minor ailments, children of students of theology living together in a village near the town, children of agricultural workers unused to contacts with many Europeans, and children who had taken part in a social-psychological study in villages near Kampala. The last groups were seen in their homes. The conditions of the examination varied from one group to the other, but the tests were all carried out by the author and the technique used was always the same. The Gesell tests were utilized not only to define the state of development but also for the study of behavior.

The results showed that the young African child was precocious in development when compared with European or American children of the same age. The precocity was usually lost in the third year and after that time the African children were usually retarded.

The advance was found to be particularly marked in the first months. The head was raised at a very early age; sitting and standing were also early. Manual development was remarkable for its precision and dexterity. The test objects, although completely new to nearly all the children—toys and objects that might have an educational value being rare in the homes—were manipulated and used with pleasure. The children showed a very lively interest, and their adaptivity was greatly superior to that corresponding to their age. Language was also highly developed, as much in expression as in comprehension. Even the very young children were interested by the examiner and attempted to communicate with her. Personal-social reactions were surprisingly good. Behaviour in front of the mirror was remarkable: from 6 weeks onwards, the child smiled at his image.

Geber finally observed that "the remarkably dynamic behavior, and the sociability of the very young children was in strong contrast with the quietness and timidity of the older children." She concluded.

The stages of development, and the alterations in behaviour, are discussed in relation to the intimate and almost uninterrupted contact that the young African child has with its mother, and to the abrupt breaking of that contact at the time of weaning. The better development of the children of the theological students, who attended a nursery school in their villages, makes it necessary to consider the possible importance of such schools in the African setting. The excellent memory for the spoken word and the manual ability that are so notable in the African, suggest the need for special educational methods enabling these qualities to be utilised to the best advantage. On the other hand, genetic factors cannot be neglected.

Many observers have commented on the effect on personality of the sharp contrast between early and later childhood experiences and have incriminated this fact as the etiological factor for the prevalence of overt anxiety in Africans. Thus some sweeping generalizations have been made, far beyond the scope of observed clinical facts, on the so-called traumatic weaning.

Growth-Relation to Stimulus and Need

The responses or activities which enter play during this time are extraordinarily complex and their interrelations are manifold, but they are themselves ruled, in a way which still remains resistant to formal interpretations, by what seem to be purely elementary cultural factors.

It is generally agreed that mental growth takes place in response to a stimulus, but it does not seem to be generally recognized that it also takes place in response to a need. It is the need of the moment that determines whether the stimulus will be accepted or not; it is the need of the moment that determines the direction, and to some extent the intensity, of all mental growth.

All along the line, the African child would seem to be exposed to a variety of experiences and situations. A loose analogy may be seen here in the field of immunology: the African child in the process of development is exposed in carefully graduated doses to potentially stressful, disease-producing stimuli, and as a result the child develops such a degree of immunity that its vulnerability to illness, especially severe neuroses, is reduced. Psychotic regression, grief reaction, and depression are examples of psychopathological phenomena that are markedly modified in the African.

Child Rearing in an Urban African Community

In many societies generally and in contemporary Africa particularly, men, as a result of their occupational roles and community participation, are more involved in extrafamilial institutions and are more exposed to influences that generate change. In this way the fathers are likely to be important mediators of change.

Several studies have been conducted to determine the pattern of mother-child relationship within an urban context in contemporary Africa. The traditional pattern, as described above, has altered considerably. In many urban centers today, the care of the child is in the hands of housemaids, many of whom are themselves under stress of transition, inadequately prepared, and emotionally immature. Many mothers in urban centers go out to work, have inadequate housing facilities, maintain tenuous or peripheral social relationships with the neighborhood. Most of the attention given to the child by the mother is physical and limited. There is very little personal relationship or emotional tie, with much more restricted physical contacts. The mother is often tired and exhausted after a long day and therefore prone to emotional difficulties herself. The social orbit of the child is restricted and he is denied access to "multiple mothering" and mother substitutes. Because of frequent change of house-servants, relationships tend to be inconsistent and not dependable.

In a detailed study of disorganized and disintegrating communities on the outskirts of Kinshasa in 1965, certain clinical observations were made about child development. The sociogenic and psychogenic features of this periurban environment were as follows:

1. Mental and emotional factors in the development of the child were not given full play—there was no consistency of relation-ships, there was an impaired balance of acting out, mastery, and love as well as the defective nature of other aspects of child rearing related to emotional security, optimal mental development, and expression of drives.
2. Stimulation and opportunity for sensory, motor, and integrative experience in the environment were considerably reduced.
3. Communication, empathy, and identification with adults were not normally fostered because of the disorganization of the family and the group, for example, through loosening of authority (children without fathers).
4. Management of fear and anxiety in their children was handled badly.
5. Expression of affection, sexual interest, and other aspects of intimate relationship was minimal, if not absent.
6. There was lack of support for coping with typical stresses in the early years.

It was reported by pediatricians that there was a high incidence of babies that were born "weak," poorly motivated, ineffective feeders; moreover, initial adjustment crisis between the mother and the infant was much more likely.

The dilemma with which we are now faced in Africa, as a result of rapid social change, is that we are moving toward a type of human development which is incompatible with human growth. In the main, social groups, in spite of fissions and cleavages, are held together by means appropriate to traditional societies. That is to say, they depend on an emotional identification and involvement, personal uncon-scious needs being expressed in the structure concerned, for example, with types of authority and traditions of child care.

In conclusion, one is tempted to state that the traditional pattern of child rearing in most parts of Africa is concerned with forestalling emotional disorders, with building specific ego functions, and it is also directed at reducing the vulnerability of the ego to specific types of psychological situations. The object is to ensure that the child's primary experiences with common affect-laden interpersonal issues, such as trust, dependence, autonomy, separation, strangeness, and cooperative play, be mastery experiences rather than disorganizing failures.

However, in the cities and periurban areas, there is strong evidence of high incidence of moderate to severe psychopathology among African children due to typical socioeconomic stresses in the early years, including interuterine, perinatal, and postnatal environmental factors, such as a history of birth and pregnancy defects. Typical stresses in the early years have also been found to include such factors as the following: high-temperature illnesses; sequelae of diseases; hemoglobinopathies (genotype); nutritional deficit; sudden separation from the mother; severe handling, including force feeding, rough bathing, and discipline for crying.

These and other factors tend to diminish the child's capacity and psychic resources for genuine emotional involvement and interaction with, and mastery of, the new developmental issues. We need to develop more refined knowledge of the early phases of personality growth, critically reexamine some of our present concepts and techniques to enable us to systematically apply principles of preventive action. At the moment, I believe that we continue to miss early signs of identifiable disorders.

Hartman, Kris, and Loewenstein's contributions have provided us with a bridge between the clinical data of psychoanalysis and observation from a critical body of data from the behavioral sciences. They emphasize concepts that describe developmental changes not directly tied to shifts in drive intensity of the ego but that may result from a changing social environment.

References

1. Lambo, T. A. Characteristic features of the psychology of the Nigerian. *West Afr. Med. J.*, 9 (3) (1960), 95–104.
2. Garmezy, N. Models of etiology for the study of children who are at risk for schizophrenia, in *Life History Research in Psychopathology*, Vol. 11, M. Roff, L. Robins, and M. M. Pollack, Eds. University of Minnesota Press, Minneapolis, 1972.

3. Lambo, T. A. Growth of African children (psychological aspects). *Conf. Rep. First Pan-African Psychiatric Conf. Abeokuta.* Government Printer, Western Nigeria, 1961, pp. 60–64.
4. Kenyatta, J. *Jomo Kenyatta: Towards Truth About "The Light of Kenya".* (George Delf) Doubleday, Garden City, N.Y., 1961.
5. Knapen, M. Th. Some results of an inquiry into the influence of child training practices on the development of personality in Abacongo society (Belgian Congo). *J. of Soc. Psychol.*, 47 (1958), 223–229.
6. Carothers, J. C. *The African Mind in Health and Disease.* World Health Organization, Geneva, 1953.
7. Biesheuvel, S. *Race, Culture and Personality* (The Hoernle Memorial Lecture). South African Institute of Race Relations, Johannesburg, 1959.
8. Kenyatta, J. *Facing Mount Kenya; the Tribal Life of the Gikuyu.* Secker and Warburg, London, 1953.
9. Laubscher, B. J. F. *Sex, Custom and Psychopathology, A Study of South African Pagan Natives.* G. Routledge, London, 1937.
10. Harlow, H. F. The nature of love. *Am. Psychol.*, 13 (1958), 673–685.
11. Ribble, M. A. *Personality and the Behaviour Disorders.* Vol. 11, J. McV. Hunt, Ed. New York, 1944, p. 21.
12. Geber, M. The Psycho-motor development of African children in the first year and the influence of maternal behaviour, *J. Soc. Psychol.*, 47 (1958), 185.
13. Geber, M. Motor development of Baganda children from birth to six years. *Schweiz. Z. Psychol. Anwend.*, 20 (4) (1961), 345–357.

Discussion

Reginald S. Lourie, M.D., Med., Sc.D.

When combining our site visits with Dr. Lambo's most comprehensive and knowledgeable survey of the positive and negative influences on the African child in a changing environment, I was most impressed by the intensity of the closeness of the mother and the baby on her back. She has become so aware of the meaning of the baby's every move, that she knows which movement means that she should remove him from his carrying scarf and let him void. Even more impressive is that when that baby is turned over to be carried on his 10-year-old sister's back, she too, I observed, is tuned-in on the young child's movements and removes him in the same way. I found myself wishing that there could be a similar kind of "imprinting" this type of sensitivity and closeness in our young girls in the Western world as part of a preparation for motherhood. Also from this point of these observations, I disagree with our African colleagues that these children are not "toilet trained." I also can think of no better way for a baby to develop a sense of trust.

Dr. Lambo's important points on patterns of vulnerability and flexibility lend themselves to being discussed together because they are so closely related. It would be useful to look at them in light of the newer information from child development research. In particular our studies of the synthetic functions indicate that underlying flexibility is the constitutionally based reaction to stress. About 25 percent of individuals tend to disorganization in one degree or another in the presence of stress in contrast to the 30 percent at the opposite extreme who do better under stress. Those who disorganize are at risk as to flexibility unless we recognize this vulnerability and help with the development of better coping methods and defenses.

As Dr. Lambo spoke of trust, flexibility is important here too. Too great trust can lead to the child being hurt as he is introduced into a more complicated environment. With flexibility it could lead to the child's becoming an optimist but under other circumstances might the child become a pessimist?

The culture that helps the development of nonaggression does not always prepare the child to be competitive when he comes from the rural to the urban areas. Similarly, when his value systems and models do not prepare him to be able to deal with a society that functions on more than one standard, he can be vulnerable. In the urban society one must learn to function on a double standard, triple standard, and even complicated systems.

The implications of this presentation are a challenge to the commonly accepted stages of psychosexual development. We hear that African children are reared in patterns that do not allow separation anxieties to develop, as well as bypassing negativism, castration anxiety, and oedipal stages. Are the "standard" stages expected in personality development applicable only to the Western world?

Another important question we must ask ourselves here is whether neurosis and severe psychosis are the costs of more advanced and complicated social and cultural systems.

In the best of all worlds I wish we could merge the early child-rearing patterns we heard about here with the methods that are necessary to prepare children for rapidly changing systems in which they are expected to function productively and happily.

Our thanks go to Dr. Lambo for providing us broad strokes with the scientific agenda of our meeting.

Theodore B. Cohen, M.D. (U.S.A.)

I have been most interested in our African colleague's observations
and impressions. It seems inevitable that many of the effects of rapid
cultural change which have been observed world-wide would also be
present in Africa. I certainly agree with Dr. Lambo that "this flux
may constitute one area of vulnerability." When the structure of
traditions and culture is disrupted, we expect to observe psychic stress
and symptom formation because egos have been deprived of the
defensive use of stability to ward off both internal and external
threats. When a large project of small-unit homes was developed in
Ivory Coast, studies indicated that the resultant loss of tribal and
extended family psychic structure caused an increase in family
breakup and mental illness.

I would like to raise some questions, from the point of view of
an interested outside observer, about the effects of some of the more
traditional, less changed, African patterns of child rearing which
Dr. Lambo describes.

He says that "most African children undergo a more prolonged
infancy period of nutritive and emotional dependency." The mother-
child symbiosis is ended with sudden weaning and multiple parental
substitutes. In American society excessive infant gratification often
results in orally fixated, omnipotent children. Unless there is object
constancy with true resolution of the separation-individuation
process, the child may develop a borderline personality, remain
immature, and tend to act out. Does the abundance of gratification in
traditional African upbringing lead to overoptimism, stimulate
primary process thinking, and result in failures in sublimation? Does
the failure to have adequate limits affect the reality principle and
increase a tendency to distortion?

Some of us who know children who have been excessively exposed
to primal scene are impressed with the early and later acting out, as
an attempt to master the overwhelming excitement. Does the early
and regular casuality about sex contribute to hypermaturity as a
defense against anxiety, or to the "prevalence of overt anxiety in
Africans," which Dr. Lambo notes? It seems a likely possibility that
splitting mechanisms would be commonly used by children growing
up surrounded by polygamous relationships.

A child whose hypermaturity is fostered by being given the

responsibility of carrying around, sleeping with, and caring for younger siblings would seem to be missing some important play and learning experiences. One also wonders about the value of the hypermaturity as a defense against the rage the child might otherwise feel toward the mother.

Dr. Lambo questions whether object substitution may provoke anxiety or alter the perceptual, affective, and cognitive apparatus. Our observations lead us to believe that whereas many normal or mildly neurotic children can successfully maintain multiple object relationships ego-defective and developmentally arrested children very much need the continuity of a relationship with one person, the structure of a consistent environment, and the security of reasonable limits. Lacking these requirements, many of our vulnerable children never reach a high level of psychic maturity. It would be helpful to know how a hyperactive, hypersensitive, ego-defective child's adaptation varies in the permissive, multiobject traditional African society.

Although there is reason to believe that we find a comparable amount of mental illness in all societies, there is obviously a cultural difference in the way it is expressed, accepted, and treated. We can learn much from a cross-cultural exchange of observations and research, not the least of which is a clearer insight into our own culture.

Sociopsychological Aspects of the Vulnerable Child, Risk and Mastery: Children of the Modern Elite in Nigeria

Tolani Asuni, M.A., M.D., D.P.M., F.R.C.Psych. (Nigeria)

Children of the elite constitute a special vulnerable group of children in Nigeria and perhaps all over the world, but they should arouse greater concern in Nigeria than they are being given. They are the ones in whom greater material benefits have been conferred and one should expect that "to whom much has been given much should be expected," but this is not so. They are relatively few in the total population. Their parents have achieved their elitist status generally in one generation, so that the contrast in their upbringing and that of their children is very sharp.

Let us first look at the traditional pattern of child rearing to which their parents have been exposed. They were born in an extended family situation when infantile mortality was very high. They were brought up in an emotionally warm environment with a number of mother and father surrogates. Their physiological and other needs were met instantly without delay. They were carried on the backs of their mothers and mother surrogates. When not carried on mothers' backs they were free to crawl all over the house or even the compound. They were weaned at 2 or 3 years. They were hardly ever left alone except when asleep.

Their toilet and social training was not limited to only father and mother but extended to the extended family constellation. The resultant effect is that they belong more to the extended family group than to just father and mother.

When they got older they were accepted by their peers, who had had the same type of upbringing in the same neighborhood where positive neighborhood feeling was very high. It was the intelligent and relatively wealthy parents who sent their children to school— even though they might be illiterates themselves. All the parents could do was to give the children encouragement and time to study. They were unable to assist them with the scholastic exercises, but these children competed in a healthy way among themselves, the older helping the younger. The father, however, took the boys out when he was carrying out his trade and the mother did the same for the girls.

Whatever weaknesses there were in their upbringing were buffered by other built-in systems in the social setup. They have developed into successful people in their various fields.

Now let us look at the child-rearing pattern of the children of the elite. They are born usually in a nuclear family setup with grandmother visiting and staying for only a short period of time. They live in houses in the new residential areas where neighborhood feeling is less. Greater fuss is made of toilet training. They are kept in cribs instead of crawling about the house. They have only their immediate family around and usually a nursemaid who is paid to look after the child, whom the mother does not carry on her back while she is pursuing her business or doing her domestic chores. Because of the low neighborhood feeling the child is sometimes not allowed to play with the children of the immediate neighbors. In this way he is more isolated than his parents were in their childhood. Their immediate friends and peers live far away so they cannot readily form a youth neighborly group like their parents did.

When father or mother chastises him in the absence of the other parent there is no other close relative around to give him comfort and solace. The children are left to their devices without much guidance and leadership and there are no close peers next door or in the immediate vicinity. There is no open and free spontaneous line of communication between children and parents. If he does not do well at school, the parents do not try to find out the reason but proceed to blame him. The family seldom eat together so that often the parents do not know how well the child is feeding.

Unfortunately the checks and balances and buffers to protect the child in times of crises are not there, because the parents, who had not experienced the same pattern of upbringing, have not realized these needs. Furthermore, the time of upbringing gears the child to be a more independent person than the parents and the society at large can tolerate.

Results

Although it is difficult or even impossible to attribute the defect in personality formation to a single factor, the result of the foregoing differences in pattern of upbringing cannot be ruled out as being at least contributory to the following problems which have been observed:

1. RELATIVELY POOR PERFORMANCE IN SCHOOL

Assuming that the parents must be intelligent to be successful, one would expect their children to be quite good academically, but they are not often so. The parents do not read much themselves, so the children do not have the example to copy. One father asked his son why he was not doing as well as less privileged kids. The son's answer was that the less privileged children knew that if they failed their examination, that would be the end of the school education which the parents had been straining themselves to provide; but if he failed his examination, he was sure the father would continue to pay his fees and if necessary to find him another school.

It appears that the awareness of the elitist status of the parents reduces the motivation of some of their children to do their best. This can partly be explained by the attitude of the parents themselves and their perhaps understandable effort to use their position to help their children get on in spite of their weaknesses.

Quite often the preoccupation with academic success to the exclusion of the emotional needs of the children goads some elitist parents to send their children to boarding schools too early and, worse still, abroad too early. Sometimes these children do badly academically, and where they do well they are frequently misfits in

the society back home and even in the country where they have had
their education.

In this connection the situation of children of African parents
studying in England can be mentioned. Some of these children are
kept with foster parents, usually of poor quality, and they are visited
by their parents once a week or once a month or at even longer
intervals. The result is that the children often do not accept them
as their parents. The parents obviously assume that the foster parents
are equivalent to relatives, not realizing the subtle and not so subtle
differences between paid white foster parents and relatives. Some of
these children become problem children and when they do return
home it takes them a considerable period of time to adjust if they
ever learn to adjust.

2. ABUSE OF DRUGS

Contrary to what is believed in Western countries, marijuana, at
least the African species, is not innocuous. It is cheap enough and
available enough to be within the reach of the less privileged child,
but it would appear that proportionately more privileged children
are involved in the use and abuse of marijuana; furthermore, some
of them have traveled abroad and are conversant with the drug youth
cult and the literature on the subject—usually the literature saying
that it is not a danger, which they quote.

While the children of the less privileged take amphetamine to
keep them awake to be able to read far into the night, the children
of the elite use amphetamine and mandrax (a sleeping tablet) to
expand their minds or to make them enjoy themselves. It is as if
they have greater need of these drugs than other children to assuage
their anxiety, or they are more exposed to these drugs than other
children.

It seems that their frustration tolerance level is very low and they
resort to drugs in conflict situations, instead of learning a more
mature way of coping with them. They very easily identify what to
them is traumatic and conflicting and make a mountain and an
excuse of these situations for their drug use. They often quote the
social alcoholic consumption of adults to justify their drug use, just
as it is done in Western countries. This suggests that their role and
the expectations for them are being patterned on Western style in a
society which is very much in a transitional stage between industrial

and traditional systems, remaining more in the direction of the traditional system.

We have found it more difficult to treat the children of the elite with drug problems than the children of the less privileged. Perhaps one reason for this is that the participation of parents in the treatment program is more intense among less privileged and the authority of the parents of the less privileged child is stronger than that of the elite.

These children do not think of their future professional career in terms of the sciences, which are badly needed, but in terms of arts. Event then their plans are vague. They have some grandiose ideas about their aptitude and competence in music and art, which they have not been able to demonstrate. They tend to drift.

It has not been possible yet to see what they will become in the future. We only hope that they will mature before it is too late.

3. IDENTITY CRISIS, RELIGION, AND PSYCHOSIS

Teenagers tend to resort to religion when they are getting disillusioned about the image of their father as omnipotent and going through a period of identity crisis. Most teenagers get over this crisis. In Nigeria we have observed a phenomenon which is limited to the children of the elite. These young people, usually males, get so deeply involved with the Grail Movement with headquarters in Switzerland, to the exclusion of almost every other interest including their schoolwork. Some have actually developed psychosis in the process. They try to justify their psychotic experiences through the book *The Light of Truth,* the Bible of the movement.

These children are emotionally detached from their parents, whose words of guidance are blatantly rejected. In fact they go against the advice of their parents in spite of the harm they do themselves in the process. Their academic performance drops because they are not interested and they have no definite plans for their future. They become withdrawn and asocial, especially at home.

On close examination of the situation, it is found that they generally belong to successful elite families where the father is very busy and does not have or find time to be with his children, show interest in their activities, and participate in some of them. The local leader of the Movement, himself a successful man, entertains these young boys in his house, spends considerable time with them, talks with them, and shows great interest in them, especially in the direction of the tenets of the movement. It is no wonder that they come to identify themselves almost exclusively with this man and what he stands for.

The question is what role has this Movement played in the development of their psychosis. Is it just coincidental—Would those of them who developed psychoses have done so even without their involvement with the movement, and would they have used other systems in their groping? If their fathers had given more time for them and established a rapport and intimate line of communication with them, would they have gotten so deeply involved and developed a psychosis? Our feeling is that the programmatic, goal-directed guidance of the parents could have helped to plant their feet firmly in the world of reality.

Why is it that the children of less privileged parents do not get involved, even though in some cases their fathers, for different reasons, do not seem to give them any more of their time than do the elite fathers? One possible reason is that the family of the less privileged are more reality oriented with the practical problems of survival, succeeding in life and striving hard to provide the means to educate their children. Another possible reason is that the social and economic distance between the elite and the less privileged operates against their involvement. Furthermore, the children of the less privileged family may not have the time, because of their expected participation in domestic and other family chores, to indulge in such socioreligious meetings.

Comments

It may be argued that this trend is universal and it is not peculiar to Nigeria. It may well be so, but the question is whether Nigeria can contain or afford it. The answer to this is indicated by the concern of parents to the extent of seeking psychiatric intervention. Even in developed countries, one wonders to what extent this trend can be contained! Even if it can be contained in developed countries, this is no reason why it should not cause concern in developing countries. The attitude of parents to their children in developed countries is a bit different from developing countries. The educational system in the latter is so crowded that it is difficult, if not impossible, for a child who has dropped out of school for two or three years to come back again. The scope of the educational system is also limited and once a child misses the boat in one direction, it will be difficult to catch another boat going a different direction. The level of unemployment is very high and it is very difficult to get a job without adequate qualifications. There is no social security in terms of unemployment benefits, old age pensions, local council or government housing schemes providing cheap accommodations. Thus parents in developing countries have legitimate reasons to be concerned for the future of their children. This is enhanced by a saying in Yoruba language, "May our children be greater than us," their parents.

This problem is not striking in the traditional family if it exists there at all. In any case survival is relatively easier in the traditional system than it is in the nontraditional system. The children of the elite have been removed and are distant from the traditional system, and it is unrealistic to expect them to fall back to a system which is alien to them and for which their upbringing has not prepared them.

The problem of these children is the failure of their parents, who do not appreciate the added and different responsibility of parenthood in a sociocultural and economic environment different from that in which they grew up.

Normality and Tribal Society

Colin M. Turnbull, D.Phil. (U.S.A.)

One of the major problems for the social anthropologist in branching out into a field such as this is that his traditional preoccupation is with culture, with social institutions and social structure rather than with people. We tend to be concerned, at least academically, with whether or not a system works, and how it works, and perhaps with why it works in that particular way. We are also concerned with what generalities can be drawn from comparative studies of this sort.

I have recently been much concerned with the question of just what is "human nature," in the sense of what is "natural to humanity," hence with the concept of normality. It is important to stress that although I do not in any way underestimate the importance of human biology and physiology as determinant or highly influential factors with respect to human behavior, they are *not* my specialty and I focus therefore almost exclusively on cultural factors.

Another problem in dealing with this topic, for the social anthropologist, is that we frequently find ourselves necessarily taking a relativistic attitude, so that my own immediate question is just how does one determine what is normal, or even healthy, and what is not. One of the two examples that I shall draw on, that of the Ik of Uganda, raises this question quite dramatically, for in those terms by which we most frequently define normal human behavior the Ik are almost to a man abnormal, if not deranged. Yet while living with them it did not take long for me to adapt and assume for myself the new "normality" and judge as insane those few individuals who behaved, for instance, with compassion, love, kindness, consideration, and trust. All of these qualities, in the Icien situation, are abnormalities, for in the present drastic context they are all qualities that directly threaten survival. The urge to survive seems to me to be as about as fundamental and unequivocal a characteristic of humanity as can be found, for unlike other animals we have the facility for concealing it, even to ourselves, under the cloak of our supposedly inherent sociability. Yet I believe it to be there, in individual rather than social terms, and the Ik show clearly how under given conditions that urge can dominate human behavior to the destruction of all those other qualities we normally ascribe to humanity. Thus for me perhaps the measure by which I judge mental health, or normality of behavior, is the measure of successs achieved in the game of survival.

The two examples I have in mind illustrate the preceding problems, but they also highlight many of the issues that perhaps more directly concern those at this conference, particularly the issue of vulnerability. Both examples concern traditional peoples at the simplest level of technology, hunters and gatherers, both faced with the inevitable problem of social change of enormous magnitude and rapidity. Yet, oddly enough, the people the most drastically affected by change, the Ik, are the people who have perhaps made the most dramatic and stable response, however abnormal and inhuman it may seem to us.

The Mbuti pygmies, whom we should look at first as a traditional people who have almost completely resisted and rejected all change, and who continue to survive in conditions approaching abundance rather than adequacy, are reacting to threats of change with a humorous skepticism. They are alert and aware, yet one by one, even band by band, they are beginning to be picked off and destroyed because of their inability to perceive that change has already come and that their traditional way of life has a limited future. At the moment the change is largely unplanned and undirected and because of this, and its relatively slow and subtle encroachment, the Mbuti do not consider it a threat and make no preparations for dealing with it. Rather than being beneficial to them, their own traditional and continued security as forest hunters, and the slow pace of change,

spell disaster. As hunters and gatherers, with very limited concern
for the future, the Mbuti know very well that even if there were a
concerted effort by the government to move them out of the forest,
or even if the large-scale commercial exploitation of the forest were
begun tomorrow, it would be years before the Mbuti felt any
significant effects. Insofar as they think of the future at all it is in
terms of days rather than weeks or months, let alone years. They
dismiss as fantasy any arguments based on long-term change.

Here again is an example of the relativity of the problem we are
tackling, and of how the areas of and causes for vulnerability are
likely to vary considerably from one context to another. Traditional
farmers, for instance, obviously have had to develop a much more
complex and future-oriented concept of time than hunters, whose
economy is so strictly diurnal. Farmers do not suffer from the same
difficulty in adapting to the notion of change for they are more
concerned with the future than the present, and they are better
prepared to consider the future implications of changes they see
already taking place around them. Further, the particular difficulties
associated with introducing traditional, tribal peoples to the notion
of progress as understood in the Western world are much less for
farmers, who habitually think in terms of growth and who have
learned to see security in things (storable food, land, crops, metal,
even money) as well as people.

Farmers also are more technologically oriented than hunters, and
their economy is one of aggression almost, a constant battle with the
natural world, with one very basic form of normality. The hunters,
on the other hand, live as a functioning part of the total ecosystem
and do not view themselves as being in a hostile world that they have
to control or dominate. Moreover, hunters, whose experience is that
each day provides for itself, have not developed a technology to
enable them to build up a storable surplus. Security is seen and
found in their role in the ecosystem as deriving from the natural
world around them (defining themselves as "forest people,"
"mountain people," and so forth), and the only form of security
they consciously cultivate in addition to this is the network of
interpersonal relationships established through marriage, bond
brotherhood, initiation, prestation, and name sharing, to mention
a few of the many forms of reciprocity institutionalized in such
societies. Herders, fishers, and farmers in the traditional African

scene establish and carefully maintain similar networks, and for them too such interpersonal and intergroup relationships remain the ultimate and most basic form of security, which they fall back on when their technology is unable to provide for the inevitable crisis.

It is significant that belief in magic, witchcraft, and sorcery and the establishment of magico/religious institutions of this nature arise with the advent of herding and agriculture, that is, with man's attempt to dominate the natural world and alter it to his advantage. This is a fair measure of the increased uncertainty inherent in these ways of life, as opposed to the hunting and gathering way that man so relatively recently, and perhaps unwisely, forsook. Again we have a problem specific to one form of culture and not another, for whereas the hunter and gatherer do not feel unduly perturbed by the lack of belief in magic and witchcraft in Western society, the herder or farmer is likely to feel bereft of a vital prop. It may take him some time to be convinced that Western technology offers greater security, and to persuade him that a belief in Western technology is an adequate substitute for a belief in witchcraft, no less reliable if no more so.

These few examples show something of the relativity of "normality" in different cultural contexts and indicate how wide ranging are the causes of vulnerability and security, concepts of time, subsistence technology, and magico/religious belief among others. The ramifications of any one of these areas are widespread, and vulnerability in any society related to all areas of social structure; domestic, economic, political, and religious. We next consider in more detail the two hunting and gathering societies I have mentioned, the Mbuti and the Ik.

The Mbuti pygmies live in the equatorial Ituri Forest in the Republic of Zaïre, and they may well be descendants of an extremely early if not original branch of homo sapiens. From historic (ancient Egyptian) sources we know the Mbuti have been in this particular area for some 5000 years, and there is no reason why they should not always have been there. The forest is a world that is in itself constantly in process of change, of course, but it is cyclic rather than linear change. As far as the Mbuti population is concerned its experience in all respects is one of stability rather than growth. It early on learned how to survive in this world, how to keep its size at the optimum economic level by various institutionalized forms of population control.

The Mbuti also learned how to play their role in the forest ecology. It seems, for instance, that among other roles the Mbuti are vital as predators in keeping down the elephant population, and their recognition of this role is clearly reflected in their overall value system. Organized in hunting bands, these bands fluctuate in size and composition from month to month, so rather like the forest itself the Mbuti population is in a constant state of flux, with no overall change of any great significance. The stability of the situation is most dramatically evidenced by their habit of referring to the forest (to which they constantly shout, talk, sing, or dance) as "mother" or "father," explaining that they do so "because, like our parents, the forest gives us all we need . . . food, shelter, clothing, warmth, and affection." The inclusion of "affection" indicates the degree of conscious awareness by the Mbuti of the extent of their own security.

Within this world, where hunting bands seldom rise above thirty or fall below three nuclear families in size, communication is virtually total. The system of kinship terminology defines everyone in a hunting band at a given moment as one or other category of kin—grandparents, mother, father, sibling, or child. Sexual differentiation is made only at the parental level, and even at that level there is no direct way of differentiating classificatory parents (such as the forest) from those we would call "real" parents. This is another aspect of both the flux and the security that are so much a part of Mbuti life. Someone you call "mother" one day, you refer to by her personal name the next day if she moves to another band. You may do this even if you came from her stomach, which is the only way the Mbuti can designate the mother who gave birth to them. If there is much habitual and frequent exchange between two bands, then the kinship terms may be extended to include both bands, in which case it is better considered as one single band divided into two segments.

This is clear evidence of Mbuti recognition of the primarily economic nature of interpersonal relationships, and the terminological system equally clearly defines the recognized areas and degrees of social responsibility. Between the band and the Mbuti as a whole there is no intermediate step, unlike farmers and herders, who recognize successive levels of social grouping and responsibility, from family through lineage and clan to tribe (and, incidentally, from there, using the same system, to "nation," as some contemporary African leaders well know). But the brotherhood of all Mbuti is recognized in the way in which they refer to themselves as *bamiki ba n'dura,* children of the forest. With typical fluidity this allows for classificatory Mbuti such as village farmers or other outsiders, including anthropologists, who elect to live in the forest rather than outside it. Beyond that vital classification there are only the nonforest people, generally referred to as animals. This reference is not as derogatory as it sounds but is rather descriptive, indicating that like animals nonforest people do not come under the system of social obligations that encompass all forest people. They are rather to be treated as prey, to be hunted, tricked, exploited at will.

In the Mbuti world of flux, centralization is obviously unworkable, therefore authority is dispersed throughout the community, using age as the prime principle. Each age level (children, youths, adults, and elders) has its own area of authority and thus its own measure of social control. Sex is not used as a divisive organizational principle except in the division of labor, and even there it is not rigid. This egalitarian organization does not imply any inherent "goodness," it is merely the most effective form of organization in that particular context. Thus there are no truly competitive games at which one Mbuti can "defeat" another. Instead their games teach the children to develop the necessary skills equally. Some allow for what seems to be the inevitable urge to excel (i.e., to be unequal) and teach that such excellence does not pay. In adult life any hunter who shows he is better than others, rather than being honored and applauded, is exiled. Thus Mbuti politics are as egalitarian as Mbuti economics, and the "family," that is, the hunting band, establishes the model for such equal behavior and relationship. It is recognized that one's obligations are to one's fellow hunters of the moment, and that theoretically these obligations could, at any other moment, include *any* other forest person, or Mbuti.

An essential part of the system is the clear boundary drawn between forest and nonforest, and a clear recognition of the cessation of all obligation at that boundary. This does not result in hostility between the Mbuti and their farming village neighbors, however; on the contrary, since it is reciprocal, it makes for an even, effective, and frequently affective relationship, allowing each people to live in close territorial propinquity yet at great social distance, each retaining its own system of beliefs and values as well as its own way of life. Thus the social unit is, ultimately, a religious unit, a unit of believers. The problems of vulnerability introduced with social change can thus be easily imagined—more easily than the solutions, alas. As long as the Mbuti can see himself as the hunter, dealing with animals (however dangerous and powerful), he can cope with the situation, mentally at least. This requires that the two worlds, the forest and the nonforest, be kept distinct, however. As long as there is the refuge of the forest into which they can retreat, the Mbuti will remain Mbuti and will easily recover from any shocks they may feel on contact with the changing, nonforest world around them.

The Mbuti will continue to come to the edge of that world, even to participate in it for brief periods (attending schools, for instance, wearing clothes, helping on farms, going to missions, even starting "model villages," paying taxes, and voting). But these are no more than temporary, calculated forays and are merely part of typical Mbuti tactics for dealing with dangerous game—get to know it but prevent it from getting to know you—and imitation when in proximity to the game is the best form of concealment.

In their traditional relationship with the forest villagers (who, because they cut the forest down to build their villages and grow their crops, are thought of by the Mbuti as nonforest people) the Mbuti have created an image of subservience, and pretend to an adoption of village culture whenever in the presence of villagers. They even submit to village initiation rites, but this is all part of the process of keeping the village at a distance, maintaining that barricade between the two worlds.

With the Mbuti, then, at one extreme of isolation and total self-sufficiency there is virtually no vulnerability within their world. This includes the Mbuti in contact with the nonforest world, at least for as long as it can be dealt with within this traditional framework of systematic opposition. But when the Mbuti are ultimately brought face to face with people who are neither forest nor nonforest people, neither hunters nor animals, then their vulnerability is as total as was their security. Their entire social system, including their value system, will not only be inadequate, it will be dysfunctional and there will be little or no chance of adaptation. Change will have to

be total and there will, then, be no more Mbuti, no more forest
people. Individual Mbuti are able to make the transition without any
apparently disastrous effects, for it is not uncommon for a village
male to marry a Mbuti wife. She then becomes part of the village
world and although she may herself return to the forest at any time,
her children by the villager may never do so. They are regarded from
birth, by both peoples, as villagers, as nonforest people. Again the
lack of vulnerability is due to the fact that there *are* two worlds, and
to the Mbuti facility for living in both of them, moving from one
to the other at will, but never blending them. Even in the heart of the
forest, for instance, on any important ritual occasion the path leading
from the hunting camp in the direction of the nearest village,
perhaps many days away, is symbolically closed by dragging across
it a branch, often so small that any child could jump over it or walk
around it.

Here is an extreme at which a people have developed a social
system that does not allow for "progress" in the sense of irreversible
change, nor even for adaptability beyond the ability to participate
in two worlds. Vulnerability is thus likely to be total rather than
partial, and it can occur at any point, in any of the four areas
mentioned, domestic, economic, political, or religious. The
introduction of "better" hunting technology could be as totally
disastrous and destructive as conversion to Christianity. An example
of this vulnerability having come to pass, resulting in total change
from extreme sociability to extreme unsociability, can be seen with a
second example, the Ik. These are a people who as recently as 1920
were living in the open grassland mountain region between northern
Uganda, Sudan, and Kenya, but otherwise employing a mode of life
and social organization very much like that of the Mbuti, and as
successful.

Due to the drawing of colonial boundaries, which became national
boundaries, a large area that once served as the hunting territory of
this small tribe was divided, and the nomadic hunting pattern of the
Ik was seriously impaired. The Ik were taken in as Ugandan citizens
since the major part of their former territory now lay in that nation,
and as long as Kidepo Valley was still accessible to them their
situation was not too desperate. For the best part of the year they
still had good hunting and for the rest of the time they were able
to survive by poaching and by various intrigues with neighboring

pastoral peoples. The final blow was when Kidepo was declared a national park and all hunting was outlawed. The Government did its best to encourage the Ik to take up farming, and indeed it had no reason to expect that they would do otherwise since other hunters at the far end of Kidepo had not only adopted farming as a way of life but were thriving in their new economy. The Ik, however, were more isolated and more conservative, and they refused to change. They retreated to the barren heights between the Kenya/Ugandan escarpment and Kidepo, an area devoid of game for most of the year and almost totally unsuitable for farming or cattle herding.

By then relations between the three nations whose boundaries had carved up the Ik's former hunting territory had deteriorated, and with the war in southern Sudan, just across the border, anything but the briefest and most inconspicuous poaching forays became impossible. The park also was increasingly patrolled by armed askaris, and still the Ik refused to accept government offers to resettle them in farming land and to teach them how to become farmers. They attempted some farming themselves, however, in what was left to them of their old homeland, the barren mountains in the north-eastern corner of Uganda. Thus evidently their reluctance to take up farming was not so much resistance to a new kind of subsistence activity as to the relocation it would have involved. On behalf of the government I took three Ik down to the plains, to an area that had been suggested as suitable for relocation, and after the first day all three became listless and complained of sickness (headaches, chest pains, nausea, and so forth), which, whether in their minds or bodies, was real enough. Again they were willing to consider the proposition of change but unable to accept it.

At this time, when I was first there in 1964, there was one of the periodic droughts that can be expected every four years. Their farming efforts had already proven next to futile, and certainly quite unreliable and unpredictable, and they had developed a vital subsidiary economy involving the cattle raiding practices of neighboring pastoral peoples. In effect the Ik became entrepreneurs, organizing intertribal raiding that reached a scale approaching international warfare, at least in the eyes of the national governments concerned. In point of fact such raiding is an essential part of the local ecosystem, but nonetheless Ik enterprise interfered with its natural order and gave the Ugandan government even more cause to wish to relocate them and put an end to such seemingly aggressive and violent activity.

The Ik had increasingly been facing a very simple situation: in their new environment there just was not enough food to go around. They either had to move out of their former homeland altogether or starve. They chose the latter alternative but developed a system of selective starvation that has enabled them to survive as a group, though drastically reduced in size and transformed in nature. In my first 18 months I saw the population reduced from 2000 to about 1200, and it was further reduced during the next year. But that period covered two consecutive years of famine. Since then the population seems to have stabilized itself at just over 1000 (an accurate population count has been impossible) and, frighteningly, they have stabilized their nonsocial survival system, keeping the population down to this workable level. I am not suggesting that the Ik consciously crop their population rather as game wardens crop animal populations in a park, but they are very much aware of what is happening to them and rationalize it forthrightly enough.

The first to be allowed to die (they do not kill) are the old, when food shortage is greater than usual. Old may be anything above 25 years of age and of course includes the infirm and sick. Regardless of the bonds one would expect in any other traditional African society, such as kinship, age, and residence, the healthy Ik merely watch the old die without comment and without any attempt to prevent that death. Even an individual who has managed to gather plenty for himself would not consider sharing it with an old person who was starving to death. The Ik say that it would be a waste of food, for the old are going to die soon anyway, and they are no longer of any use: they cannot get food for themselves and can no longer get children. They are right, for even if an individual had food enough to share one day he is not likely to have it the next, so systematic sharing patterns are impossible. Further, the sense of dependence that sharing would encourage itself becomes dysfunctional. The criterion as to whether a person *should* be alive or dead is simply whether or not he can supply himself with enough food and water and adequate shelter.

If there is still not enough food to go around the Ik let the children die next, with the argument that their survival is in any case questionable, whereas the adult survivors, who throughout remain

relatively plump, can always get more children, and by surviving
have demonstrated their ability to get food and water. Thus the
breeding group is kept alive and healthy, which is sound biology.

From our more comfortable, well-fed standpoint, we inevitably ask
ourselves: How can human beings behave this way? How can a
mother stand to see her child die of hunger when she has food to
offer, even at sacrifice to herself? That is because the norm, for us, is to
be well fed, if not gorged. It is because up to the present the norm for
mankind has been one of adequacy, under which norm sociability has
had great survival value, particularly at a relatively low technological
level. In our present "civilized" condition of abundance, however,
sociability is being replaced increasingly by individuality as a survival
mechanism and organizational principle, and we may well be heading
in the same direction as the Ik, at their opposite extreme of
deprivation.

It is of course impossible to say what the first Ik thought or felt
when they saw their children or their parents die and were powerless
to help. I have, however, seen an old lady cry when she was reminded
by the "kindness" (in their evaluation, and perhaps rightly,
"stupidity") of my colleague and myself when we helped her out of
a ravine, tended her wounds, and gave her food and water to help her
continue after she had been abandoned by her fellows. She said she
cried because we had reminded her that there had been a time when
children had helped their parents, and parents had cared for their
children. But Lo'ono died anyway, a few weeks later, and now there
is not one Ik left alive who has such uncomfortable memories.

Everyone alive today is alive because they have been brought up in
a system that has, from birth onward, taught them that the road to
survival is through rigid individuality. The Ik mother, not having
access to plastic bottles, must perforce feed her reluctantly born infant
at the breast. The infant thus learns dependence upon another
individual for food and warmth and shelter and may, if not taught
otherwise, conceptualize this as love, that luxury we so arrogantly
believe to be an inherent part of human nature.

The Ik mother, with better sense, teaches the infant otherwise.
By the time the child reaches the age of 2 she begins to wean it in a
seemingly heartless and cruel fashion. I have seen Ik mothers watch
their children crawl into smoldering fires and laugh as they burn
themselves. I have seen them watch as their children fall off low

ledges; and I have seen them out in the hot fields or open country take the children off their backs and simply lay them on the ground and return hours later, seeming almost to hope that the burden would have been removed either by death through sunstroke or by one of the many predators that are as hungry as the Ik. I have seen both these things happen, but I have never seen remorse, regret, sorrow. The only positive reaction I can remember was one of pleasure since the death of the child led to the discovery of a sleepy, well-fed leopard that could be, and was, easily killed and consumed, baby and all. In these and other ways the mother is in a sense being perfectly normal; she is teaching her child (and reminding herself) the essential lesson that in their particular world survival is an individual game. Occasionally an Ik may be seen helping another, but help generally is interpreted as an aggressive act and is frowned upon, for it invariably is a demand, motivated by self-interest.

At the age of 3 the child is turned out of the house, though it may be allowed to sleep in the open courtyard, within a stout protective stockade. Unable still to fend for themselves entirely on their own in such a competitive world, children organize themselves into age gangs of two distinct levels: from 3 to 7 years old, and from 8 to 12. These age gangs are not to be confused with age *sets*, in which members of a set establish and maintain bonds of reciprocity throughout life. An Ik enters an age gang as an individual, alone, and leaves it as such. Within each gang there is no mutual assistance in food getting. As they scavenge the ravines and fields it is the swiftest and strongest who is likely to see a source of food and get to it first, and he will try to consume it all rather than share it. Thus the swiftest and strongest, usually the oldest, gets thrown out of the junior gang and is forced to join the senior gang as the slowest and weakest and youngest, and once again as the least likely to survive. Within the gang cooperation only exists in that they jointly roam their given territory; there is thus a bond of territoriality. There is also the bond of mutual protection against other predators, particularly adult Ik.

By moving through the age gangs until one is finally thrown out, at 13 or so, as an adult, entirely on one's own, the Ik children learn that cooperation may, under certain circumstances, have advantages for the individual. They learn, however, that it is purely contextual and that permanent bonds are unworkable. They also learn to allow the others the same courtesy and consequently the Ik are not a violent people, either in thought or deed. Rather are they a passionless people, coldly calculating and assessing each situation in terms of their own individual survival. It is a system that works equally well in times of plenty and in times of deprivation, but plenty is recognized as posing a threat since it makes mutuality *possible*, and allows for the establishment of such bonds as affection and trust and dependence, which, in the norm of deprivation, are dysfunctional. So in the third year when I saw the Ik fields laden with food, or when the government tried to help them with famine relief, they destroyed the abundance. They let the fields rot, each individual merely getting what he wanted for the day each day, and the healthy Ik who collected the famine relief prudently gorged themselves on it once out of sight, consuming it all rather than carrying it back to share. This was not greed, nor was it the ignorance, stupidity, or idleness with which we usually dismiss ways foreign to our own; it was factual recognition of the dysfunctionality of sociality.

The one Ik I saw that was referred to by others as mad was a 12-year-old girl who had not been properly cared for by her mother. Her mother had loved and cared for Adupa beyond the age of 3, and Adupa had consequently learned to conceptualize this as love, and responded in kind. However, there inevitably came the time, when I was there, that the mother could no longer manifest her love for Adupa in the form of food and water. Had she taken Adupa with her on a foraging expedition both would have died, for frequently in a day's search for food there will be no water, and a hole dug in the sand at the end of the day may yield a cupful, barely enough to keep one person alive, let alone two. Adupa, alas, because of this poor upbringing, had not learned to fend for herself, and even if she did find food she did not swallow it hastily and in secret, so that she became prey of other children. As she got weaker and weaker she kept returning to her parents and demanding help, a most un-Ik-like thing to do. They finally let her into the family compound, when she was almost too weak to stand, then left it, walling it up behind them so that Adupa could not get out. They went off on a foraging expedition and returned a week later and threw out the rotting body. Everyone laughed at me and said, "You see, we *said* she was mad."

Rather than try to isolate specific areas of vulnerability in these two situations I will try to draw some general conclusions of a more anthropological nature, which, as a social anthropologist, I see to have significance in this search for vulnerability in any society, but especially in a society in the process of emerging from the tribal state to that of participation in nationhood.

I think we should be aware that tribal organization, partly because of its technological level, is generally one of adequacy rather than of abundance or inadequacy. In a subsistence economy the rewards for labor are seen very directly and immediately and felt in the fullness of the stomach (a phrase which the Ik use as their definition of "goodness"). This has profound implications for their assessment of the kind of changes generally introduced with a more elaborate technology, a surplus economy, cash, centralized and remote government, and grossly expanded social/political horizons. The latter is of particular importance since tribal politics are the politics of kin, where the tribal horizon in a sense defines a "grandfamily," sharing a common ancestor and hence a common system of belief. This is the source of the common morality that is so strong a feature of tribal organization. Plurality of belief, a characteristic (including lack of belief) of the modern nation, is a constant source of uncertainty and instability, since social obligation then has to be learned rather than felt and enforced through physical coercion rather than religious belief.

Tribal organization rests on various principles, including territoriality, age, kinship, and religious belief. By religious belief we must be careful not to associate tribal religion with what we lightly dismiss as magic or superstition. It is a belief that is spiritual in the truest sense of the word, that is intimately bound up with the concept of identity and with that other organizational principle, kinship. It has the enormous strength of being felt as an individual belief by the individual, yet in fact being a shared belief because it is taught. It is taught from the day of birth to the day of death by daily action, ritual and otherwise, and in speech. It is a part of daily life, and as practical as any other part.

The family, in all its many forms, is the most basic social unit, and the tribal form of family establishes a model for all social relationships, being expanded ultimately, as I said, to conceptualize the tribe as a grandfamily descended from a common ancestor. Kinship terms indicate social rather than genealogical connections and define social obligations. And of course it is highly significant that kinship terms in such societies are classificatory and can actually be used to establish a specific form of social obligation regardless of actual kinship. We would make a disastrous mistake if we interpreted any tribe's particular kinship terminology to correspond to our own concepts of mother, father, brother, sister, and so forth.

Kinship as a model establishes social bonds in a vertical manner, however, through common descent (actual or fictitious) and thus can be as divisive as well as cohesive. To counteract this the principle of age operates to cut horizontally across the vertical bonds, uniting agemates regardless of kinship. We saw how the Mbuti used age rather than kinship as a prime organizational principle, in fact. And finally territory plays a vital role in establishing yet another set of boundaries for society. Again with the Mbuti we saw how they draw the boundaries of social obligation around the hunting band to include all those who are hunting together in the same territory at any given moment. But the Mbuti, like the Ik, are nomads, and have a very special concept of territory and the same principle among sedentary farmers may be just as strong but take a different form, and be associated with a less fluid concept of kinship and perhaps with a more rigid system of age classification.

These are some of the major principles that bind a tribe together, that give it order and cohesion, and it is worth noting that although the tribal individual is no paragon of virtue, order is nonetheless maintained effectively and nonviolently without the existence of organized physical coercion. There is no police force in the tribal society. But as the nature of society changes from the fluidity and smallness of that of the hunter and gatherer to the increasingly rigid and complex structure of the agricultural society, physical coercion becomes increasingly institutionalized until, with the traditional nations and empires, we get true legal systems and penal codes, at which point sociality as well as society take on a very different aspect.

Thus we can see a wide diversity of causes for vulnerability. Relocation from one environment to another; emergence into a plural society; introduction by national education and by conversion to Christianity or Islam to new systems of belief and values, more divorced from the practical run of daily life and with less immediately evident relevance; broadening of social horizons beyond the possibility of conceptualization as within the family model; introduction of new social divisions and classifications such as class; replacement of one concept (and form) of family with another, with totally different structural implications; change of language, with the possible loss of original significance at a symbolic level—these are

302 The Dakar Conference

some of the more obvious areas of danger. And because of the omnipresence of religious belief in tribal life, even a change in diet could have drastic consequences in a child's (or adult's) sense of security. All tribal organization is highly integrated, and anything affecting one part is going to affect the whole. An innocent change from breast feeding to bottle feeding could well have far-reaching consequences, for it is surely at the breast where sociality is first learned, by direct participation and experience. And such sociality and the "morality" that derives from it in conjunction with all the principles of social organization mentioned is of a very different quality from any sociality learned intellectually in classrooms or Sunday schools.

But then again, recognizing the relativity of values, we should look to the future and ask if, for the sake of increasing their survivability, we should not encourage the loss of the old forms of sociality and consciously teach the new solitary individualism that is such an inevitable corollary of the modern technological society, which defines security in terms of bank balances rather than people, and where it is possible to establish solitary security in the form of cash— a possibility totally inconceivable in tribal subsistence economies. It seems to me, indeed, that this is the critical transition we have to consider, and one that we ignore because we insist that our civilized form of society *is* social, because of our failure to recognize that consistent changes have been taking place in our own sociality, in both degree and quality. Thus to teach and preach sociability may, in fact, be to introduce a new and all-encompassing area of vulnerability. It is certainly to my mind the most significant area of vulnerability that any African child has to face, with the immense power of a still vital tribal (and therefore social) tradition behind it, yet with the brave new world of unsociality ahead of it. To suppose that we can maintain those old social values merely by teaching them is a tragic fallacy; either they or the contemporary Western way of life must change to coincide with the other. The choice is ours.

References

Further details on the two peoples mentioned may be found in the following reports, formal and informal, of my field work:

The Forest People (New York: Simon & Schuster, 1961), a descriptive account of the Mbuti.

Wayward Servants (Garden City, N.Y.: Natural History Press, 1964), a more
    formal detailed account of the Mbuti and their relationships with the
    villagers.
The Lonely African (New York: Simon & Schuster, 1962), a general account of
    problems of alienation facing tribal Africa emerging into a world of
    Western concepts and technology, with specific examples and biographies
    from a single village in Zaïre.
The Mountain People (New York: Simon & Schuster, 1972), a descriptive
    account of the Ik of northern Uganda and of the process of social
    degeneration.
    French translations of the above are available as follows:
Le Peuple de la Foret (Stock, 1963).
L'Africain Desempare (Seuil, 1965).
Wayward Servants and *The Mountain People* are in the process of translation
    and publication.

Familial Influences on Infant Development in an East African Agricultural Community

P. Herbert Leiderman, M.D.* and
Gloria F. Leiderman, Ph.D.* (U.S.A.)

Introduction

We have reported in a previous paper [8] that psychological test performance of Kikuyu (Kenya) infants selected from the population of a periurban agricultural village is related to certain familial, economic and demographic variables. These variables include economic resources available to the family; the number and age distribution of persons living within the household; the presence of simple modern amenities such as calendars, books, and radios within the household; and the sex of the infant. In this chapter we shall examine how these variables might be related, particularly emphasizing the degree to which the economic level of the family influences child-rearing practices in an East African agricultural community undergoing rapid modernization.

In general it appears that major characteristics of sub-Saharan African communities which are undergoing modernization and urbanization are the rapid shift in economic status, family values,

---

* Child Development Research Unit, University of Nairobi, Kenya, and Stanford University.

family structure, and child-rearing practices. In many families newly involved in the cash economy, women frequently bear a greater burden of responsibility for household management in addition to their child-rearing activities, partly because the traditional male roles are less meaningful in the changing society. This is particularly true in those families where, in order to move into the cash economy, husbands live in urban areas distant from the family household. Although these changes in family relationships cannot be attributed solely to an increase in the affluence of the family, changes in the family structure and in child-rearing practices frequently accompany increased family affluence.

Description of Community

Before proceeding to a detailed account of the daily routine of the typical family in our sample, we shall first describe the village in which our study was done. This is a Kikuyu-speaking community of some 4500 individuals, located about 25 miles from the urban center of Nairobi at an elevation of approximately 7500 feet in the Kenya highlands. The highlands, extending out from Nairobi, consist of gently rolling hills and ridges, covered by the luxuriant foliage of trees, shrubs, and grass nourished by the 35 inches or more of rain per year. The lands which had formerly been heavily forested have been largely cut, and rows of trees or shrubs now mark the limits of the rectangular-shaped plots of land.

The village is approximately four miles from the nearest paved road, which leads to Nairobi. The roads into the location are made of clay or dirt and frequently become impassable during the season of heavy rains from April through June and light rains in October and November. The village center is located about three miles from the area of the Kenya highlands settled by Europeans (British), but this proximity has had relatively little influence on the village itself, since the European community was, and remains, chiefly oriented toward Nairobi.

The community covers an area of approximately 10 square miles. The village center consists of a market and meeting place, surrounded by a series of small shops in well-constructed stone buildings. Most of these sell a variety of goods, although several are specialized, in that there is a tinsmith, a bicycle repair shop, and a cloth and tailoring shop. We identified three sections within the community, differentiable on the basis of distance from village center, type of family structure, and size of family plots of land. The one nearest to the village center consists of small households, generally on small plots of land usually less than one acre in size. The houses are made of rough-sawn wood with tin roofs, though dispersed among them are some modern houses and occasional traditional Kikuyu circular houses made of mud and wattle with a thatched roof. Households in this central section are located on small lanes and paths aligned along the larger mud roads. The homes are partially screened by trees, separating the families visually from the roads though not auditorily from one another. Some of the families in this central section have plots of land adjacent to their houses; many others have small plots a distance away. The major crops grown are maize, beans, and millet. A few chickens are kept, and very rarely a cow.

A second section of the community consists of traditional Kikuyu compounds, which are typically occupied by polygamous families. Here the houses are of traditional circular construction, with thatched roofs, arranged in groups of four or five structures on plots of land of generally at least two acres, and in some cases more than four acres. Families in this section have sufficient land to keep cows and chickens, and more land than those in the village center on which to grow staple crops.

A third section of the community is made up of families living in modern rectangular houses, of somewhat better construction, on plots of land greater than two acres. Like the families in the traditional compounds, several of these have outbuildings for storage of maize. Frequently adjoining plots belong to members of the same lineage. Most of the individuals in this section therefore generally have extended family relationships, with husband's brothers' families and grandparental generations living in other houses on the same plot or adjoining houses on separate but contiguous plots of land.

Water could be bought at one of two pumps or taken from the river. Families with greater economic resources are able to obtain tin rainbarrels to collect water from their roofs, thereby saving the cost of water from the pumps. Some families are affluent enough to have taps in their home compounds. None of the homes had electricity or cement floors at the time of the study. There are only four private vehicles within the community, none owned by individuals included in the study. There was one telephone located in the village center. Contact with outside communities is made generally by walking, although there is bus service available to Nairobi several times a day from the village center.

Fuel for cooking and warmth is obtained by the women in the household. Sometimes accompanied by their young daughters, they would walk from one to five miles several times a week to cut wattle trees and carry loads of wood to their homes. If the family had sufficient cash resources, fuel could be purchased from "charcoal burners," who would deliver to the village center or, in some instances, to the homes directly.

Cash crops consisted mainly of pyrethrum, which is grown cooperatively within the community. A few families keep sufficient chickens to sell eggs commercially, although none of the families in the sample did so on a large scale. A few families with cows are able to sell surplus milk to a milk cooperative.

Health services are provided by means of a mobile health team that comes once a week from a distant community. More generally health care is obtained at a community health center manned by a medical assistant, located five miles away. Our research project provided medical attention to members of the sample on a half-day per week basis.

Familial Economic Level and Infant Development

Although there appear to be considerable economic and status differences within the community, it should be obvious that a concept of social class as used in Western studies cannot be transferred to a vastly different culture with different value orientations. In United States studies [5] concerned with the role of social class in child development, familial income and father's education are used as indices of social class. In our previous study, we did not find that the amount of parental education was predictive of infant's psychological development and therefore decided to use only the economic level as a simple variable to describe differences between families. It should be understood that social class is not an explanatory variable but rather a means of identifying different groups of families to search for specific factors that might influence child development. Thus family economic level, as used in this study, merely provides an index of economic resources available to the family and cannot be construed as equivalent to the Western concept of social class or socioeconomic status. At some future period, if an index of Kikuyu socioeconomic status is needed, it might serve as one element in such an index, providing as little or as much to African studies of infant development as has the concept in studies of child development in the United States.

There are obviously many ways in which family economic level may influence a child's psychological development, ranging from the purely physical, such as malnutrition, to the purely social, such as variety and intensity of social experience. In any given study, however, it is possible to include only a small portion of the variables involved in determining a child's growth and development. For example, we did not examine the role of maternal nutrition in this study, nor did we evaluate through laboratory tests the infants' nutritional status, although nutrition might seem an obvious choice in studies relating to familial economic level and child development. However, those studies which have examined the effect of maternal nutrition during pregnancy [11] and infant nutrition in the first year have not found this a powerful influence in psychological growth. In this particular study, all infants were breast fed and survived through 1 year of age. Clinical examinations of the infants before, during, and at the end of the study did not reveal evidence of gross nutritional abnormalities. Therefore it is reasonable to conclude that malnutrition did not play a major role in the relationship of familial economic level to infant test performance.

Economic level and infant test performance can also be affected by the size and composition of household, but it cannot be assumed that the larger the family, the greater the drain on total family resources and hence the greater the burden on family members responsible for providing the basic resources. Indeed, larger families offer the possibility for greater help in household chores. More important than size, however, is family composition. As we reported in our earlier paper [8], infant test performance was higher if the household contained adolescents and individuals over age 40 and fewer children under the age of 3. These findings strongly suggest that additional assistance for the mother in her farm and household chores or a decrease in her caretaking responsibilities enhances infant development. Thus the degree to which a mother may share

responsibility for the infant with a caretaker is obviously of great
importance in the development during the first year. The main
thrust of this chapter then will be to contrast maternal and caretaker
behaviors, related to familial economic level, as influences on
infants' development during the first year of life.

Description of Daily Activity of Mother, Caretaker, and Infant

To better understand the data collected and analyzed, it might be
helpful to describe a typical day for mother, caretaker, and infant in
this village. We start with the mother. The activity of the vast
majority of women in the sample centers about the household, the
agricultural fields, the market, and, on weekends, the church.
Typically a woman arises before dawn, kindles the fire, and prepares
food for the day. Food consists of ground maize, millet, and
occasionally beans, served with hot tea mixed with milk and
sweetened with sugar. The food prepared in the morning frequently
lasts for the entire day and is sufficient to provide for the entire
family's needs. In a home with an infant, the mother nurses him
while performing her household tasks. Frequently by 6:30 or 7 AM,
she is on the road, with or without her infant, to fetch water or wood.
Usually accompanying her on these journeys is an older daughter,
anywhere from 5 years to early adolescence, who helps the mother cut
wood and carry water. If the infant accompanies the mother, he may
be strapped on her back, by means of two towels, with his head
uncovered if the weather is suitable or covered if not. Support for the
infant's back and neck is provided by the second towel. On the return
journey from the water source or the forest, the infant may be carried
against the mother's chest or, if carried by the daughter, strapped to
her back.

On those days when mother goes to her fields to cultivate her crops
or perform other seasonal tasks, young girls, occasionally the boys,
assist the mother. Whether the mother takes her infant to the field
depends on the infant's age, the season of the year, the availability of
a caretaker, and perhaps her own inclination. In general, mother will
take her infant regularly to the fields until he is 3 or 4 months of age.
She may have a caretaker with her to watch the infant while she
works but stops her work to nurse him. In the early afternoons mother
frequently returns home from the fields to manage the affairs of the

other children and proceed with household tasks, such as grinding maize, washing clothes, or directing the older children in household chores. However, depending on the amount of work that she has to do in the field, she might remain there for the entire day but come home at least once during the day to observe her infant if he was left at home. At the end of the day mother and children gather for an early evening meal which consists of the maize and millet prepared in the morning as well as the usual hot tea and milk. In the evening, the husband might spend time with the mother and children, or he might prefer to socialize with his male friends in the village center.

Most families retire fairly early, usually shortly after dusk. The infant sleeps with his mother, and the other young children sleep in special places within the hut or very near the mother. Depending on the size of the house and the observation of traditional practices by the family, the husband generally sleeps in a separate hut or separate room. Older boys sleep in separate huts or in their father's room if there are no separate sleeping quarters.

Two days a week the mother visits the central market within the village or, depending on the amount of produce she has available for sale, she might move to a more distant market. The market, of course, provides the opportunity for socializing with other women, and it is used for this purpose as well as for commercial transactions. Frequently the infant accompanies mother on these journeys to the local market. An older sibling of the infant might accompany the mother to a more distant market to help carry him, or he might be left at home with a caretaker.

If the mother holds an outside position, the routine naturally is different. Such a woman might be a nursery school teacher or work in a tailor shop in the village center. She would go off to her small shop or to school, usually returning at midday to take care of the infant who had been left with a caretaker. These women tend to be more educated and hence less involved with the traditional practices of the community, and even though they are away from home more, they are inclined to spend more time with their children and husbands when they are at home. Husbands of these women generally have cash incomes. Although such fathers do not necessarily spend more time with their children during the day, they might very well do so in the evening.

The role of infant caretaker and mother's helper is an important one for the infant. Typically, the mother's principal caretaker is a young girl aged 10 to 12 years, occasionally a young adolescent, and rarely a male sibling and/or a paternal grandmother living in the household. Most typically, the young caretaker is the older sister of the infant, but if there were no older female sibling available, children might be recruited from the mother's natal family or from other families in the village. The caretaker may have completed at least two years of "nursery school," finishing by the age of about 8 years and, if fortunate, may have had from three to five years of primary school, finishing by age 11 or 12. Her education in most cases was terminated for lack of funds or lack of family interest in schooling of female members. She would be old enough to know the responsibilities of the household, yet young enough to want to be included in the children's games and activities.

In her typical day, the caretaker gets up with the mother and helps with activities about the house. She frequently accompanies mother to collect fuel and water, usually taking responsibility for the infant during these journeys. If needed, she accompanies her to the fields where she may assist in cultivating and planting or care for the child while the mother performs her chores. If the infant is left at home in the care of this young girl, she is solely responsible for his care and arranging for his feeding and other needs. She provides food if he is old enough to take supplemental food, or, if he is still nursing, she might carry him to the mother in the fields. Depending on the interest and sense of responsibility of the young caretaker, she may watch the infant extremely carefully or she may do so in a more desultory manner, giving in to the temptation of playing with her friends and sibs while overseeing the activities of the infant. However, most of the caretakers take their responsibilities very seriously, and many are genuinely interested and involved in the young infants in play as well as in caretaking tasks.

From the typical infant's vantage point, his first year might be considered as the halcyon period of his life. He spends the first 4 months in almost constant contact with his mother. He is fed on demand, accompanies her on journeys, sleeps with her, and is comforted at night by the warmth of her body. By 4 months of age he has seen or heard most of the activities in the household and has been stimulated tactically and kinesthetically by being carried by his mother and his many sibs. He probably has not had much social interaction with his mother, at least in the form of verbal communication, but has probably had a considerable amount with his sibs and other children. His father has most likely looked at him but has not held him nor played with him, though this pattern might be changing as fathers in the more modern group take more direct interest in their young infants.

By 4 months of age, the infant has been introduced to his caretaker. By 5 to 6 months, the infant is with his caretaker almost half of any day, although for much of that time she might be distracted by playmates and household chores. Mother continues to nurse him on demand but occasionally, by 6 months, she will not be immediately available so he is fed other foods or must wait to be nursed. By 6 or 7 months of age he is allowed greater freedom. He is put on the ground to move about, and usually crawls by 7 to 8 months and walks by 10 to 12 months. Mother is still the central figure in his life, though she clearly shares her caretaking activities with other individuals. As the infant grows older in the first year, his caretaker and other sibs become an increasingly important part of his social life. Routine caretaking is still mostly the responsibility of the mother, but in most other activities he is guided by his own wishes, under the direct supervision of a caretaker and the indirect supervision of his mother.

Although this description typifies the mother-infant interaction, as the infant goes through the rapid changes of the first year, there is considerable variation in the amount of time and attention he receives from other family members. The father, however, may remain only distantly involved. Although children are highly prized both for themselves and for the social status they may bring their parents, the weight of tradition and outside obligations limit his direct contact with the infant during the first year.

Sample

Our sample consisted of 67 infants and their mothers. Originally 90 families were selected out of an estimated population of 100 families in which infants were born during the period of 1 July–31 December 1969. Of these infants 18 were used as controls and will not be reported. Five infants and their families were lost to the study when they moved away, or they were dropped after missing two or more tests or interviews.

Table 1 Description of Sample ($N = 67$)

	Mother (%)	Father (%)		Mother (%)	Father (%)
Age			**Language spoken**		
15–20	01		Kikuyu only	37	14
20–25	25 ⎫		Kikuyu and Swahili	29	27
25–30	21 ⎬ 17		Kikuyu and English	02	00
30–35	24 ⎫		Kikuyu, Swahili,		
35–40	13 ⎬ 38		and English	32	59
>40	16	44	No information $N=1$		8
No information $N=0$		10			
Birth order			**Church membership**		
1	11	22	PCEA	44	29
2	18	24	Baptist	06	05
3	27	17	Catholic	19	16
4	18	16	Anglican	11	13
5–6	20	17	African Greek		
7–8	06	03	Orthodox	18	10
No information $N=1$		9	None	02	27
			No information $N=2$		8
Education			**Nairobi travel**		
None	41	18	Daily	03	55
Standard 1–4	25	25	Weekly	11	11
Standard 4–6	10	02	Monthly	38	14
Standard 7–8	13	42	Yearly	35	09
Teacher training			Never	13	11
or Form 1–11	07	13	No information $N=4$		11
Technical training	04	00			
No information $N=0$		12			

The description of the sample is presented in Table 1. It shows that the group is a relatively diverse one in terms of age, education, household arrangements, amount of land, occupation, languages spoken, and contact with urban centers. All of the individuals within the sample were members of the Kikuyu tribe. Most of the men and about half of the women had lived in the community since it moved from a former site one mile away at the end of the "Mau Mau rebellion" in 1958.

Information about the families was obtained by means of interviews with mothers and observations of the homes undertaken by two University of Nairobi undergraduate students fluent in Kikuyu and English. Demographic information and ethnographic data were collected on both the mother and father, as well as information on age, education, current employment, household density, and

Table 1 *(continued)*

	Family (%)		Family (%)
Years married		Land	
Unmarried	08	None	14
1–4	22	< 1.9 acres	43
5–9	25	2–3.9 acres	29
10–14	17	4–9.9 acres	07
15–19	10	> 10 acres	07
20–24	10	No information $N=9$	
25	08		
No information $N=8$			
Family structure		Occupation of father	
Monogamous	68	Job with salary (trained)	42
Nuclear	32	Job with salary (nontrained)	09
Paternal	29	Business	09
Maternal	07	Part-time work	02
Polygamous	12	Subsistence farmer, < 2 acres	14
Divorced, separated,		Subsistence farmer, 2-4 acres	06
widowed	12	Subsistence farmer, > 4 acres	04
Unmarried	08	Unemployed	14
No information $N=2$		No information $N=9$	
Children in family		Educational materials in household	
Study child only	18	None	24
2	16	One	12
3	10	Two	07
4	12	Three or more	57
5	12	No information $N=0$	
6	10		
7	06		
8 or more	16		
No information $N=0$			

economic resources available to the family. In addition, home observations were made on the availability of modern amenities such as calendars, books, and playthings. Approximately two-thirds of the sample were identified with three lineages residing within the community; seven of the nine traditional clans were represented by either the mother or father of the infant. All of the sample were personally acquainted with the senior investigators and were volunteers to the study. They understood that we were particularly interested in how children grow and develop.

Infant test performance was determined by means of the Bayley Test of Infant Development [2] given in standardized form by a

specially trained British-educated Kenyan nurse. Pilot testing of
infants not involved in the study yielded reliabilities of 85 percent
agreement between the investigators and tester on the final two of
ten infants.

Infant Testing

Infant testing began in January 1970 and continued through
September 1970. Of these infants, 23 were born between 1 July and
30 September 1969, and they were tested at intervals between the
ages of 6 and 14 months. Another 44 of the infants were born between
1 October and 31 December and were tested between ages 1 and 9
months. All infants were tested at least three times and those tested
most frequently eight times, at approximately 2-month intervals.
Additional testing was done of a subsample at 1-month intervals,
accounting for the larger number of tests for control purposes. Of the
infants, 65 were tested at least four times and 2 were tested only three
times. Testing was conducted in either the morning or afternoon at
times when infants were judged to be alert and awake. Transportation
was provided from the infant's home to the testing site within the
village to minimize fatigue of mother and infant and to maintain
schedules.

As a first step in attempting to elucidate the relationship between
infant test performance and familial economic level, we took
advantage of the fact that each infant was tested several times in the
first year, thereby providing us with the opportunity to determine the
rate of development as well as the level of performance. To do this,
a straight line was fitted to the log of items passed on each test against
the age of the child for both the mental (perceptual-sensory) and
motoric (neuromuscular) portions of the test. This statistical approach
yielded a slope representing the "rate" of psychological development,
and an intercept representing the "average level" for the child. These
fitted curves were a reasonable approximation to the actual scores
obtained, in that they reduced the variance of the simple mean by
over 70 percent for all but two infants. Performance at 6 months was
the point selected for determination of the intercepts since all infants
in both groups had scores at the 6-month age point. It should be
emphasized that all scores for these infants were related to the Kikuyu
sample and not to United States norms.

Economic Level

We determined the economic level of the family by selecting five demographic items from the interview questionnaires which were thought to best characterize the varying economic circumstances of families within the village. They were (1) the amount of land available to the family; (2) the presence of cash income; (3) the number and type of cows owned by the family; (4) the number of chickens kept by the family; and (5) the source of water supply. This choice of items is based on knowledge of the criteria used by individuals within the community in determining differences in economic level. An additional advantage of these particular items was that they could be determined by observation or by direct report by the mothers.

Each of the five demographic items was scaled to obtain an index of familial economic level. The sample was divided into three groups of approximately equal numbers based on these composite scores. A typical family in the lowest group can be characterized as having little land or no land to farm, no cash income, no cows, few chickens if any, and water obtained from the river or perhaps from the village pump. A family in the middle range might have two to four acres of land, no cash income, no cows, perhaps a few chickens, and water obtained either by purchase from the village pump or from a neighbor who could afford a tap. A family in the upper group would typically have a farm of at least two acres, and generally more than four, with cash income, one to four local cows or one grade cow, several chickens, and water obtained from the village pump or from a home tank or outdoor tap.

Familial Economic Level and Infant Test Performance

The relationship between infant test performance and familial economic level was determined by correlating the slope and intercept for the mental and motor tests with the index of economic level. For the total sample of 67 infants and their families the correlation between mental intercept and economic level was +.39, correlation for the slope was −.32, both significant at the $p < .01$ level. The data suggest that a positive relationship between economic level and infant test performance on the mental test is found utilizing the *level*

Table 2   Relationship between Familial Economic Level and
Infant Test Performance during First Year (*N* = 67)

	Intercept	*r*	Slope	*r*
Mental	61.4	+.39**	.12	−.32**
Motor	27.7	+.25*	.12	−.22

**$p < .01$.
*$p < .05$.

of performance rather than the rate of development. Indeed, rate of development is inversely related to the economic level, suggesting that environmental influences occurring after birth are such as to bring the scores of the infants from different economic levels closer together over time.

Our interpretation of these data is that the difference in performance level between these infants is either present at birth or begins very early postnatally. It might be inferred that genetic or prenatal factors are of crucial importance in determining these scores, since social influences had little time to manifest themselves. The negative correlation for slopes suggests that the later postnatal influences detract from the superior performance of the upper groups within this sample.

For the motor scores, the correlations between familial economic level and motor intercept is somewhat lower, +.25, $p < .05$, whereas the correlation for slope, though negative, is not significant. Findings for the motoric test performance parallel the findings for the mental test but are less powerful, suggesting that the motor test performance is relatively unresponsive to postnatal influences, or that perhaps the test itself is a less differentiating one for this population group.

These same data are illustrated in Figures 1 and 2. Means were obtained for the slope and intercept for the three economic level groups separately, and as can be seen they are consistent with the correlations obtained for the total sample. The middle and upper level groups have very similar mental intercept and slope scores, as can be seen in Figure 1. The lower economic group is distinctly lower on mental intercept and slightly higher on slope. The middle economic level group scores highest at the 6-month intercept point in the case of the motor tests, as seen in Figure 2. Differences between the middle and higher economic groups are small and approach statistical significance only in the case of the motor score. The observation that the middle group scores highest in the motor test is

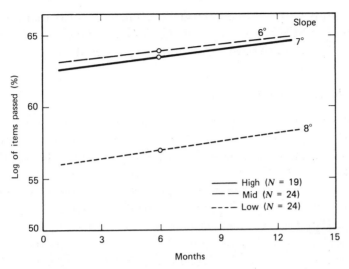

Figure 1 Familial economic status and infant test performance—mental test.

noteworthy if we refer to the findings of Geber [4], who reported that higher socioeconomic groups actually perform less well on motor tests than lower groups. If we assume that our sample distributes over a lower economic range than did hers, and her upper economic group was at a higher income level, then our positive relationship between economic level and test performance and her findings of a negative

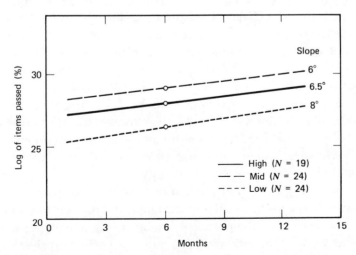

Figure 2 Familial economic status and infant test performance—motor test.

relationship are more easily reconciled. The possibility that the relationship between test performance and familial economic level is curvilinear rather than linear should be considered.

Caretaking Behavior

Before proceeding with the determination of how maternal caretaking might influence infant development in relation to familial economic level, it is important to determine who actually does the caretaking for the Kikuyu infant during the first year. To obtain information on the behavior of the caretaker, whether the mother or another individual, we adapted a method developed by Munroe and Munroe [10]. Unscheduled periodic visits were made to the household by a research assistant who observed the activities of the mothers and other household members in relationship to the infant. Each of these observations lasted 5 minutes. Observations of the infant included sleep, caretaking, playing, walking, moving, feeding, and social interaction. Those of the mother included instrumental caretaking tasks, holding, carrying, socializing, and proximity to the infant. If in a given 5-minute period the behaviors were rapidly changing, then the initial observation was recorded. The mothers were not apprised in advance of the visit. Three high school level village residents, trained in the observation techniques, were responsible for the observations.

Every mother or caretaker and infant were seen in the course of daytime activities between 8 AM and 6 PM. Each household, over a period of 9 months, was seen at least 8 and at the most 23 times with an average of 15 observations per home. Scores for maternal and caretaker behaviors were determined by frequencies as a percentage of that particular behavior observed in relation to the total number of observations made in the same household. In three households no caretaker was ever observed, and in two households the mother was never observed taking care of the infant. Agreement between observers using this technique was greater than 80 percent for a series of ten observations done simultaneously.

The data (Figure 3) indicate that the mother is the primary caretaker of the infant until about 5 months of age. From that time she is observed to be the principal caretaker less than 50 percent of the time while other caretakers take more responsibility. For the rest

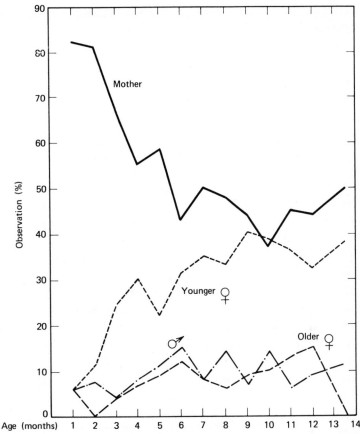

Figure 3 Identification of caretaker.

of the infant's first year, the young female caretaker is observed with the infant about 40 percent of the time and a young male or older female (grandmother) for the remaining 10 percent or more of the time.

The question of what the mother or caretaker actually does in relationship to the infant is clearly important. Because of the relatively few observations on older women and males, we examined only the behavioral relationship referable to the mother and younger female caretaker. The data are shown in Figure 4, and are summarized for the entire year ignoring developmental changes occurring with the infant's increasing age. Therefore these data should be considered only as trends until a more definitive analysis can be made.

The major differences between caretaker and mother are in social interaction with infant, carrying infant, and proximity to infant. Mothers spend a greater proportion of their daytime activity than caretakers near their infants, a smaller proportion in socializing and carrying them, and about the same proportion in instrumental caretaking activities and carrying them while doing other tasks. These findings suggest that mothers spend much of their daytime function in overall supervision of their infants, but they rely to a considerable degree on the caretaker for many infant care functions such as carrying and social interaction. Many of mother's caretaking functions are shared with at least one other individual. Despite the frequently reported observation [6] that the African mother is with her infant almost constantly during his first years, this is not accurate for this community. The mother is not free to be with her infant constantly and must rely heavily on others for infant caretaking in order to accomplish the multitudinous task in managing her household. Most definitely she is a "working mother" with more or less full-time help. Whether this multiple mothering influences later psychological development must await further empirical study.

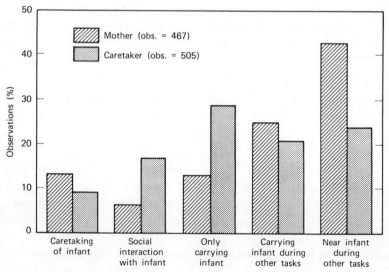

Figure 4 Summary of maternal and caretaker behavior during infant's first year.

Economic Level and Caretaking Activities

The next step in the data analysis is to examine the relationship between familial economic level and caretaking activities. Table 3 shows that the presence of mother is negatively related to familial economic level. This indicates that mothers in the highest economic group spend less time with their infants. When maternal presence is subdivided into specific caretaking activities, only carrying behavior is negatively related to economic level.

When maternal behavor is partitioned for the three economic groups, carrying by mother is seen to be less and social behavior greater for the highest economic group, although the second finding is not statistically significant. These data suggest that mothers of the highest level, when present, did less carrying of their infants and more social interacting with them than did mothers in the other two economic groups. The sample size is too small for these data to be statistically significant, but considering the possible importance of social stimulation in the psychological development of the child, then this finding may serve as a lead to future studies.

The equivalent analysis for caretaker behavior is presented in Table 4. The presence of the caretaker is correlated $+.57$ with economic level, the obverse of the findings for mothers and predictable since either the mother or the caretaker was present at any given time. None of the specific caretaker behaviors was significantly related to familial economic level.

Examination of the data differentiated by economic groups indicates again that the caretaker behavior was somewhat different in the high group when compared to the low groups. Caretaking behavior was greater and carrying behavior was lower for the

Table 3 Maternal Behavior and Economic Level

| | Total ($N=67$) | | (Observed %) | | |
	Observed (%)	r	Low ($N=24$)	Mid ($N=24$)	High ($N=19$)
Mother present	53	$-.57**$	70	49	35
Social activity	6	$+.11$	6	5	8
Caretaking	15	$+.09$	14	14	16
Proximity	37	$-.01$	38	38	16
Carrying	38	$-.31*$	43	43	28

$**p < .01.$
$*p < .05.$

Table 4   Caretaker Behavior and Economic Level

	Total ($N=67$) Observed (%)	r	Observed (%) Low ($N=24$)	Mid ($N=24$)	High ($N=19$)
Caretaker present	47	+.57**	30	51	65
Social activity	16	+.11	12	20	16
Caretaking	8	+.22	6	7	13
Proximity	23	+.21	19	19	34
Carrying	47	−.17	50	53	35

**$p < .01$.

highest economic group. This finding seems to imply that caretakers for the highest economic level group behaved differently from caretakers in the lower economic groups. Whether these caretakers received different instructions or whether the infants elicited different behaviors from caretakers is not known. On the basis of what we know of the community, we would lean toward the first explanation rather than the second. It is likely that caretakers in the families of greater economic means have fewer household chores to perform while caring for the infant and thus can attend more directly to the infant's needs rather than having to carry him while doing other household tasks. Again, more definitive analysis and additional observations are required before a conclusion can be drawn.

Maternal Behavior and Infant Test Performance

The final step in the present analysis is an examination of the relationship between maternal and caretaker behaviors and infant test performance. In this chapter we can only indicate trends in these data. Future analyses will be performed to relate specific maternal and caretaker behaviors to specific cognitive and psychomotor behaviors of the infant.

Maternal and caretaker presence was plotted against time for each infant for all observations. A best fit straight line was calculated for each individual. The slope and intercept of maternal and caretaker presence were correlated with the slope and intercept of the mental and motor performance of the infant (see Table 5). The average (intercept) level of infant's performance at 6 months was positively related to caretaker behavior for both mental and motor performance, suggesting the importance of the caretaker in determining infant's performance at this point in his development.

Table 5   Relationship between Caretaking Behavior
and Infant Test Performance

	Mental		Motor	
	Slope	Intercept	Slope	Intercept
Mother present intercept	+.37	−.42	+.25	−.26
Caretaker present intercept	−.37	+.42	−.25	+.26

However, since caretaker presence is positively related to familial economic level, this finding may merely indicate the influence of other variables associated with caretaker behavior.

More intriguing perhaps, because it lends support to maternal stimulation theories of precocious infant development, is the finding that mother's presence is positively related to the rate (slope) of mental and motor test performance. Thus despite the wide differences between infant's performance, the rate of psychological development is positively associated with the presence of the mother. At this point in the data analysis, specific maternal behaviors, such as social interaction, carrying, or caretaking, contributing most to this association cannot be differentiated.

In both of the analyses done thus far, mental performance yielded higher associations than did motor performance. This finding implies that the Bayley mental test is more sensitive to social influences, reemphasizing the point that performance on the motoric test may be more a function of innate biological factors than is the mental portion of the test.

To summarize, these data are supportive of other work indicating that the presence of mother is important for the infant's psychological development during the first year [3]. Her presence appears to affect the *rate* of development and appears to have very little effect on the average *level* of the infant's performance at 6 months. Her presence has less effect on the *level* or *rate* of motoric development, perhaps suggesting that performance in the motor test is more closely related to biological or constitutional factors than is the mental test performance.

Conclusions

The major findings in this study are (1) familial economic level is related to the "average level" of infant test performance and not

the "rate" of development; (2) caretaking behaviors vary with
economic level of the family; (3) infant caretaking involves "multiple
mothering," especially after 5 months of age; and (4) mother's
presence is positively associated with the rate of psychological
development during the infant's first year.

To understand the relationship of mental and motor test
performances to the economic level of the family, a genetic
explanation may reasonably be invoked. It can be argued that the
level of performance is determined by the time of birth or very
early in the course of the infant's development since social
environmental factors have not yet been operable. This conclusion
must be tentative since we did not specifically control nutritional
factors, nor did we directly assess genetic component in the infants,
their parents, grandparents, or sibs. Nevertheless, the findings are
consistent with such a hypothesis.

One possible explanation for the mechanism by which such
genetic differences could have arisen can be found in the bride-
wealth system of the Kikuyu [7]. This system has been in effect for
at least 300 years since the Kikuyu became intensively engaged in
agriculture, and it may have been the practice before that time when
the Kikuyu were still a mixed agricultural and pastoral people.
Under the bride-wealth system, the father of the prospective groom
was traditionally obliged to provide the father of the prospective
bride with one to three cows, or ten to thirty sheep or goats. More
recently, cash has been substituted for stock in order to complete
the marriage contract. Although the amount of bride-wealth was
fixed within certain limits, it could vary depending on the wealth
of the groom's father and the desire on the part of both families for
the marriage. The number of cows, goats, or sheep available for the
bride-wealth within the groom's family depended in part on the
number of married or marriageable daughters, in part on the prowess
of the father's family in acquiring cows through raiding neighboring
groups or through trading, and in part on the amount of land
available for grazing and farming.

The amount of land owned by the Kikuyu was carefully defined,
since land was not held in common but belonged to individual
families or lineages. Thus the amount of land that a family might
acquire would depend on the strength and drive involved in clearing
the forests, or the skill in trading and retaining it through dealings

with one's neighbors. Further, the acquisiton of strong and healthy wives to cultivate this land was not an inconsiderable factor. Thus the size of the herds and the amount of land would be important criteria in determining selection of brides. If there was selection pressure over many generations, encouraging the marriage of wealthy and clever men to strong, hardworking, and long-lived females, then the progeny of such unions might well be biologically superior. This superiority might be reflected in infant test performance, especially when assessed in the first year of an infant's life, though one might expect it to hold for motoric as well as mental test performance.

Having presented this hypothesis as a plausible one, we readily admit that it is based on many unproven assumptions. The important point to emphasize is that genetic factors cannot be discounted in these findings and, in fact, may be crucial in evaluating the early postnatal development of the infant.

The second finding of this study concerns the variation in infant caretaking by familial economic level. This should be no surprise to Western observers making observations in their own cultures who recognize economic class differences, and it is not unexpected in studies of non-Western cultures undergoing relatively rapid social and economic changes. This finding merely underscores the necessity to include assessment of subgroup variation, even in societies that superficially appear to be relatively homogeneous. In areas where change is occurring rapidly, such variables as economic resources may be indicators of involvement in a changing life style, and they may also provide the opportunity to examine the relative influence of social, psychological, and biological factors as they influence infants' growth and development.

The third major finding of this study concerns the relative contributions of mothers and caretakers in caretaking functions during the infant's first year. The myth of the ever-present, ever-devoted African mother is simply not borne out in the Kikuyu case. The Kikuyu mother, on the average, spends only about half of her daytime activities involved with her infant after he reaches the age of 5 months. A considerable proportion of daytime infant care is undertaken by a caretaker, generally a girl or young woman between 6 and 16 years. The mother has far too many obligations to provide necessities of life for the family to be involved in direct care of the infant, except for feeding. She is generally without any help in physical tasks from another adult. If she is particularly fortunate, she may have an older daughter to help her; a grandmother might be available; or she may have the resources to hire a caretaker. Depending on the skill of this caretaker and the mother's managerial skills, the infant may or may not receive the direct attention that the Kikuyu mother might like to provide her infant if her other obligations permitted.

The major implication of this observation is that care of the Kikuyu infant is polymatric rather than monomatric. Although some observers of sub-Saharan African infants [1] have assumed the primacy of mother in infant caretaking, these data, along with the observations of others [9], indicate that this generalization is unwarranted. In this study we have provided a semiquantitative assessment of the mother's and caretaker's contributions to caretaking during a period when it is expected that mother is pre-eminent in the infant's life. Whether this shared maternal role is characteristic of agricultural people, whether it is of recent origin even among the Kikuyu, must await further historical and ethnographic reports from other cultures.

As the Kikuyu family undergoes further modernization and assumes forms more characteristic of Western societies, the shared maternal role may give way to the single caretaker model. If such a shift occurs, it may place an additional burden on the mother, who may be quite unprepared for the major responsibility for her infant, apart from the possible advantages to the infant of polymatric versus monomatric caretaking. This issue may not be dissimilar to problems facing urban groups in transition in Western society. Anticipation of the problem in those societies undergoing rapid change might help avoid some of the less constructive effects on mothers, and possibly on infants, that we have discovered in our own society.

On a more theoretical level, the study of shared caretaking in the early years is particularly valuable for understanding the development of social attachments. In the Kikuyu case, the mother is almost solely responsible for feeding the infant in the first year. She shares most other activities with other female caretakers. How does this shared nonfeeding caretaking behavior affect social attachments? Does the Bowlby-Ainsworth [1, 3] thesis concerning the primacy of mother in mother-infant bonding hold for this group of mothers and infants? Does the intensity of attachment to mother differ from the attachment to the more socially interacting caretaker? If the very early attachments are triadic, what effect does this have on psychological and social development of the child and the family structure? These fascinating theoretical issues, of course, must await more thorough study of societies and individuals varying in early attachment relationships.

The last finding concerns the role of the mother. Does she have any influence on the infant's cognitive and motoric development in the first year? Our finding indicates that maternal presence is associated with the *rate* of mental and motor development of the infant. Given the particular behavior observation techniques employed, however, this finding must be considered with reservation. We were able to measure only a few influences of the mother on her infant. Clearly there was a consistent bias in times of observations, leaving a lack in our knowledge of mother-infant interactions occurring at night and on weekends. In addition, we have not reported on specific cognitive and social behaviors of the infant as they relate to mother or caretaker behavior. These additional analyses are undoubtedly of considerable importance, and although in progress, they must be completed before conclusions can be drawn.

Our analyses to date indicate that the mother's presence, whether in direct contact with her infant or in supervision of others caring for the infant, facilitates his mental development during the first year. Motor development is relatively independent of maternal influences during this period.

Current Kikuyu society demands a great deal from the mother but, on the other hand, provides her with a support network for the care of her infant. This polymatric arrangement is based on family bonds and may have a very differential impact on the developing infant from either a traditional kibbutz caretaking institution or our currently controversial United States day care centers. Thus the study of such a system may provide insights for planning alternative mothering for infants in Western society as well as understanding infant development in rapidly modernizing societies.

Acknowledgment

Ths work was supported by Carnegie Foundation grant to Professor John Whiting, Harvard University, and by Grant Foundation grant to P. H. Leiderman, Stanford University. We wish to thank Dr. Helena C. Kraemer for statistical analyses, Barbara Andersen, Adrienne Lindstrom, and Rosalind Revell for research assistance, and Tome Tanisawa for typing of the manuscript. We are particularly grateful to Beatrice Babu for infant testing, Violet Gatheru, Eunice Mutero, Arthur Ngiritta, Florence Waithira, and Irene Njeri for data collection. Our special appreciation to Professors John and Beatrice Whiting who in many ways made this study possible.

References

1. Ainsworth, M. D. S. *Infancy in Uganda. Infant Care and Growth of Love.* John Hopkins Press, Baltimore, 1967.
2. Bayley, N. *Bayley Scales of Infant Development.* Psychological Corp., New York, 1969.
3. Bowlby, J. *Attachment and Loss.* Hogarth Press, London, 1969.
4. Geber, M. In *Growth of Normal Child in First Three Years of Life,* Vol. 7, A. Merimond, Ed. Karger, Basel, 1962, p. 138.
5. Hess, R. D. Social class and ethnic influences on socialization, in *Carmichael's Manual of Child Psychology*, Vol. 2, P. H. Mussen, Ed. pp. 457–558. John Wiley & Sons, New York, 1970, pp. 457–558.
6. Jeiliffe, D. B. and Bennett, F. J. Aspects of child rearing in Africa. *J. Trop. Pediat. Environ. Child Health*, 18:1 (1972), 25–43.
7. Kenyatta, J. *Facing Mt. Kenya, The Tribal Life of the Kikuyu.* Martin Secker & Warburg, London, 1953.
8. Leiderman, P. H., Babu, B., Kagia, J., Kraemer, H. C., and Leiderman, G. F. African infant precocity and some social influences during the first year. *Nature*, 242:5395 (1973), 247.
9. Levine R. In Psyche and environment, by W. Muensterberger. *Psychoanalyt. Quarterly*, 38 (1970), 191–216.
10. Munroe, R. H. and Munroe, R. L. Household care and infant care in an East African society. *J. Soc. Psychol.*, 83 (1971), 3–13.
11. Stein, Z., Susser, M., Saenger, G., and Marolla, F. Nutrition and mental performance. *Science*, 178 (Nov. 17, 1972), 708–713.

Nutritional Factors in the Vulnerability of the African Child

Adewale Omolulu, F.R.C.P.I., F.M.C.P.H., D.P.H., D.C.H. (Nigeria)

Maternal undernutrition is the rule rather than the exception in Africa. The American Academy of Sciences recently reviewed the problems of maternal nutrition in pregnancy in the United States [3], but the problem in Africa is much worse than the findings of this report. The intake of the rural nonpregnant Nigerian woman is about 1850 calories, and this intake is not increased during pregnancy. The average gain in weight during pregnancy is 6 kilos, as opposed to the 12 kilos expected in developed countries. The child is at birth mature but "small for age" with an average birth weight of 2.8 kilos. The percentage of babies below 2.5 kilos at birth is nearly 20 percent (as opposed to 5 percent in developed countries). These small for age children have a high neonatal mortality; in one of our studies in rural Nigeria, the neonatal mortality rate was ____ per thousand singleton births.

Widespread and long-lasting breast feeding in all areas has been the saving grace of the African child. With adequate breast feeding, the rate of growth of these children has been shown to be more than that of children of developed countries. By the time he is 3 months old the African child has caught up in weight.

It is unfortunate that the sophistication of Western civilization, the indiscriminate high-powered salesmanship and advertising of the babyfood manufacturers, and the modern tendency of mothers having to go to work in offices and shops where there are no facilities for continuing breast feeding are resulting in a movement toward artificial feeding. In a recent survey in Nigeria [1] it was found that most mothers in big towns were using both the bottle and breast milk. Of the highly educated elite women interviewed 96 percent used both the bottle and breast feeding; of the middle-class working women, 88 percent, and of the illiterate townswomen, 45 percent. Only in the rural villages was 100 percent breast feeding reported— but even here there were signs that this state of affairs would soon change. In the clinics, village women with adequate breast milk flows are seen changing to bottle feeding and bringing up their children with marasmus, failure-to-thrive, and gastroenteritis. These conditions result from inadequate milk formulas due to low economic status and inability to buy enough milk powder for the formula, lack of understanding of sterilization of bottles and feeds, and poor environmental sanitation. There is an urgent need for governments to take an interest in this move toward artificial feeding on the continent, since most countries in the developing world do not produce milk powders. If the move to artificial feeding is not slowed, governments will have to find the foreign exchange needed to import large quantities of milk powders and formula that will be needed. The strain on the already inadequate health services is also great. Most hospitals and health centers in the towns have had to set up rehydration units to cope with the large numbers of children brought in with gastroenteritis and dehydration.

The mother-child relationship is made much closer in African surroundings by the act of breast feeding, the mother carrying the baby on the back and the child sleeping with the mother on her mat or sleeping place. Traditionally, the mother is not allowed to leave her house or do any work for 40 days after delivery. During this time she is well fed, bathed, and all her wants and needs supplied by her husband, her parents, and her in-laws. She can thus recover from the stress of childbirth, devote her whole attention to the baby, building up a good and lasting rapport. The provision of food, fuel, and money for these 40 days lying-in period was one of the main responsibilities of the husband. Unfortunately, urbanization as well as the need to work has cut down and in some cases prevented the observance of this traditional practice. The child as well as the mother has been the worse for it.

The act of breast feeding is looked upon as a normal process all over the continent. Whenever a child cries it should be breast fed. Thus breast feeding takes place in the bus, in the market, during meetings and discussions, with no feeling of shyness by the mother nor of repugnance by others. On the other hand, Western civilization teaches that the breast should not be seen by other people. This teaching has been learned by the educated, sophisticated elite and is slowly spreading down the line. In urban areas it is now rare to see mothers breast feeding their children. They prefer to breast feed at home, undercover or even in their bedrooms. A hungry, screaming child may be carried unfed for a long distance till a "safe" place is found for breast feeding. Medical personnel are also advocating special sleeping places for the baby, away from the mother because of the fear of the mother overlying the child. This separation of the child from the mother will have both nutritional and psychological results. During a recent survey of child-feeding practices in a village in Nigeria [2] it was found that in some cases the child got most of its breast feeds from the mother during the night. These mothers fed water to the children most of the day because they were busy working; they offered the breast in the evenings, during the night, and in the mornings.

After the fourth month, yields of breast milk are inadequate to supply the nutritional needs of the child. Unfortunately, in most African countries traditional weaning foods are low in both calories and protein. Gruels or paps, made from cereals like maize, sorghum, or millet, are the main weaning foods in most parts of the continent. These gruels and paps contain over 90 percent water, with protein contents of 1 percent or less, and they supply only 30 calories per 100 milliliters (cf. breast milk with 1.2 percent protein and 70 calories per 100 milliliters). In almost all cases the rate of growth of the child slows down after the fourth month of life. By the end of his first year the child is fed primarily paps or gruels, getting only a few sucks from the breast. During this time, too, the child starts crawling on the ground, picking up ova and cysts of intestinal parasites. The child is also now left with the older children, thereby coming into contact with their childhood communicable diseases like whooping cough, polio, measles, and smallpox. All these insults coming over a relatively short period of time and falling on an undernourished child result in an almost continuous period of fevers, coughs, and gastroenteritis.

In some areas of the continent the child is not given solid food until he is walking—any time from 12 months to 18 months—or until he starts grabbing food during adult feeding times. The average African child is thus nutritionally famished from about the ninth month of life till he starts eating the adult diet, about the twenty-second to twenty-fourth month of life. The fevers and illnesses make him irritable and unable to respond to love, which puts a great strain on the mother-child relationship. Traditionally, the mother is not allowed to become pregnant till the child is weaned at 22 to 24 months. Mother can thus devote her whole attention to the child. With urbanization and the breakdown of tradition, it is now not unusual to find mothers being pregnant when the child is only 12 to 16 months old. The result is usually disastrous for the child. As soon as the mother finds herself pregnant, she stops breast feeding, believing that the breast milk would harm the child. The weaning has of necessity to be abrupt and sudden, thereby creating great psychological stresses on both mother and child. Nutritionally, the child, who had not been introduced to adult diet, is now suddenly deprived of its main source of protein—breast milk—and forced to either subsist on paps and gruels or start taking the peppery, "hot" adult foods.

With all the preceding stresses, it is understandable that the highest incidence of protein calorie malnutrition (PCM) in most parts of the continent occurs during the second year of life. In Nigeria the highest incidence of PCM is seen about 18 months. In a few countries of North Africa, where breast feeding is stopped at the age of 3 months, marasmus is seen during the second half of the first year of life. The position in most countries of Africa is like that of Nigeria, where kwashiorkor, marasmus, and other forms of PCM are seen in the second year of life. The incidence of PCM in most countries of Africa is around 4 percent of children at risk. In Nigeria 50 percent of cases are obvious kwashiorkors and the other 50 percent marasmus. Apathy is one of the important signs of kwashiorkor and is present throughout the condition. The lack of interest in the surroundings, inability to eat or play, and lack of response to motherly love and care create a great strain on the mother and make both treatment and rehabilitation of kwashiorkor cases long and difficult. By the time most cases of kwashiorkor come to hospital, their mothers have lost interest in them due to the apathy of these children.

Apart from medical treatment, the restoration of the mother-child relationship is one of the problems in the rehabilitation of cases of kwashiorkor. This apathy affects the awareness of the surrounding and in most cases has repercussions on training, intelligence quotient, and book learning. Due to the acute shortage of beds in most African countries, doctors cannot afford to keep these patients until they are fully rehabilitated. Cases are therefore sent home before they are fully recovered. It is hoped that the setting up of Nutrition Rehabilitation Units, where the mother and child are looked after on discharge from hospitals, will fill this gap and hasten full recovery as well as the return of mother-child rapport.

The ambulant African child is normally the responsibility not only of his parents but also of his extended family and, in rural areas, of the whole village. He is welcome in all homes; relations and friends of his parents are always ready to receive and look after him; he is allowed to partake of any food that is available in any home he visits. Thus, although he may not be adequately fed in his own home, the older child soon realizes that he can eat in other homes and he makes use of this facility.

Once the child is on the adult diet, he has to conform with the eating practices of adults. In areas where eating is from a common bowl, he has to learn to fill his stomach in competition with the others. In some rural areas only two meals are taken in a day. Father leaves home early to get to his farm without breakfast so mother does not prepare breakfast. If there are no leftovers, the child counts himself lucky to get money to buy food from the food vendor. The main meal in rural areas is in the afternoon, when father returns from the farm. Since the preparation for cooking does not begin until father's arrival, food may not be ready until 4 PM or later. After this heavy meal, the adults may not have the evening meal until 9 PM, by which time the child may be asleep.

Most African countries and their governments now realize the importance of formal education and allocate 30 percent or more of their budgets to the provision of this amenity. In some states, compulsory primary education has been introduced, and children of 5 to 6 years must start schooling. Schools are sited so that no child has to travel more than three miles to get to his school. One of the important causes of the high failure and dropout rate is the lack of attention to the nutrition of the children. In rural areas, the child has to walk the distance to school. This may take an hour and he therefore leaves home by 7 AM. Since breakfast is not usually prepared at home, he gets to school hungry. He is then made to sit down to lessons till 11 AM or later, when he gets a break to buy food! The conditions in the big towns are not better. In Lagos (Nigeria), due to the traffic bottlenecks, parents and children must leave home by 6:30 AM to get to work and school at 8 AM. After this long strain of traveling, the child does not get a break to eat until 11 or later.

In the sedate noncompetitive life of yesteryear, the African child was able to withstand these nutritional upsets and emerge victorious. The fast life of urbanization, formal education, and competition are placing extra strains and stresses on these nutritionally starved children. There is a need for us to take a good look at these children and work out ways of alleviating some of these stresses.

References

1. Breast Feeding in Nigeria, *Children of the Tropics*, No. 82, 1972.
2. Food Science and Applied Nutrition Unit, University of Ibadan, unpublished material.
3. *Maternal Nutrition and the Course of Pregnancy*, National Academy of Sciences, 1970.

A Note on Kwashiorkor as Anorexia Nervosa in Infancy

Henri Collomb, M.D. and Simone Valantin (Senegal)

Since the initial description by Williams in 1932–1935, kwashiorkor
has been generally regarded as a consequence of protein deficiency
occurring at the time of weaning. However, since all African
children suffer from some degree of protein deficiency at this time,
the question arises as to why only a few of them develop kwashiorkor.
It occurred to us, arguing along the lines of Spitz's work on
hospitalism [1], that there may be a psychological aspect previously
overlooked.

The symptoms of kwashiorkor include anorexia, behavior
disturbances (aggressivity, seclusiveness, emotional lability),
psychomotor regression, loss of speech, and skin lesions.

To investigate our hypothesis, we carried out an extensive
sociodemographic survey on 1000 cases, and a psychological study
focusing particularly on the family dynamics.

We arrived at the following conclusions. Kwashiorkor is more
frequent in urban than in rural settings, although protein deficiency
is more severe in rural areas. It is also more frequent in districts
undergoing recent and rapid urbanization where the socioeconomic
level is not remarkably low. It seems to involve selectively the oldest
sibling, occasionally the second, and only exceptionally the later
offspring. Curiously enough, the illness does not receive the usual

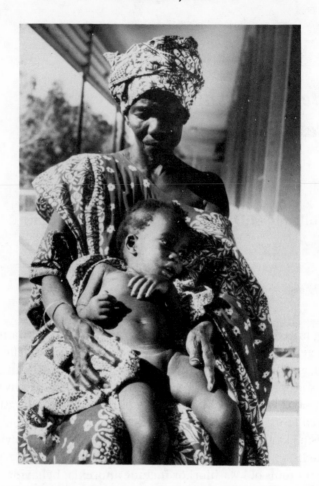

traditional explanation placing the blame on some antagonistic
force in the outside world or ancestors.

    The most significant facts are the association with recent
urbanization and the occurrence at the time of weaning. This
suggests that the mothers under the stress of a new type of life may
find it difficult to care adequately for the child once weaning has
been completed and there is preoccupation with the new baby.
When kwashiorkor develops, the causal factor is located in the child,
who is accused of hostility toward his future sibling and of drinking
the milk of the pregnant mother that is being reserved for the new
baby. His aggression is punished by the development of the illness,
and his resentment of the future sibling speaks against him.

The word itself, kwashiorkor, has some interesting derivations. In the language of Ghana it means "first-second," indicating the jealousy of the oldest child to the siblings that follow, and in Rwanda in East Africa the word used for the disease means "to be abandoned." The psychological implications seem well understood. For instance, if an adult sees a child crying in the street, he might very well ask: Is your mother pregnant, and did you catch the kwashiorkor?

In our study at Dakar, we observed that cases followed for three or four years no longer show any differences from the normal population of children, although this is based on observation and not on any systematic psychological investigation. Furthermore, the mothers in this group have reported separation problems with regard to their own mothers during their childhood.

A very tentative explanation therefore is that there is a psychodynamic factor involved in the causation of kwashiorkor and that this involves the projection of aggressivity by an anxious mother exposed to the stresses of recent urbanization, a mechanism of which she herself is unaware. Initially this finds expression through the child's symptoms, but later on, in the second stage, it becomes organized around him in a number of traditional explanations. There is therefore some dynamic similarity to anorexia nervosa occurring much later on.

Reference

1. Spitz, Rene. Hospitalism—An inquiry into the genesis of psychiatric conditions in early childhood, in *The Psychoanalytic Study of the Child,* Vol. I. International Universities Press, New York, 1945, p. 53.

The Black American Child in School

James P. Comer, M.D. (U.S.A.)

From the beginning, the United States has been concerned about the education of its youth. But it has been a differential concern. The children of the most powerful and most privileged people in most communities received the best education. They were groomed for leadership and control of the nation's governmental, business, industrial, and educational institutions. They, in turn, established social policy which maintained the status quo.

Less privileged groups and individuals were forced to fight for educational opportunities, which, because of industrialization, soon became critically linked with economic opportunities, which, in circular fashion, affected educational opportunities. As the nation changed from an agricultural society with a low level of scientific and technological knowledge through a moderate level to a high level of such knowledge, reflected in products and tools, the level of educational and social development needed to be secure in the nation's job market changed accordingly.

The application of science and technology dramatically changed the demands on most workers from physical strength to educational, social, or relationship skills. Before the turn of the century a man could be uneducated and unskilled and still find a job that would enable him to care for himself and his family. In the generation that followed into the 1940s, a person needed a moderate amount of education and skill to be reasonably secure on the job market.

From the 1940s into the decade of the 1970s, a person needed a
relatively high level of education and skill to be secure in the job
market. Today even a high level of education and skill is not always
protective, as is evidenced by the plight of engineers, schoolteachers,
and other occupation areas where there is an oversupply.

People who were able to gain and hold jobs which enabled them
to provide for the basic needs of their families were in a better
position to provide family members with emotional security and a
good foundation for educational and social development than those
who were not able to gain and hold such jobs. Children from
inadequate income families were at greater risk from the standpoint of psychological, social, and educational development.
Certainly some children from inadequate income families developed
well and some children from adequate income families had
developmental difficulties. Nonetheless, numerous studies show a
positive relationship between adequate income and adequate social,
psychological and educational functions and vice versa [6, 8, 13].

Since America was a land of new immigrants and former slaves
during the crucial industrial development years between 1865 and
1915, there was always a new and vulnerable group being closed out
of educational and economic opportunities. Each immigrant group
had to gain political and economic power to force the society to
provide the education and training opportunities its members
needed to keep up with changing job and social demands.

The former slaves, Black Americans, were more vulnerable to
exclusion from adequate opportunities than any other group. Anti-
Black sentiment ran higher than antagonistic feelings toward
immigrants and religious minorties for a number of complex
reasons [4]. Blacks, fresh from an experience of forced dependency
and extremely limited personal and group opportunities, lacked the
group cohesion, "know-how," and institutional supports other
groups brought with them. Most important, Blacks were not
protected by the laws to the extent of other groups. Through
violence, fraud, and racist politics it was possible to deny Blacks
access to political or policy-influencing power.

Because Black rghts were not protected, Blacks were closed out
of meaningful participation in the labor unions. Not only did the
unions provide many people with some job protection and training
opportunities, but they provided them with experience in

organization, politics, and policy negotiations. Unions provided
many people with a sense of power and influence in a societal climate
that, without question, put production needs ahead of the developmental needs of most people. Without power—at the ballot box or
through unions—Blacks were closed out of adequate income jobs
and social and educational opportunities more than any other group.

As a result the Black American child was and is at greater risk of
social, psychological, and educational difficulty than most other
children [3]. Yet many Blacks have developed mechanisms to reduce
the risks, indeed, to enable their children to thrive in families, in
school, and in adult society [1]. Today the school remains an
important institution. It holds the key to the Black American
future. But too many efforts are made to understand the problems of
Black children in school without paying attention to the nation's
record with regard to Black education. Because of this, too many
programs miss some of the "necessary ingredients" for improving
Black education.

The Record

Before the 1915 northward migration of Blacks, more than 90
percent lived in the South. Public education for White southerners
did not exist to any great extent until the 1870s. (Ironically the fact
that it existed at all was due in large part to legislation enacted by
Black influenced Reconstruction legislatures.) From the earliest date
of public education in the South, what was available to Blacks was
of a lesser quality and quantity than what was available to Whites.

As late as the 1930s the nine states containing almost 80 percent of
the Black-population had expended two to four times as much
money on the education of a White child as it did on the education
of a Black child. In areas where Blacks were in a sizable majority,
the disparity was even greater—more than twenty-five times in some
cases. In 1931–1932, Georgia spent $9.50 per pupil for Black
education compared with $41.02 per pupil for Whites; Alabama,
$10.72 for Blacks, $40.90 for Whites; Louisiana, $12.86 for Blacks,
$62.21 for Whites; North Carolina, $18.08 for Blacks, $41.12 for
Whites; Florida, $17.33 for Blacks, $48.71 for Whites; South
Carolina spent $8.08 per Black student, $53.00 per White student [2].

A further indication of the lack of interest the society had in

Black education is reflected in school enrollment figures, median years of school completed, and the percentage of illiteracy in the population. In 1850 1.8 percent of the Black population was enrolled in school as compared with 56.2 percent of the White population. Most Blacks were still in slavery. In 1870 9.9 percent of the Black population was enrolled in school as compared with 54.4 percent of the Whites. It was not until 1950 that the Black student population came within five percentage points of Whites enrolled in school [9].

The median number of school years completed by Blacks in 1940 was 5.7 as compared with 8.7 for Whites. As late as 1967, the median completed by Blacks was 9.1 years compared with 12.1 for Whites. In 1940 1.1 percent of the native-born Whites were illiterate, 9 percent of foreign-born Whites and 11.5 percent of Blacks. In 1959 7.5 percent of the Black population was illiterate compared with 1.6 percent of the Whites [8, 14]. The enrollment figures do not tell the whole story. It must be remembered that Blacks were often in school for one or two months a year compared with eight or nine months for Whites. Until very recently the physical plant of Black schools was always less adequate than that of White schools. Before 1900 Black teachers were often high school graduates whereas White teachers were graduates of normal and four-year colleges. Until the last two decades, most of the teachers in Black schools were less well trained than those in White schools. Yet the record shows there was and still is a desperate desire for education among the Black population.

What was true of elementary and public school education was also true of college level education. Because the states refused to provide sufficient money for Black land-grant colleges under the first Morrill Act in 1862, a second act was passed which required states to provide equal funds, even if the schools were segregated. In spite of this legislation, the states were slow to form Black schools and they received an unequal share of the funds once established. In 1930 Blacks made up 23 percent of the total population of the 17 states maintaining racially separate institutions. Yet Black colleges, as late as 1936, received only 6 percent of the funds given to each state for the support of land-grant colleges. The federal government was not much better. In 1955, 52 land grant colleges for White students received 25.7 percent of their budget for education and general purposes from federal grants. Seventeen Black institutions received only 3.1 percent for the same purposes.

In a 1964–1965 survey of college and university endowments, only three Black institutions—Hampton Institute, Tuskegee, and Fisk—reported endowments above the average $9 million level of the 882 institutions reporting. Well-known institutions—Howard, Lincoln, and Meharry Medical College—were among the 28 Black colleges in the study. Predominantly White Harvard had an endowment of nearly $600 million—now over $1 billion. Its predominantly Black counterpart, Howard, with only one-third fewer students, had an endowment of just over $5 million. In fact, the 1964–1965 endowment of all 100 Black colleges was about one-half that of the 1964–1965 endowment of Harvard [11].

Equally troublesome as inadequate financial support was the attitude about Black education reflected in the despair of the missionary Daniel Earl of North Carolina writing in 1761: "the Planters urge it a sin and politick to enlarge the understanding of their Slaves, which will render them more impatient to slavery" [11]. A similar concern existed through the 1950s. Many Black colleges and even public schools were formed simply to pacify Blacks, with no intention of making them first-rate institutions providing first-class education. These institutions often were controlled by racist school boards that did not encourage creative and scholarly inquiry, particularly in areas that might affect the status quo.

More important, Black colleges and universities were closed out of the mainstream of academic life. Black scholars often were denied admission into professional associations and even when admitted, could not expect to receive recognition for outstanding work. Because of inadequate funding, teaching loads were excessive; thus research and professional development were difficult. Blacks were not on national academic policy-making or certification boards. Black scholars did not flow between educational, business, and government institutions, gaining knowledge, money, and contacts that would benefit their institutions and their students. Motivation for a high level of scholarly work and progressive curriculum programming was not possible under these conditions. The detrimental impact of this situation on educators in Black schools and, in turn, on the students themselves can never be fully measured.

The Consequences

Inadequate funds, undereducated personnel, inadequate facilities,
a school board acting to oppose rather than support progress, and
exclusion from the academic mainstream did more than result in
undereducation. These conditions were a message to Blacks: "You
are not valued or wanted in society. You are not expected to fully
participate as first-class citizens." This message had an extremely
adverse psychological impact. If dramatic changes in the nature of
the American economy and job market had not been taking place,
this situation would have been immoral and a psychological trauma
but not a major social catastrophe.

It is now more clear than ever before that education begins at
home; parents and early caretakers are the first and most important
teachers or child developers. Listening language, concept formation,
abstract thinking, and strategies for learning are well on their way
toward full development by the time a child is 5 years of age.

Such development occurs best in environments of safety, care, and
affection, with parents able to understand and respond to a child's
needs and desires in a way to stimulate the learning processes. It
occurs best where parents can set reasonable limits to protect children
from their own aggression, channel it, and convert the aggression
into the energy for learning. Such development occurs best where
parents are good behavior and learning models for children.

Such conditions occur least often in high conflict families, in
depressed and apathetic families. Low-income families without, or
with a conflicted sense of belonging, direction, and purpose—
regardless of race—are more often affected in this way. For historical
reasons, a disproportionate number of Blacks are so affected.

A 1973 report by the Twentieth Century Fund Task Force shows
that more than 30 percent of young Black males, the age of starting
families, are unemployed in many cities [12]. Many others are
barely earning a living wage. Although the problem receives more
attention today, it is not new. Since slavery, many Blacks have just
barely earned a living. Thus many Black males or heads of households who had little or no control over the fate of their families in
slavery, for economic reasons, often had and have little ability to
provide for themselves and their families after slavery and until this
day. The psychological and social consequences of this situation for

the Black family, community, and child development have been the focus of many studies.

The resultant adult, often male, displacement of anger and frustration onto family and friends in many cases has been described. Excessive child neglect and abuse is often reported. Frequent family breakups and movement in search of better conditions are much discussed problems. Conflict and insecurity, as well as the resultant acting out, apathetic, and depressed behavior of many adults appears to hamper the cognitive, social, and psychological development and behavior of too many Black children. This, in part, leads to underachievement and troublesome behavior in school. It must be remembered that this is not the outcome for a majority of Blacks.

Compensatory Mechanisms

Efforts to compensate for educational underdevelopment among many Black children have focused on individual deficit. This is understandable. The deficit appears to be individual, definable, easily modifiable. Individual deficit suggests that the problem is not in families, institutions, or societal attitudes and arrangements. It is a less guilt-provoking focus for those who, in one way or another, identify with persons or systems responsible for unjust and handicapping attitudes and arrangements.

Because of the focus on individual deficit, the successful, adaptive and compensatory mechanisms of the Black community have received less study and attention than needed. This is unfortunate because it is here that one should look when one is trying to fashion appropriate compensatory programs. Such studies should show who "makes it" and why. They should suggest better institutional and societal arrangements and attitudes than we now employ.

The major adaptive mechanism was religion and/or the Black church and the subculture that formed around it after slavery [7]. The Black church became a "substitute society" for a people excluded from the total society. It enabled many Black families to protect themselves from the adverse impact of economic and social exclusion as well as extreme psychological trauma.

It fostered an important and necessary value system—honor in work, cooperation, fair play, love of family and fellowman. It promoted a delay of immediate gratification through the promise of a reward in heaven and recognition and approval from fellow church members here on earth. It was a place where Black people could experience the leadership or executive functions they were denied in the larger society. Leadership skills were developed here in a way similar to (but not the same as) the way they were developed by immigrants in labor unions. (The Black church trustees were very much like city council members.) It was a place where people ignored in the larger society could exercise their talents and experience a sense of belonging, value, and worth.

Most of all, the Black church was a place where Blacks could have a sense of psychological ownership in a social system. This permitted a better than should be expected outcome for many Black families living under the oppressive and stressful conditions of societal rejection and economic marginality.

The distinguished Nigerian psychiatrist Dr. Thomas Lambo pointed out that an important spiritual force has sustained oppressed African peoples everywhere. It is my impression that Africans brought to America borrowed a foreign institution—the White church—modified it to meet their spiritual and organizational needs, and made it their own—the Black church. It was the spiritual orientation of Africans that made this adaptation possible. Once the church became an important institution, it produced and sustained the spiritual force to which Dr. Lambo refers.

Many White families gained direction, motivation, and purpose by accepting the values of the larger society, being accepted by the society, and experiencing a sense of belonging. Adequate income and participation opportunities in the larger society rendered the White church less important. Inadequate income and participation opportunities in the larger society made the Black church a very important institution and the major source of direction, motivation, and purpose.

The church permeated all of Black community life. Colleges, businesses, and social organizations such as lodges and clubs often emerged from it, greatly influenced by it. Studies of Blacks and Whites by job, income, and occupation which ignore the Black person's status in the church miss a crucial variable. Because Blacks were closed out of the economic mainstream, more Blacks will have less education and poor jobs. But that was less predictive of motivation and potential than a Black person's status in the church.

Many of the most successful Black families—even though they are no longer involved with the church, or even reject and condemn it—can trace their roots to this "substitute society." The importance of this background is reflected in the makeup of a compensatory education program for which I was a consultant in 1966. Of 125 Black students from 10 southeastern states picked for the program on the basis of academic promise, 95 percent had one or both parents who were regular churchgoers, deeply involved as organizers and leaders in the church community [5].

This situation is rapidly changing as mainstream opportunities increase for some Blacks. Yet many Blacks are still very much involved with and rely on the Black church for social and psychological sustenance.

I am aware of the criticism of the Black church. With only a few exceptions the church leadership failed to recognize that the Black church was a "substitute society" as much as a spiritual enrichment center. While the threat of psychical violence and economic reprisal was there, it could have become more of a political and economic force in behalf of Blacks than it did. On the other hand, without the church the Black community would have suffered greater fragmentation, greater family and individual social and psychological trauma than it did.

I discuss this matter here only to point out that the church provided Blacks with what is universally necessary for good human development and functioning—a sense of belonging and ownership in one's social system. It is this need that has not been considered or met often enough in social and education programs in the Black community.

Obviously the church and every other adaptive effort made by Blacks were not enough. Far too many Black families were adversely affected by destructive circumstances in the total society. Families which were not able to protect themselves from the impact of economic deprivation, with resultant adverse social and psychological consequences, were and are least able to prepare their children for school. There is another area of the problem. Many Black parents provide their children with an excellent emotional experience, but because of the exclusion from the mainstream of American life they are not able to provide some of the social inputs or experiences needed to maximize cognitive development. Despite the past, it is my impression that most Black children receive a family and community experience that would enable them to make it in school. The problem for many begins in school.

The Black Child in School

Today political and economic influence needed to develop social policy are not simply matters of numbers at the ballot box or jobs. Science, technology, and social policy have forever changed the way that people come by wealth and power, power and wealth. Mineral finds, land grants, providing goods and services in a rapidly expanding economy, and so on, are much less possible now. Academic, work and social skills, and expertise are needed to influence the political and economic system—to bring about programs that will enable families to gain stability, programs that will maximize the opportunities of the Black child in school. This requires a school program that is not only good, but tailored to the needs of the community.

Unfortunately in the Black communities most in need, school programs are neither good nor tailored. The blatant inequities in financing prior to the 1950s and their detrimental consequences relative to personnel skills, motivation, facilities, and programming have been mentioned. There has been positive change in all these areas in the past few years. But these gains are limited by a subtle process of neglect and abuse that continues to hamper the progress of the Black child in school.

For many years now the problems of cities have been neglected or managed in a way that was least troublesome in the short run but extremely problematic in the long run. Public school systems—the second most critical institution in our society—usually receive attention after other municipal concerns have been attended. As a result school systems are too often forced to respond to "the squeaky wheel." Until the late 1960s the middle-income population, more often White, squeaked most.

Capital improvements went to schools in middle-income areas. Equipment and supplies often made their way to middle- and upper-income areas in greater quantity. Support personnel—aides, social workers, and others—were often assigned equitably by school but not by need, the greater need being in the low-income schools. Troublesome personnel were often shifted to the community of least resistance, usually overwhelmed Black communities. As a result, schools serving children and families with a greater number of problems were often "strapped" with the least able personnel, less support personnel, and less equipment and supplies. Most important, the school staff—even very able staff—is usually not trained to deal with the special problems of children, families, and communities in trouble.

Children, some with experiences and life styles different from those of the staff, presented the usual relationship questions: How much do you care? How much do you value me? How competent do you believe me to be? What will you tolerate from me? What are your expectations of me? Some—a minority, but more than in communities under less stress and in less trouble—presented beyond the average learning and behavior problems. Aggressive physical behavior, impulsive behavior, and other disturbing behavior on the part of some children is often viewed as "bad" behavior rather than the product of a less than desirable developmental experience.

A response by school staff that seeks to "crush out the badness" by harsh or punitive discipline only continues an undesirable relationship pattern too many children from difficult home situations already have with adults. It does not lead to a channeling of aggressive energy converting it to "the stuff" of learning. Skills—listening, language, abstract thinking, and so on—missed or underdeveloped the first time at home are missed the second (and often last) time at school. School underachievement or failure often leads to behavior problems. When many children are so affected schools develop poor learning climates, often chaotic, with a staff spending more time trying to keep order than it spends providing a learning experience.

The staff has been frustrated in its mission and the understandable reaction in "these kids." Too often poverty, blackness, and badness are associated as factors to explain underachievement. Negative attitudes and expectations of the children develop, even when they were not present in the first place. In a variety of ways, conscious and unconscious, such attitudes and actions promote more undesirable behavior. Management of the difficult problems often brings staff and parents into conflict.

Already aware of the fact that their schools are least well serviced.

negative attitudes and actions by the staff are simply additional proof of this to parents and community. Angry and distrustful relationships or apathy and hopelessness often pervade the community-school interaction. Racial, class, and income differences complicate this situation. As a result, even children who come from desirable family relationship experiences and have enjoyed good personal development before beginning school will not function well in such schools.

The strength or weakness of a community is its people. When they feel an institution in their setting to be foreign or antagonistic toward them, they can withdraw, attack, or ignore it. In the case of a school, there is ambivalence. Most recognize the school as the hope for the future of their children. Thus a double message is often sent to children in communities alienated from the school: The school is your friend and hope for the future; the school is your enemy.

It is more difficult under these conditions for children to identify fully with the staff, work, and direction of the school. The anger, the sense of powerlessness and hopelessness of parents and affected communities, can directly affect—adversely—the self-concept, motivation, sense of purpose, and achievement of their children.

Intervention must address at least three problems on at least two levels. Change must take place at the national social policy level. Intervention must take place at the level of the individual local school. Social policy must permit and enable more families to function well: must permit more parents to be better "first teachers." Schools—if not the society—must permit more people to have a sense of psychological ownership in them.

There is no way around the fact that better school functioning for more children will require adequate family incomes for more people. Certainly adequate financial support for all schools is needed. Programs to improve the training and selection of teachers and administrators for schools are needed. But much can be done now— at the level of local schools—with existing personnel.

One of the necessary moves is to reduce the conflict between schools and the communities they serve, or try to serve. To do this a mutually supportive alliance must be established between home and school. To establish such an alliance schools must involve parents in a meaningful way and make the school culture less foreign to the community subculture. A few schools have moved to share decision making with local communities. When done carefully, this addresses a long-standing Black community problem—a sense of exclusion, powerlessness, devaluation, and alienation. The involvement of parents in staff selection, curricular and extracurricular program development, workshops, and so on, goes a long way toward reducing staff-community antagonism and distrust. It goes a long way toward mobilizing the strength of a community—its people.

The community is engaged in a variety of religious and social activities. These include church choirs, banquets, and fashion shows. Through parental involvement in extracurricular activities such events move right into the school. This reduces the "foreign" nature of the school. The skills, work, and play habits involved in these activities can be integrated into the regular school program. A critical emotional link can be made between home, community, and school. With this development the values, work, and ways of the school can be taken on by parents and children who have ways that limit or interfere with good school performance.

Parents so involved begin to have a sense of psychological ownership of the school. But even more important, they come to see themselves as important contributors with regard to the future of their children. I have seen some parents so involved come to realize that they could better control their own lives and destinies. I have seen school staffs so involved develop more positive attitudes about children and their parents.

Finally, but most important, I have seen the changed or more positive attitude or climate of the school transmitted directly and indirectly to children. Then the process becomes circular. Children relate and achieve better in a climate where they sense that they are respected, belong, and are valued. Their academic and relationship performance improves. In return they are more highly valued and respected and around again. It is in this climate that preschool deficits can be compensated for and fewer school deficits occur.

There is an important lesson in such outcomes for national social policy. Critics of social reform programs often have said that money is not enough. It is often said that adequate family incomes would not help many people become better parents. Money is not enough. The missing ingredient is the opportunity to belong to an institution or group with supportive values, a sense of purpose, and a productive style as well as an opportunity to sense belonging and being valued.

National social policy—in addition to providing adequate money— must also bring about such outcomes.

There is less of a problem in this regard in middle-income communities. Middle-income, largely White parents feel less alienated from the school and the culture of the school. The staff is of the same or lower income group and style as the parents. Parents feel less powerless with regard to what goes on in the school and in the larger society. Compensatory education programs that do not attempt to address these problems where there is staff-community conflict "miss the boat."

I am not suggesting that low-income people or that Black people be forced to change their life style. In fact what is called the culture and life style of Black people and of poor people is often not of their making or their choice. It is often the result of being closed out of opportunities—educational, social, psychological, and so on. I am suggesting that the school that recognizes this and modifies its program to meet these needs can provide a choice. They can provide a place where parents and youngsters can gain the skills and styles necessary to function within the mainstream of the society, as well as within their own subculture. And after all, that is one of the functions of education.

References

1. Billingsley, A. *Black Families in White America.* Prentice-Hall, Englewood Cliffs, N. J., 1968, Chap. IV.
2. Blose, D. and Caliver, A. Statistics on the education of Negroes, 1929–30; 1931–32. U.S. Department of Interior, Office of Education, Bulletin 13. Washington, D.C., 1936, p. 16.
3. Clark, B. *Dark Ghetto.* Harper and Row, New York, 1965, Chap. V.
4. Comer, J. P. *Beyond Black and White.* Quadrangle Books, New York, 1972, Chap. IV.
5. Comer, J .P., Harrow, M., and Johnson, S. Summer study-skills program: A case for structure. *J. Negro Ed.,* Winter 1969, 38–45.
6. Deutsch, M. The role of social class in language development and cognition. *Amer. J. Orthopsychiat.,* 35: 1 (1965), p. 78–88.
7. Frazier, E. *The Negro Church in America.* Schocken Books, New York, 1962.
8. Gagne, *The Conditions of Learning.* Macmillan, New York, 1966.
9. *Historical Statistics of the United States, Colonial Times to 1957.* U.S. Bureau of the Census, Washington, D.C., 1960, pp. 213–214.
10. Letters from Missionaries (1761–1763), in *Social History of American Education, Vol. I. Colonial Times to 1860,* Rena L. Vassar, Ed. Rand McNally, Chicago, 1965, p. 47.

11. 1964–1965 Voluntary Support of America's Colleges and Universities. Council for Financial Aid to Education, New York, 1967, pp. 3, 21–59.
12. Twentieth Century Fund Task Force. *The Job Crisis for Black Youth.* Praeger, New York, 1973.
13. U.S. Department of Health, Education and Welfare, *Perspectives on Human Deprivation: Biological, Psychological and Social.* U.S. Government Printing Office, Washington, D.C., 1968, Chap. I.
14. U.S. Department of Labor, Bureau of Labor Statistics, The Negroes in the United States, Their economic and social situation. Bulletin 1511. Washington, D.C., 1966, p. 194.

The Risk of Going to School

Reimer Jensen (Denmark)

It seems almost provocative to speak of the risk of going to school at a time when many children in the world are unable to attend schools because there are no schools and when governments in many countries are making increased efforts and investments to build up or expand their educational systems. It has become a human right in the developed parts of the world to go to school, and schooling provides an important tool in raising the economic, technical, and cultural standards in developing countries. With these considerations in mind, is it at all realistic to talk about the risks of attending school? But risks there are and these should be investigated.

The positive aspects of schooling are fairly obvious. The school acts like a booster in the child's developmental process. It widens the child's experiential world and gives him a feeling of belonging to a larger group than his family or neighborhood. It opens up perspectives of history and possibilities for the future. It is a melting pot where individuals are mixed and transformed into homogeneous groups by the process of acculturation mediated through the teachers and crystallized in the curriculum. In some ways the school can be compared to a factory where children are taught to use tools that help them tackle the tasks that lie ahead in adult life. It carries out this role by utilizing the inborn capacities of the children and its own knowledge of the learning processes to generate an educational system within the individual child. Once again we have to ask ourselves how a positive subsystem of this kind can prove a hazard in certain cases.

The school is something like the family. We know how important it is for a child to grow up within a family to develop into a capable person with a well-functioning personality. Severe disturbances can result when he is deprived of family contact or some kind of substitute arrangement or when the family or its substitute fails to function adequately.

But even if the family, or its equivalent, is absolutely necessary for the development of the child, it can also prove a danger for the child, interfering with his development, with the functioning of his personality, his life experience, and his capacity to realize his innate potential as a human individual. It can also conduce to severe psychopathology.

In a similar way, the school may not only not fulfill its functions with respect to a certain child but may actually distort his development or direct it into channels at variance with his own natural line of development. It may make premature demands on the child when he is far from ready for them.

In short, the school can expose a particular child to experiences that may be detrimental to him in different ways. For example, it may create a feeling of inferiority or a tendency to avoid problems or of depending on other people to solve them. A teacher's evaluation of a child's performance often may help the child in building up his confidence; on the other hand, it may have a totally negative effect in undermining his enthusiasm and belief in himself. It may inculcate group attitudes, values, and behavior that create conflicts for the child in his adjustment to his family and community. He may have resources to cope with this complex situation and even to profit from it in the long run, or it may prove too much for him and force him into increasingly inadequate modes of response to the point of pathology.

It is a fact that communities offer schooling to their children not purely for the sake of the children but to secure their own future existence and development. They want their values and norms transferred to the new generation and in this sense it means that the children are sacrificed to the existence of the society. In the ordinary way, the school tries to find a balance between the needs of the child and the needs of the society, but there are, unfortunately, many examples where this balance is not obtained and the children become victims of a training that pays little or no attention to their special interests and needs. (Some educators, like Illich, are so sensitive to this aspect that they are in favor of abolishing the traditional type of school altogether as a major source of hazard for the development of children.)

Since there are no absolute standards or goals in child development, the school may become, at times, a battlefield reflecting the conflict of ideas in the society as a whole. Although in a democratic setting, it is not directly used as an instrument for political or religious persuasion, the educational system might react to situations in society in ways that exert undue influence on the child. The school cannot help but mirror society since it prepares the child for living in society and rewards and punishes according to society's standards.

Even when the school builds up a system of first aid and treatment facilities for nonconforming children, the fact cannot be disguised that children come out of school with very different experiences. Some profit from it and some suffer from it; some like to attend and others dislike it. How they look upon school has been investigated at many places and in many ways.

In a Danish-American study on adolescents in secondary schools a questionnaire was administered to the students regarding their attitudes to school, to home, to their peer group, to their further education, and to themselves. A large sample was used and interesting data were obtained, some of which have already been published (*Youth in Two Worlds*). It confirms the viewpoint presented here that going to school is a complicated process—at times a challenge but at times a risk to which the vulnerable children gradually succumb.

Competence and Biology: Methodology in Studies of Infants, Twins, Psychosomatic Disease, and Psychosis

Donald J. Cohen, M.D. (U.S.A.)

When Descartes separated mind from body, he left us with the central question of the philosophy of mind: How do physiology and experience interact? Those of us who are practically concerned about the lives of children require models of development which give appropriate status to both mind and body, and which are sufficiently explicit to guide research and action.

Without explicit models and shared understanding of how to conceptualize the organization of behavior or use basic concepts such as stress and vulnerability, child psychiatrists are themselves vulnerable to disciplinary difficulties. We may wander into conceptual roundhouses or unnecessary muddles; we may misinterpret data already available or fail to see connections; and we may overlook promising leads from other fields of inquiry.

This paper sketches a multivariate model or viewpoint which emphasizes biological endowment in interacton with psychosocial forces. The examples of empirical studies are drawn from my own work, often done with collaborators, and I try only to suggest the scope, without attempting to review, the literature that is relevant to this type of synthetic approach.

Congenital Organizaton of Behavior: Sucking to Reduce Distress

During the first day or two of life, when infants are given an empty rubber nipple on which to suck, they often mouth it, bite down, or emit sucks of irregular amplitude and uneven rhythm. As Wolff has demonstrated, within several days sucking behavior of healthy infants displays a well-defined organization. Children emit bursts of eight to ten even-amplitude sucks at a rate of about two per second, with pauses of several seconds between bursts [47, 96].[1]

When environmental events other than the delivery of milk were made contingent upon a child's sucking—for example, when sucking was followed by a loud noise or bright light—the sucking rate, once stabilized (in sucks per second), did not usually change. Instead, pauses between bursts tended to shorten. If the intensity of environmental stimulation increased even more—for instance, if the noise was made quite loud—the amplitude of the sucks altered and, finally, the entire sucking pattern tended to become as disorganized as during the first day or two of life. The child ceased sucking and cried. Thus increasing stress appeared to increase sucking until a point when an individual child's threshold was exceeded and his sucking system was disorganized.

The sucking rate and rhythms of about 25 2- to 5-day-old boys were measured during the acute stress of circumcision. A pacifier connected to a pressure transducer and recording apparatus was placed in the child's mouth. The child's heart rate was monitored by electrocardiography, and his behavior was observed. Two broad patterns of response to circumcision were explicated. In the first the infant continued to suck throughout circumcision, with shortened pauses between bursts of sucking and decreased pressure or amplitude of individual sucks. These boys tended to show only moderate increases in heart rate (up to about 160 beats per minute) and to have only transient upsets in their feeding and sleeping during the following day. The second, and more common pattern involved some degree of disorganization of sucking with biting and irregular sucks interrupted by long periods of crying and kicking. Many of these boys developed extreme tachycardia (up to 220 beats per minute) with occasional

---

[1] Dr. Peter Wolff, with whom the work on sucking reported here was initiated, has studied in detail the general role of rhythmic organizers and has illuminated their theoretical significance for understanding early development [95].

inversion of T waves on the electrocardiogram indicating a high degree of physiological activation. In contrast with the boys who continued to suck, those whose sucking disorganized tended to go off feedings, sleep more fitfully, and be irritable during the hours following circumcision.[2]

Such observations of stressed newborns provide material for constructing a simple model in which sucking is seen as a congenital capacity that functions to modulate distress and inhibit physiological overreactivity. Clinical use is made of this capacity when a colicky infant is given a pacifier on which to suck. In this model the basic sucking pattern and increased sucking with stress are congenitally organized and universal, whereas the threshold beyond which stress leads to disorganization (rather than to more sucking) is seen as individualized [26, 48]. Later, after introducing current biological ideas about the regulation of pleasure, we may speculate about the neurophysiological basis for this arousal-modulating system. But it should be underlined here that sucking is probably not the only arousal or distress-modulating mechanism available to the infant. Other active processes such as the redeployment of attention may also be operative. Sucking, however, is obvious and easily measured, and it serves as a convenient prototype.

In another study newborns who were lustily crying because of hunger were given a pacifier to suck while their total bodily movement and amount of crying were measured. After they were quiet, the nipple was quickly withdrawn. With increasing experience, newborns quieted more quickly when given the nipple and started to cry more quickly when it was withdrawn. This accommodation to the nipple could be observed even in 1-day-old infants with no postnatal experience with nutritive sucking. Although there were marked individual differences in the speed of quieting and the latency to cry after nipple removal—with the most comfortable infants quieting quickly but waiting to cry on nipple withdrawal—all infants showed the capacity to learn or accommodate to the use of the pacifier as a way of decreasing the distress and physiological upheaval of hunger and hunger-crying [13].

[2]For further discussion of the relation between autonomic changes and arousal, as well as for individual differences in autonomic responsivity, see Richmond and Lipton [73]; Richmond, Lipton, and Steinschneider [74, 75]; Graham and Jackson [36]; and Hunt, Lenard, and Prechtl [43].

Thus the sucking of healthy newborns seems congenitally organized to have a more rapid onset and fewer pauses in order to modulate distress. Because of genetic, intrauterine, or other factors, some newborns have significantly greater capacity to modulate internal distress by sucking than do others. For the newborn less able to modulate distress, major stresses such as circumcision and minor, daily, unavoidable stresses of frustration and discomfort are more likely to overwhelm the child's ability to maintain physiological homeóstasis and to remain experientially calm [6, 7]. Such episodes of being overwhelmed, in conjunction with the congenital endowment that leads to being easily overwhelmed, may be seen as the biological-experiential matrix for emergent, individual differences in the predisposition to anxiety.

In this simplified theoretical scheme, parents can be pictured as exerting their influence in three ways: by contributing the child's genes; by protecting the child from potential stress; and by comforting the child when his own defenses against overarousal are unequal to the challenge.

There is an extensive literature on the enduring impact of early experiences in animals and even in humans. The endocrine environment during gestation [58], early mothering in the premature nursery, obstetrical medication [8], and other experiences may have long-term impact on development. For example, infant rats who receive stimulation, handling, and increasing control of their environment show less anxiety when tested in an open field situation several months later [45]. Presumably, early infantile experiences shape the organization of early adaptations and also the ways in which a child will later respond to new situations. Optimal conditions for a newborn child involve enough stimulation to allow for the unfolding of functions such as the accommodation to the nipple and, at the same time, sufficient protection to prevent the child from repeatedly being overwhelmed by stress which he is unable to modulate.

Clinicians often observe that irritable children have sensitive, anxious parents. This correlation may represent the resultant of several forces. First, the parents' anxiety may represent their own genetic and unfolding endowment marked by disturbances in the modulation of anxiety. Second, anxious parents have difficulties in preventing a child from experiencing stress and in comforting him when he is overwhelmed by stress (which may be borne more easily by other children). Third, the child who is easily upset—as a result of his genome and his endowment—is more difficult to care for and thus is more likely to elicit parenting, from any adult, which is complicated by guilt, tension, and ambivalence. The parents of children with colic, general irritability, hyperactivity, and childhood autism—to name only some conditions in which the modulation of stress is impaired—are likely to be sensitive individuals themselves and to be very much upset in their attempts at parenting.

Stress Which Cannot Be Modulated: Childhood Eczema

What happens when stress cannot be modulated? Severe, unremitting childhood eczema provides a natural experiment on the impact of prolonged, internal distress in the first years of life. Childhood eczema is a skin disease that usually appears between the third and tenth month of life, starting as a mild rash on the face which then spreads to include the pressure surfaces of the baby's arms and legs. After a relatively benign course marked by limited periods of discomfort, the disease often remits by age 5 years. For a small minority of children, childhood eczema follows a more severe, devastating course, marked by months and years of unremitting rash, often covering the child from head to toe with an oozing, crusting, terribly itchy eruption from which he can find no rest.

Severely afflicted children have been treated with a variety of topical agents (such as coal tar, steroid creams, and lubricants), systemic medications (antipruritics, sedatives, and sometimes corticosteroids), and environmental maneuvers (hand restraints, bandaging, and avoidance of various objects suspected to be allergenic). Often a combination of treatments offers some relief [39, 86].

To study children who cannot comfort themselves or be comforted by parents, I cared for about 80 children severely afflicted with eczema. Most were referred by pediatricians, allergists, and dermatologists who had failed with the usual medical treatment. Thus the children were an unusual sample of very disabled treatment failures.[3]

[3] The study of eczema extended over four years and was conducted at Children's Hospital Medical Center, Boston, Massachusetts. Dr. Robert Griesemer, Chief of Dermatology, supported the research and shared his unsurpassed understanding of physical and psychological features of childhood skin diseases.

The pathophysiology of eczema involves a circular chain reaction in which vigorous scratching leads to a bloody, maculopapular rash, which in turn stimulates more scratching. Within minutes, a paroxysm of scratching may turn a child who has the tendency to severe eczema from being relatively free of rash into being covered with eczema, blood, and excoriations. Children with eczema appear to be born with the disposition to develop a vasculitis, characterized by edema and perivascular cellular infiltration, during the first months of life. This tendency presumably is based on the genetic endowment for hypersensitivity or physiological vascular instability in which biogenic amines in the skin have been implicated [51, 72, 81]. A child or adult without the tendency to eczema who scratches may develop lichenification or excoriations, but he will not develop eczema.

For a particular child with eczema, proximal causes of occasional scratching often can be identified: skin irritation, woolen clothing, temperature change, sweating, and the like. But such proximal causes are often weak, transient, or predisposing stimuli, paled by the most important initiator of the pathophysiological scratch-rash cycle: emotional arousal, anxiety, or stress.

For a normal toddler frustration or scolding may lead to crying, a temper tantrum, or externally directed aggression. For the 3-year-old with a history of severe eczema, the result of emotional arousal or stress is most often a paroxysm of scratching. The normal toddler may be relatively unmoved by adversity such as separation and discipline, and he is capable of modulating much distress before becoming very upset. One with eczema seems particularly vulnerable. Thus the eczematous child not only expresses distress by acting inwardly, but he is also more sensitive, fragile, and prone to experiencing even minor family upsets as disorganizing. And for him scratching leads to more rash, which leads to more scratching. The result of a paroxysm of scratching is an exhausted, bloody child who has literally torn away at his own skin to reduce incessant itching, and has succeeded only in making it worse. The paroxysm comes to an end when the child is finally distracted or exhausted, or when his itch perception is disordered by skin trauma.

The difference between a child with benign eczema and one whose eczema follows the severe course which I have pictured often appears to consist of the nature of the family's response to the child's distress, rash, and scratch-rash cycle, as much as in the child's physiological predisposition to the underlying vasculitis. Children with limited eczema often come from families which can be called "supportive." These families accept the child's first rash with relative equanimity, remain available throughout the course of the tendency to develop eczema, protect the child from undue stress, and comfort him when overwhelmed. Children with years of severe, unremitting eczema tend to come from families where this supportive system has not been available or maintained. Here the parents have reacted to the child's rash with tremendous anxiety or worry, and then often with ambivalent caretaking and withdrawal. For such parents the rash may arouse many types of personal meaning: as an indication that they are inept; as a satisfaction of an unconscious need for punishment for felt wrongdoing; or as a source of arousal of concern about bodily contact and sexuality. Moreover, the rash and the parents' subsequent unadaptive responses may become locked into already established interpersonal conflicts in the marriage or extended family. In short, the rash of the child with very severe eczema is often far more than a rash.

Children with severe eczema for many years direct much of their energy and attention to caring for their own bodies. Cracking and uncomfortable skin, unsightly appearance, and irritability often prevent them from acquiring age-appropriate social or motor skills. Thus by age 3 or 4 years afflicted children may present a clinical picture of severe developmental retardation which affects speech, social skills, and muscular coordination, and they may show a diffuse lack of interest or capacity for establishing warm, friendly relations.

In the course of treatment, the eczematous child's energies can be redirected from his body to the outside world, and he and his parents can be helped to reestablish mutually satisfying, pleasant relationships which can then be extended to include peers and other adults. Over many months almost the complete picture of developmental retardation may be erased, even in the presence of a continued, although never so severe, series of exacerbations of the rash. The key to such a transformation lies in the clinician's success in reducing the child's distress through appropriate psychoactive medication, protection from undue stress, and skin care, and the physician's simultaneous success in modifying the parental distress and anger through appropriate counseling, personal availability, and willingness to share responsibility for months, and especially during times of crisis [17].

This study of children with eczema and their families was in the context of clinical care lasting for months and years. In many ways it elaborated the model that originated in the laboratory study of sucking and distress, the time-base for which was hours and days. The natural history of eczema is a function not only of the underlying vasculitis but of the child's threshold for disorganization, his ability to modulate distress, and other channels in addition to scratching that remain open for the expression of his distress [56]. Often in the presence of a supportive family the rash remains benign, although recurrent; occasionally a family's capacity to remain available, affectionate, stimulating, and yet protective is limited. The people who carry and contribute the genes to the child for the vascular diathesis underlying eczema, as well as contributing to his lowered ability to modulate distress, are the very same people who will be faced with the parenting responsibilities posed by the distressed infant. Such parents may be genetically ill-equipped for their role, endowed as they may be for heightened sensitivity and arousal. Constitutional factors are expressed not only in children, but in the adults who are their parents.

The description of the life of a child profoundly afflicted with eczema requires an important counterpoint. For some children with milder eczema, and even some whose disease is severe, life and development may be not at all bleak. Impressively active, thoughtful, alert, and inquisitive, these intelligent children take in people and objects with special awareness of details. They seem very alive to family events and sensitive to nuances of feeling. And although they often, or even usually, appear to be high-strung and temperamental, their heightened appreciation of feelings and their subtle social relations create an impression of precocious deepening, an impression which I believe to be clinically valid. One might be inclined to view this type of maturation as a pattern of response to illness, intense bodily sensations, gratifying special care, and the resultant tuning-in or attuning of attention. And all of these factors play important roles. Yet the positive developmental trends noted sometimes may be seen in children whose eczema has been relatively mild; and even for some with more severe eczema, the psychological adaptations which are, in fact, primarily responsive to the illness seem also to be embedded in a more pervasive, psychosomatic complex.

Keeping in mind that speculation is just that, perhaps we can pursue this concept of a psychosomatic complex somewhat further. Confronted by a sensitive and perhaps trying child with eczema, an experienced and not too busy pediatrician might very well ask himself: Is there more here than meets the eye? Is it possible that some qualities of this child's inner life or overall development reflect not only the skin disease, and its psychic consequences, but also are more directly reflective of the child's general neurophysiological endowment? Such an endowment might operate simultaneously in what may be called, for convenience, two "domains": in the physiological realm of autonomic instability, low threshold for elicitation of the scratching reflex, and the vasculitis and biogenic amine diathesis which underly eczema and, at the same time, in the realm of higher nervous functioning concerned with the regulation of arousal, attention, and the experience of anxiety. If so, the actual experience of eczema would be compounded with the psychological potential for difficulty with the modulation of anxiety. Then both the rash and aspects of the child's mental life would be, in the deepest sense, a psychosomatic whole.

Rash and mental states represent the two domains Descartes tried to neatly separate and then struggled to unite. And it is the fluidity or, rather, absence of boundaries between these two domains which leads us, as clinicians, to speak of the initial unity of feelings and bodily states, of the infant as psyche-soma [91, pp. 243–254].

In this construction of intertwining physiological and psychological processes, in which eczema has served as our model disease, there may be a suggestion about a general phenomenon: a continuum between health and disease. As we have seen, a heavy weighting or loading for the neurophysiological substrate of eczema—affecting both the skin and mental regulation—may lead to developmental crisis or catastrophe. From the vantage point of the new line of speculation, we might also wonder if there is an evolutionary advantage to being endowed with a more limited "dose" of this polygenically determined biological substrate. Would such a more fortunate individual, even if mildly afflicted with eczema, benefit from increased awareness, attentiveness, and sensitivity, and from the opportunities for forming rich mechanisms for coping [30]? We will return to this theme in the discussion of the biology of autism.

Genetics, Endowment, and Competence: Discordance in Twins

These studies on congenital organization and the unfolding patterns of response to stress have been considerably amplified by the opportunity of studying twin development during the first years of life. There are many approaches to the use of twins in developmental and psychiatric research [34, 76, 88]. Pollin has been a leading exponent of the value of twin studies in generating new hypotheses and testing critical ones concerning the origin of individuality.[4] In an important series of papers, he and his collaborators (J. Stabenau, J. Tupin, L. Mosher, A. Hoffer, M. Allen, S. Cohen, and the author) have explored the roots of vulnerability to psychopathology [59, 66–69, 83].

In the National Institute of Mental Health twin longitudinal study, eight sets of monozygotic twins and two sets of dizygotic twins were followed from the time of the diagnosis of pregnancy to about age 5 years using a variety of different techniques to assess over-lapping areas of functioning [14]. The careful observation of the 20 children under high levels of magnification indicated the ways in which genetically identical children were different from the first days of life. Detailed clinical studies of individual families revealed patterns of identification and relationship between parents and children based on these small differences. Even minor experiential or physical differences—for example, differences in weight or the early appearance of an illness—seemed to have impact on the ways in which some parents related to the children.

Although the enduring impact of differences between monozygotic twins was the major focus of this work, we must be careful not to overlook the uncanny similarity in development and experiences of children in monozygotic twinships. Without high magnification,

[4] To provide direct observational information on the early development of twins complementary to that obtained from the retrospective studies on adult twins, Pollin initiated a longitudinal study of twin development. The twin material described here is based on this longitudinal study, directed by me for two years, and on a large-scale epidemiological study (initiated in collaboration with Dr. Eleanor Dibble and Dr. Pollin) aimed at testing hypotheses derived, in part, from earlier work on adult twins and the longitudinal study [23, 24].

often only these similarities are evident. Thus monozygotic twins provide the investigator with the most dramatic type of personal evidence about genetic programming as well as the opportunity to study the subtle and not-so-subtle nongenetic determinants of development [46, 61, 76].

To more precisely assess congenital endowment during the first week of life, we devised a rating scale called the First-Week Evaluation Scale (FES). Whereas the Apgar score relates to only the first minutes of life and is highly dependent on labor and delivery variables with occasionally only transient significance, the FES relates to a child's general functioning over the first week of life and appears to reflect more fundamental dimensions of early functioning. The FES consists of six variables: general health; attention; vigor; physiological functioning and adaptation; calmness; and neurological performance. Each variable is rated on a 5-point rating scale, with 1 for very poor functioning and 5 for excellent functioning in that area. For example, being calm in general and easily calmed when stimulated is rated 5. Being fussy, irritable, and easily startled is rated 1. A normal neurological examination is 5; one with clear-cut disturbances, 1. A perfectly endowed newborn has a rating of 30.

In the longitudinal study of 10 sets of twins, the children's first-week endowments ranged from a low of 18 to a high of 30, with a mean of about 22. The mean intrapair difference in FES was 6, an indication of nongenetic determinants of endowment. In this population the FES scores agreed well with the characterization of the children using the Thomas, Chess, and Birch system [87].

At age 3½ years each child was studied in a research nursery school setting, in which measures and observations were made of the child's general behavior, play, relationship to mother, and reaction to the teacher and strangers. The FES correlated well with nursery school measures of general competence. The most well-endowed newborns became toddlers who engaged in more thematic play, spoke more maturely, and showed more originality. The less well-endowed newborns became toddlers who were more fearful and distractible.

At about the same age the children were visited at home by a psychologist who interviewed them in a novel situation. Reactions were rated using a scale for attention, speech, originality, distractibility, social relatedness, and other aspects of social competence. Scores correlated with nursery school measures and

Stanford-Binet IQ. Again children with the best first-week endowment emerged as socially mature, competent children. The mothers' responses on the Vineland Social Maturity Scale and on the Childhood Personality Scale, a questionnaire about general personality (described later), correlated well with relevant measures from the nursery school and psychological interview.

Thus a confluence of observations on early endowment and personality development indicates that the more competent newborn develops into the more competent toddler. We have been impressed in these longitudinal studies and in cross-sectional studies involving over 20 more sets of twins during childhood by the special importance of differences in arousal and attention patterns in shaping development. Such differences between children in a twinship were often noted very early by parents, just as they are by parents of atypical children who are familiar with normal infants.

Bell [4] has found that coping as a toddler is associated with two characteristics in infancy: (1) a long latency before starting to cry when a nipple on which the infant is sucking is withdrawn and (2) a high threshold to tactile stimulation. Wolff and White [94] have demonstrated that the optimal time for eliciting visual following in infants is during the period after feeding when the child is attentive and calm. Moments of comfort when the child can scan his mother's face and the mother can enjoy his relating are probably important for the formation of positive early attachments. The high FES, well-endowed newborn is more likely to have many mutually satisfying times.

The attentive and comfortable infant is more easily consoled, and although he may need and receive less caregiving from his mother, his moments with her are likely to be pleasant. Caring for this well-endowed baby arouses less guilt, anger, and subsequent ambivalent feelings than caring for the fussier infant. Finally, in a myriad of transactions, children and family reciprocally reinforce perception and self-perceptions of competence (or incompetence), assertiveness (or passivity), and dominance (or submission), which, within a twinship, can easily lead to persistent dichotomization and stereotyping. The initial advantages of a better early endowment may thus be amplified and crystallized [9, 83, 89, 91].

Even for traits for which there is a heavy genetic loading—such as cleft lip and palate or dislocation of the hip—monozygotic twins are more often discordant than concordant [5, 11]. It seems that newborn competence is another such trait: whereas there is a clear genetic loading and high degree of similarity between monozygotic twins, our studies and those previously reported by Pollin and others [68] indicate, and it is reasonable a priori to assume, that even monozygotic twins may be born with very different newborn competencies, as reflected in such areas as their abilities to attend, remain calm, and adapt physiologically. The basis for discordance in such traits as cleft lip and palate—for which the concordance rate in identical twins is only about 30 percent—is not definitely known, but minor differences in circulation and *in utero* position have been hypothesized as interacting with sensitively timed maturational processes [5]. Similarly, the basis for differences in competence cannot be completely determined, although some suggestions will be offered later.

To understand better the basis for competence and vulnerability and to put clinical hypotheses to a more vigorous test, we have undertaken a large, epidemiological study of twins from ages 1 to 6 years. The major methodology of this study consists of mothers and fathers of over 400 sets of MZ and DZ twins completing specially designed questionnaires.

A common problem in twin research relates to the assignment of zygosity to a twinship. Mothers of 155 sets of twin children completed a questionnaire with 10 times about the degree of physical similarity between the two children and if, and by whom, the two children were confused. For physical similarity in height, weight, facial appearance, hair color, eye color, and complexion, the mothers rated the two children on a 3-point scale (exactly similar, somewhat similar, or not at all similar). For confusion, the mothers answered on a 2-point scale (Yes or No) whether the children were as alike as two peas in a pod, were confused by parents, other members of the family, or strangers. The twins were bloodtyped on 22 antigens to determine zygosity. This biological method for assigning zygosity allows for clear assignment in 97 percent of cases, but, as with other methods of zygosity determination, there are always a few sets about whom a decision is difficult or impossible.

Parental perceptions of identical and fraternal twins were extremely different and highly reliable, with 98 percent agreement between zygosity assigned by the mothers' responses to the questions and zygosity determined by bloodtyping. The results raise questions about an assumption which underlies many behavior genetic investigations using twins: that the life experiences of both types of twin are comparable. This is doubtful. For example, 78 percent of parents confused their MZ twins; 99 percent of MZ twins were confused by strangers. In contrast, only 10 percent of DZ twins were confused by their parents and only 16 percent by strangers. The calculation of heritability coefficients, such as those on which Jensen and others have so heavily relied, or comparison of intrapair correlations requires the assumption that the experiences of MZ and DZ twins are identical [15]. This assumption now appears untenable.

The 400 sets of twins in our epidemiological study were classified using this new method for assigning zygosity. Mothers and fathers completed questionnaires about the children's gestation and delivery; personality and behavioral differences during the first years of life; and current personality patterns and behavioral problems. Each parent completed questionnaires describing his or her characteristic style of relating to each child and his or her perceptions of the type and degree of stress to which the family and each child is exposed.

In interpreting twin research it must always be remembered that the biology of twins differs from that of singletons, and that of MZ twins differs from DZ twins. For example, MZ twins result from a genetic accident, perhaps related to hypoxia during the first days of implantation; during gestation, MZ twins are often exposed to markedly inequitable blood circulation. DZ twinning, in contrast, results from transient endocrine disturbances, often associated with increasing maternal age and environmental stress; the placentas of DZ twins may be unequal but they are never fully united [11].

The statistical data reported here are based on analyses of the first 210 sets of twins on whom we had complete information, and results must be considered preliminary. In our series a large proportion of the twins were born prematurely (about 40 percent), and the mean length of gestation was 35–36 weeks (standard deviation ± 2 weeks). Mothers gained a mean of 28 pounds (± 11 pounds). They learned they were having twins only about the eighth month of gestation and about 25 percent of the mothers learned only at the time of delivery. Labor tended to be short (3–6 hours). The mean weights of both the firstborn and the secondborn twins were the same (92 ounces)—but there was greater variance for the secondborn (SD ±40) than the firstborn (SD ±19).

The mothers took many drugs during pregnancy, having a mean of four drugs, ranging from 0 (0.9 percent of mothers) to 11 (3.8 percent of mothers). Medications included iron (57 percent), vitamins (95 percent), diuretics (58 percent), pills for nausea (36 percent), tranquilizers (14 percent), female hormones (13 percent), aspirin and other analgesics (40 percent), antibiotics (19 percent), and blood pressure pills (4 percent). The impact on developing embryos of some of these drugs—such as the antiemetics and diuretics, used by about half of the mothers—is not known. In addition, twin pregnancies were often complicated by medical problems such as varicose veins, vaginal staining, and pressure symptoms, and mothers and fathers frequently reported that they were very anxious about the economic and social burdens posed by the twins.

Clearly, when we say that a newborn child's endowment is a function of his genetics and prenatal and newborn experiences, we must keep in mind, especially for twins, how variegated, and often "unnatural," these gestation and delivery experiences may be. Environmental forces are important in the etiology of twinning and the list of drugs alone indicates that the environment is by no means silent or benign during gestation. We have many questions about the impact of drugs on twins. For example, is the larger twin more stressed by drugs ingested by mother because he receives more blood flow and hence more medication, or, to the contrary, is he less vulnerable because of his larger size and physiological maturity? What is the impact of the medication on central nervous system maturation? We are now aware of the enduring behavioral effects of exposure to sex hormones during gestation [35, 57, 101] and of the teratogenic effects of other drugs such as Thalidomide. What are the enduring and cumulative effects of all the drugs to which twins, born small and premature, are exposed?

The Childhood Personality Scale is an instrument for describing a child's general personality. It consists of 48 behavioral items rated on a 7-point scale according to the degree to which the item accurately describes the child. Factor analysis has yielded five dimensions: behavior activity level (sample item: Does things vigorously); attention (Can pay attention for long times); social uninvolvement and irritability (Would rather be left alone); extroversion-introversion (Tries to strike up friendships); and positive verbal and emotional responses (Talks and acts happily and with excitement).

The Parent's Report is a complementary attitude instrument for description of the way a parent relates to a child. It also consists of 48 items rated on a 7-point scale according to the degree to which a behavioral description corresponds to the parent's perception of how he or she relates to the particular child. Factor analysis has led to five dimensions of parenting: respect for autonomy (I am aware of his need for privacy); child-centered (I think of things that will please him); control through guilt and anxiety (I keep reminding him of past bad behavior); enforcement of discipline (I see to it that he obeys what he is told); and control through anger and withdrawal of affection (I avoid talking to him after he displeases me) [24].

Parents' descriptions of a child depend on both the sex of the parent and the sex of the child. There were highly significant differences between mothers' descriptions of all children (boys and girls combined) versus fathers' descriptions of all children; mothers' descriptions of daughters versus fathers' descriptions of daughters; and mothers' descriptions of sons versus fathers' descriptions of sons. Generally girls are described as more person-oriented and talkative and boys as more vigorous and active. And fathers tend to see their children as extreme, either very active or very passive, whereas mothers see their children as concerned with feelings.

Mothers and fathers also differ in their descriptions of their relationships with children. Mothers tend to feel close and child-centered, fathers, oriented toward discipline and punishment. It appears to us that these statistically significant differences in descriptions of fathers and mothers of their sons and daughters may reflect not only cultural adaptations but biological phenomena associated with the greater comfort and attentiveness and the better health of the girls.

The First Month of Life Scale, a measure of a child's newborn competence, is an elaboration of the First Week Evaluation Scale. It consists of six variables scored by parents about the child's attention, calmness, vigor, physiological adaptation, general health, and overall development. The First Month Endowment score correlates very well with birthweight ($r=.481$, $p<.001$) and length of gestation ($r=.347$, $p<.001$), indicating that more mature and heavier infants are better endowed during the first month of life. As would be predicted, length of gestation and birthweight are also correlated ($r=.484$, $p<.001$).Taken together, First Month Endowment score, weight, and length of gestation are a powerful triad of predictors of later competence.

The First Month Endowment score correlates with a range of childhood personality characteristics (as derived from the Childhood Personality Scale) and parental patterns of behavior (as reported in Parent's Report) completed about the twins whose ages ranged from 1 to 6 years. For example, first-month competence correlates positively with ratings of attention and negatively with both hyperactivity and social uninvolvement and irritability. Birthweight is also negatively correlated with hyperactivity. Fathers use little control through guilt and anxiety in disciplining children with poor newborn endowment. Mothers are strict in their enforcement of discipline with the children who were healthier newborns. And parents rate themselves as being more child-centered in relation to children who were born prematurely than they do for younger children.

The relationships between early measures of competence and later differences in functioning are most apparent when the two children in a twinship are compared. Parents of twins can describe subtle differences between two children who share the same social class, family, age, and other variables, and thus who can serve as each other's matched controls. The repeated measures, analysis of variance, is well suited to statistically handle such intrapair comparisons. Generally in a twinship the best endowed newborn becomes the more attentive preschooler, whereas the less well-endowed newborn becomes the more hyperactive. This natural history, clear even in MZ twinships, is most obvious when the effects of sex are compounded with those of early endowment in a boy-girl twinship where the girl is more healthy as a newborn.

The results with twins can probably be extended to singletons: newborns who are well endowed appear to become those preschoolers who are attentive and for whom parents are consistent in the enforcement of discipline. Poorly endowed infants are likely to become preschoolers who are hyperactive and with whom parents see them-

selves as using control through guilt and anxiety. These results are
easily integrated with studies on the origins of severe psychopathology
done by Lidz, Fleck, Wynne, Jackson, and the National Institute
of Mental Health group cited previously.

Experience and Physiology: Metabolic Studies of Disordered Development

Concepts such as endowment, arousal, and stress have been used
to bridge psychological and biological research [62]. Crossing this
bridge has been made increasingly comfortable and attractive by
recent advances in neurophysiology, biochemistry, developmental
endocrinology, and physiological psychology [29, 49, 52, 55, 57, 64,
80]. These advances suggest ways in which models for relating
endowment, as observed in clinical and psychological studies, can be
understood in molecular terms. Since the empirical work to be
discussed here focuses on the role of biogenic amines in childhood
psychopathology, this area will be emphasized in the discussion. But
it would be naive to assume that the search for biological understanding of endowment, especially in relation to the modulation
of distress and the deployment of attention, will end with this one
group of chemicals.

As currently understood, central nervous system (CNS) neural
activity involves the release by nerve cells of different neurotrans-
mitters, which cross the synaptic gap and stimulate other nerve
cells to fire [3, 20]. Following release, the neurotransmitter either
undergoes active reuptake (by the presynaptic neuron) or is
metabolized into an inactive substance by an enzyme. The neuro-
transmitters that have been most studied are biogenic amines:
catecholamines (norepinephrine, NE, and dopamine, DA) and an
indoleamine (serotonin or 5-hydroxytryptamine, 5-HT). These
biogenic amines are widely distributed in the brain, and norepinephrine and dopamine are most concentrated in the hypothalamus.

In the 1950s reserpine was found to make certain individuals
depressed and to lower the levels of biogenic amines. In the 1960s
monamine oxidase inhibitors, which increase amines, were found to
be useful in the treatment of certain depressed patients. Related
studies led to the biogenic amine hypothesis of affective disorders:

manic states are the result of increased biogenic amines, depressed states, of decreased [79]. This hypothesis has broad heuristic value [21]. For example, amphetamines, which are useful in the treatment of hyperkinetic behavioral disturbance in children, generally increase arousal, inhibit neuronal reuptake of norepinephrine and dopamine, and also release norepinephrine. The effect of amphetamines can thus be understood as the result of increasing the availability of biogenic amines in brain centers concerned with attention.

Monamine oxidase (MAO) is the major enzyme involved in the degradation of biogenic amines and thus plays a central role in the regulation of neurotransmitter activity. Abnormalities of MAO have been found in psychiatric patients. For example, MAO appears to be reduced in both individuals in a twinship discordant for schizophrenia. In the schizophrenic individual, however, levels are lower than in the normal co-twin [99]. Reduction of MAO may thus represent one aspect of genetic vulnerability to severe psychopathology.

Dopamine beta hydroxylase (DBH) also plays a regulatory role as the enzyme which converts dopamine (DA) to norepinephrine (NE). Elevations of DBH occur during stress as a reflection of increased autonomic activity [90, 98], and the enzyme appears to be reduced in the brains of adults with schizophrenia [92]. Assay of DBH offers a direct method for estimating nervous system arousal, an individual's perception of stress, or possibly an individual's susceptibility to severe psychopathology. The potential of such a biochemical probe is only recently being exploited with children.

Metabolic breakdown products of biogenic amines can be measured in the cerebrospinal fluid (CSF). Most is known about 5-hydroxyindoleacetic acid (5-HIAA), the derivative of serotonin, and homovanillic acid (HVA), the metabolite of dopamine. The concentration of amine metabolites in the CSF represents a state of balance between formation of the metabolites and their active removal from the CSF [7a]. This active transport can be partially blocked by probenecid administration. As the CSF probenecid concentration increases, the levels of biogenic amines in the CSF become increasingly independent of the level of probenecid and probably increasingly reflect the actual rate of biogenic amine formation. Analyses of CSF amine metabolites following membrane blockade by probenecid thus provide a measure of brain amine turnover and, distally, of brain function.

As part of an intensive study of physiological and behavioral disturbances in children with neuropsychiatric disorders, we have analyzed the biogenic amine metabolism of about 40 children from the following subgroups: childhood psychosis (autism and atypical development); severe hyperkinetic behavioral disturbance (with and without what we call motor control system dysfunction or minimal cerebral dysfunction); epilepsy; and movement disorders. Although I use these clinical labels out of necessity, a major motivation for the research is the sense that in fundamental ways several of the clinical disturbances may eventually best be understood as representing one or several continua of developmental difficulties affecting primary neural mechanisms or organization.[5]

In our studies children with these various clinical syndromes are intensively studied as outpatients and during research hospitalization. Detailed neurological, psychiatric, and psychological assessment; endocrine, genetic, and ophthalmological evaluation; and a broad range of screening tests are performed. After 12-hour probenecid blockade, CSF is obtained (by lumbar puncture) for routine analysis and determination of amine metabolites (5-HIAA and HVA) and probenecid.

We have separated children with psychotic conditions with onset during the first years of life into two related subgroups: autistic (10 children) and atypical (10 children). The autistic children are distinguished from atypical children by their much greater disturbances in social relatedness and language use and comprehension, and they meet Lotter's major criteria for autism [40]. In addition, the atypical children have been found to have more markedly abnormal electroencephalograms, more gestational problems, and more stressed families. The children (10) with epilepsy all have severe grand mal seizure disorders. Those with movement disorders (5) have Huntington's chorea and other diseases of the basal ganglia.

---

[5] These biological studies represent a close collaboration with Dr. Bennett Shaywitz, a pediatric neurologist. Analysis of cerebrospinal fluid biogenic amine metabolites is performed by Malcolm Bowers, Yale University School of Medicine, and MAO by Dr. Richard Wyatt, National Institute of Mental Health, Bethesda, Maryland.

At school age there appears to be a significant difference between autistic and atypical children's HVA and HIAA. Autistic children have lower values for both biogenic amine metabolites. Children with epilepsy have lower levels than both groups of psychotic children. Multivariate analysis statistically suggests that these are three distinct groups.

Although the number of children with motor diseases and minimal motor control system dysfunction (MBD) we have studied is still small, it appears that there is a progression of biogenic amines from severe epilepsy, through severe motor diseases, autism, atypical development, and then minimal motor control system dysfunction (MBD) [18, 82].

The CNS biogenic amines of autistic and atypical children cover a broad range, with considerable overlap, as one would predict if these two conditions represent two regions on a spectrum of developmental disability [28]. There are individual children whose biogenic amines markedly deviate from the mean in both directions. Similarly, MAO in these children spans a broad range, from quite low to very high.

There are numerous technical and methodological problems in studies such as these. Such problems include the definition of syndromes and states; the interaction between syndrome or condition and treatment or treatment history; the ambiguity involved in deciding on an appropriate diagnosis for an evolving condition (as for the familiar case of a child who was classically autistic but who at the time of being studied appears as a verbal, odd child with severe obsessive compulsive symptoms and a pervasive, schizoidlike personality pattern disturbance); and the artifacts introduced by the stress of the research. Yet chemical and physiological facts may help clarify questions about diagnosis and sharpen clinical classification and observation.

It will be difficult to define normal values for some parameters because the need for lumbar puncture raises ethical and practical limitations. Thus we rely on data from small numbers of children (e.g., on values obtained from the rare child who has a spinal fluid examination without any central nervous system symptoms or disorder) and on the use of relevant contrast groups (e.g., contrasts involving autistic, retarded, or brain-damaged children; autistic children with no motor lag or gross brain damage; atypical children;

children with late onset psychosis; children with hyperkinetic behavioral disturbance with and without signs of motor control system dysfunction). The necessary control and contrast group information, just as the other basic data, will have to be acquired within the field of child psychiatry. Developmental changes make it unwise to rely on values from adults, and techniques have to be adapted to fit our special circumstances and the fascinating, but perplexing, developmental issues presented by childhood disturbances [2].

Recently Stein [84] and Wise [92] have hypothesized that progressive deterioration of central noradrenergic pathways may be the basis for adult schizophrenia. These pathways are vitally involved in the autoregulation of pleasure and thus in the direction and drive of intentional, goal-directed behavior [63] as well as in the regulation of physiological functions such as eating [1; 55, pp. 717–737]. Dopaminergic pathways have also been linked with schizophrenia. Stevens has suggested that these pathways, by serving as a central "gating mechanism," are involved in preventing an individual from being overwhelmed by excessive internal or external stimulation [85]. Dopaminergic dysfunction, she hypothesizes, may lead to excessive fearfulness, feelings of unreality, and alterations in attention and perception.

These noradrenergic and dopaminergic neurophysiological models may be relevant to the understanding of clinical observations discussed earlier, such as the infant's modulation of anxiety by sucking. Sucking, as we have seen, is an innately organized capacity in which regular, rhythmic motor activity reduces arousal or raises the threshold to stimulation. The capacity shows marked individual variation and may be much diminished in brain-damaged and other developmentally disabled children. Because of their prominence in the autoregulation of pleasure and modulation of stimulus strength, dopaminergic and noradrenergic pathways may play central roles in the process by which feedback from the neurologically organized sucking system modulates activity in another organized system, the control of attention and arousal. The reverberating itch-scratch circuit of the infant and child with severe eczema is perhaps an illustration of a feedback system run amuck. Here, as with normal sucking, paroxysmal motor behavior (scratching) briefly reduces anxiety and produces pleasure. However, in contrast with sucking, the relief produced by scratching is transient and is followed by increased drive, distress, and arousal.

Based on studies of animals [63] and adult schizophrenics [84], on the theoretical considerations developed about anxiety or arousal in relation to sucking, eczema, and individual competence, and on our observation of apparently reduced biogenic amines in at least some autistic children, it may be useful to hypothesize that noradrenergic, dopaminergic, or a combination of biogenic amine systems, may be involved in the etiology of childhood autism and other severe developmental disabilities. To a greater degree than adults with schizophrenia, children with autism display profoundly disorganized behavior, disturbances in learning and the appreciaton of pleasure and pain, unreasonable anxiety, oddities of appetite, abnormal arousal [42], and perceptual instability [65]. If biogenic amine disturbances are involved in autism and atypical development, it would be particularly interesting to analyze the response of these children to loading with the precursors of important amines (such as DOPA or tryptophan). Metabolic studies of this type may be more revealing in elucidating the psychoses of early childhood, which in some ways resemble inborn errors of metabolism, than they have been in the study of psychosis in adults [100].

The interactions between developmental trends involving biogenic amines and concomitant alterations in other domains (such as the endocrine system) are of particular interest to child psychiatrists. Two theoretically intriguing observations have emerged from our studies. First, we have been surprised by the apparent liability of serum thyroxine in autistic and atypical children. Changes of over 100 percent, from hypothyroid to hyperthyroid levels, have been observed in several children who show no obvious signs of endocrine disorder. Second, it appears that the level of plasma thyroxine is inversely correlated with the rate of production of biogenic amines in the CNS, a finding which is consistent with the concept that one physiological function of thyroxine is to sensitize neurons to the effect of biogenic amines (see [20], pp. 365–430, esp. pp. 365–369; [25]).

Similarly, the therapeutic effectiveness of imipramine—a tricyclic antidepressant useful in treating certain forms of adult depression, nocturnal enuresis in children, and narcolepsy—may be related to its effect in blocking the reuptake of biogenic amines and making more biogenic amines functionally available. Interestingly, thyroxine potentiates the action of imipramine in the treatment of depression, just as amphetamine potentiates the action of imipramine in the treatment of narcolepsy [19, 70, 102]. Triiodothyronine has been used, with encouraging results, in the treatment of childhood autism [12]. It is interesting, however, that amphetamines, which may be very useful in the treatment of hyperkinetic behavioral disturbance, almost uniformly make children with severe atypical development such as childhood autism, much worse [27; and our observations]. This effect of amphetamines, and of methylphenidate, appears similar to their effect in adults with psychosis [44]. Apparently in individuals already operating at a high level of arousal or already quite anxious the addition of amphetamines may lead not to increased attention and alertness but to disorganization. The efficacy of thyroxine therefore must result from activity in a localized area or subsystem as distinct from a more generalized effect on biogenic amines produced by amphetamine. Or, as one might predict from animal studies and clinical observations of patients with hyperthyroidism, there may be complex, dose-response relationships. At high doses, thyroxine, like the stimulants, may lead to overarousal, hyperacuity, anxiety, and behavioral disorganization.

At this point we are already well into the arena of speculation. But cautious that we do not mistake fantasy for reality, perhaps we could hypothesize several steps further. Could it not be possible that some children with severe atypical development suffer from a complex imbalance affecting both biogenic amines and the hypothalamic control of thyroxine? Our data suggest that there is a reciprocal relation between the rate of formation of brain biogenic amines and levels of thyroxine, a finding which is consistent with physiological evidence [50]. Thus children may be able to tolerate fluctuations or even abnormally low functioning in one system if there are compensatory adaptations in another. Might such adaptive mechanisms be aberrant in autistic and atypical children? For example, if labile levels of serum thyroxine are not accompanied by appropriate alterations in biogenic amine formation, is it possible that there may be transient or prolonged disturbances in brain function and psychological processes involved in perception, thinking, or the regulation of anxiety? There are some suggestive clinical and experimental data related to this possibility.

Abnormal hypothalamic-pituitary findings have been reported in conditions such as psychosocial-deprivation dwarfism and anorexia nervosa, two conditions concerned with modulation of anxiety, organization of behavior, and regulation of appetite [93]. These perhaps also involve the noradrenergic pathways discussed previously. There are many sensitive relationships between endocrine function and catecholamine metabolism, and endocrine-biogenic amine interactions may be of profound importance in understanding autism and other severe disturbances of development. (As an example of the influence of hormones on norepinephrine formation, see ref. 50; see also ref. 32). We should expect to find disturbances throughout the neuroendocrine axis: in the pituitary-adrenal axis, because of its sensitivity to stress [54]; in the regulation of growth hormone, which is sensitive to hypothalamic and high cortical control involving biogenic amines, and whose actions are extremely diffuse [53]; and in the sex hormones, which have important behavioral significance from early pregnancy [35, 57, 71]. These last hormones provide an interesting example of the complexity of the systems of behavioral disability with which we are concerned. Severe childhood eczema, colic, hyperkinetic behavioral disturbance, and childhood autism are all found in much higher incidence (three or four times higher) in boys than in girls. Such a profound sex difference must arouse curiosity about the interactions between androgens and biogenic amines and the enduring effects on development of early exposure to high doses of sex hormones. To understand these hormonal systems in atypical development requires study of dynamic functioning of the hypothalamic-pituitary glandular systems in these children and not just determination of static levels of hormones.

Finally, would it not be consistent with our current understanding of human behavior genetics if the parents of children with severe atypical development—on the basis perhaps of metabolic disturbances which create increased arousal and tendency to anxious disorganization—where themselves at the upper end of the curve in relation to the same phenomena? If this were so, one might expect that the parents of autistic children would be unusually sensitive, alert, and intelligent, perhaps as a reflection of their abnormal regulation of biogenic amines (or whatever other complex biochemical subsystems eventually emerge as underlying the children's developmental disabilities) and their resultant defenses and coping mechanisms. Such increased sensitivity and arousal may have important adaptive significance, which may account for the continuation of the genotype in the population, but an "overdose" of the gene or genes (as in a homozygous individual or one with heavy polygenic loading) or the combination of the genotype with other predisposing vulnerabilities (such as neonatal stress or abnormalities affecting other systems) may lead to the expressed disease. In fact, the parents and siblings of autistic children do appear to be of more than average intelligence [77]. And it is interesting that similar clinical observations have been made about families of patients with dystonia musculorum deformans, another condition which has been linked with biogenic amine metabolism.

Pollin and Stabenau [67] intensively studied adult twins discordant for schizophrenia. In their series, the sick twin was distinguished by two major physiological findings: the sick twin had lower levels of thyroid hormone (as measured by protein-bound iodine), and the sick twin was the lighter child at birth. These observations about the vulnerability to schizophrenia close the circle of our considerations and return us to twins, competence, and our main theme: What model can now guide us in our clinical investigations? How do physiology and experience interact?

Mind and Body: Model for Investigators

As researchers, we are interested in models that give coherence to isolated observations and guide us into fertile fields. In this essay, I have introduced dimensions or components of a multivariate model which, although broadly appreciated, seem only rarely to be brought together in the study of vulnerable children. Let us quickly review some of these main components in the model.

The model's starting point is the child's *genome*, the sum total of his genetic inheritance, which always contains far more potentiality than is ever expressed phenotypically. The true reaction ranges for most traits—the range of values permitted by a genotype—are really not known, and any estimates about the degree of genetic programming of complex characteristics such as intelligence thus are quite hazardous. Yet studies of twins provide compelling evidence of how powerful genes may be in human development [41].

As a result of the genome and prenatal and neonatal experiences, children are born with differing *congenital endowments*—the constellation of processes underlying equanimity, attention, vigor, physical health, and neurological functioning—and thus differing thresholds for the elicitation and disorganization of *congenitally organized behavior*. In basic and still unclear ways, congenital endowment and the congenital organization of behavior are patterned by complex biochemical interactions involving biogenic amines, hormones, and enzymes. In turn, the *early experiences* of a child—including nutrition, infection, drugs, and trauma of delivery —lead to enduring patterns of behavior encoded in central nervous system metabolism. For example, appropriate stimulation and optimal stress—as reflected perhaps by increases in dopamine beta hydroxylase, norepinephrine metabolites, and elevated thyroxin— may condition the nervous system in such a way that later novel situations are neither too overwhelming nor totally blocked from attention. Even short-term exposure to some hormones at certain developmental phases—such as testosterone during gestation and early infancy—may lead to enduring patterns of behavior which contrast with those encoded in the genome. And long-term exposure to hormones—such as testosterone in XY chromosomal males with end-organ insensitivity and thus completely female external appearance—may lead to enduring patterns of behavior which contrast with those shaped by the environment [35, 78, 101].

Arising from the *match between the child's endowment and the environment's provisions* are early adaptations and patterns of response and perception. These *persistent early adaptations*—such as the habitual fear or anxiety of the child with low threshold for disorganization—shape the child's later adaptations and style of approach to new developmental tasks. Behavioral patterns and hierarchies of action patterns in this way assume a type of autonomy which may become *crystallized characteristics of behavior* through social reinforcement [10].

Stress can be defined two ways: from the nature of the objective changes in the child's environment and from the nature of the child's responses. Seen in the latter way, the concept of stress signifies the type and degree of functional disorganization produced by either environmental or internal stimulation (e.g., separation, discipline, or persistent itch). What for one child may be *optimal stimulation* leading to the *unfolding of congenitally organized behavior*, such as accommodation to the nipple or the mastery of new skills such as sharing with a peer may, for another child, with even the identical genome, be a stress leading to disorganization of behavior and inhibition of intentional activity.

The *threshold for perception of stimulation as stressful* or the *capacity to modulate distress* appears to be a basic dimension that cuts across or unites physiology and psychology, a dimension which underlies the disposition to experience excessive anxiety and to develop maladaptive defenses against it. The molecular foundation for this dimension may lie in the functional relationships between biogenic amines, hormones, and enzymes, systems which both affect experience and are affected by it [33, 38]. The interactions between genes, amines, and hormones (such as sex hormones), which are apparent in the personality differences between boys and girls and men and women, may become most clearly visible as we study the onset of adolescence and the frequent emotional upsets of this developmental phase [16].

Parental impact on development occurs in many ways, including the following: contribution of genes; provision of prenatal environment; and structuring of the postnatal environment, including care, stimulation, and affection. Parents of children with disturbances in the modulation of distress may themselves suffer from similar disturbances, with both the parents' and the child's endowment reflecting similar processes involving the interaction between biogenic amines, hormones, and enzymes. In certain situations and when not present in too high a degree, there may be adaptive value for this increased sensitivity, which, when present at too high a level or in the combination with other predisposing conditions, may lead to severe developmental disabilities.

It would be pleasant to be able to organize these and other social, cultural, and biological determinants of development into a more tightly ordered model. And it would be important to be more explicit about the detailed processes involved in learning and cognition, to spell out the relations between such domains as genetically controlled maturational processes and what is acquired through conditioning and to clarify the social context of development. Yet even from the perspective of the fragmentary discussion and model presented here, I think it does seem likely that we will eventually be able to predict, for a population of children, the general shape of personality development and potential vulnerability based on equations containing expressions for genome, endowment, stress thresholds, experiences, early adaptations, and central nervous system dynamics. For the moment, however, the appetite for full clarity cannot be satisfied, and perhaps the major value of partial models such as the one I have sketched will be to guide us in designing studies containing a sufficiently broad array of relevant variables and to protect us from overenthusiasm in accepting any univariate equation or simple social intervention. That the model I have suggested appears to return to Freud's viewpoint on the central roles of anxiety, early structuralization, and disposition in human development should not be too disheartening for those who desire progress [37]. Freud himself offered us consolation when he knowingly wrote [31], "One should never tire of considering the same phenomena again and again (or of submitting to their effects), and one should not mind meeting with contradiction on every side provided one has worked sincerely."

Acknowledgments

I am very grateful to Dr. Albert Solnit, Professor of Psychiatry and Pediatrics, Yale University, for his guidance and support, and for the opportunity he has provided for this work, and to Dr. Edward Zigler, Professor of Psychology, Yale University, for his critical questioning and friendship. Ms. Margrethe Cone, my secretary, and Mr. Warren Johnson, Ms. Barbara Caparulo, and Ms. Jane Grawe, research associates, have all contributed to this work. The research was supported in part by Public Health Service Research Grant HD-03008.

References

1. Ahlskog, J. E., and Hoebel, B. Overeating and obesity from damage to a noradrenergic system in the brain. *Science*, 182:4108 (1973) 166–169.
2. Anthony, E. J. The state of child psychiatry. *Arch. Gen. Psychiat.*, 1973.
3. Axelrod, J. and Weinshilboum, R. Catecholamines. *New England J. Med.*, 287: 5 (1972), 237–242.
4. Bell, R. Q., Weller, G., and Waldrop, M. F. Newborn and preschooler: Organization of behavior and relations between periods. *Monogr. Soc. Res. Child Devel.*, No. 142, 36:1–2 (1971).
5. Benirschke, K. and Kim, Chung. Multiple pregnancy: I. *New England J. Med.*, 288: 24 (1973), 1276–1284; II. 288: 25 (1973), 1329–1336.

6. Benjamin, J. Further comments on some developmental aspects of anxiety, in *Counterpoint: Libidinal Object and Subject.* H. R. Gaskill, Ed., International Universities Press, New York, 1963.

7. Benjamin, J. Some developmental observations related to the theory of anxiety. *J. Amer. Psychoanalyt. Assoc.,* 9 (1961), 652–668.

7a. Bowers, M. Heninger, G. R., and Gerbode, F. Cerebrospinal fluid 5-hydroxyindoleacetic acid and homovanillic acid in psychiatric patients. *Int. J. Neuropharmacol.,* (1969), 255–262.

8. Bowers, W., Brackbill, Y., Conway, E., and Steinschneider, A. The effects of obstetrical medication on fetus and infant. *Monogr. Soc. Res. Child Devel.* No. 137, 35: 4 (1970).

9. Brody, S. and Axelrod, S. *Anxiety and Ego Formation in Infancy.* International Universities Press, New York, 1970.

10. Bruner, J. Organization of early skilled action. *Child Devel.,* 44: 1 (1973), 1–11.

11. Bulmer, M. G. *The Biology of Twinning in Man.* Clarendon Press. Oxford, 1970.

12. Campbell, M., Fish, B., David, R., Shapiro, T. Collins, P., and Koh, C. Response to triiodothyronine and dextroamphetamine: A study of preschool schizophrenic children. *J. Autism and Childhood Schizophrenia,* 2: 4 (1972), 343–358.

13. Cohen, D. J. The crying newborn's accommodation to the nipple. *Child Devel.,* 38 :1 (1967), 89–100.

14. Cohen, D. J., Allen, G., Pollin, W., Inoff, G., Werner, M., and Dibble, E. Personality development in twins: Competence in the newborn and pre-school periods. *J. Amer. Acad. Child Psychiat.,* 11: 4 (1972), 625–644.

15. Cohen, D. J., Dibble, E., Grawe, J. M., and Pollin, W. Separating identical from fraternal twin children: A new clinical method. *Arch. Gen. Psychiat.,* 29: 4 (1973), 465–469.

16. Cohen, D. J. and Frank, R. *Between childhood and adolescence: Growth, tasks and problems in the preadolescent phase of development.* A technical report submitted to the Office of Child Development, DHEW, 1973.

17. Cohen, D. J. and Nadelson, T. The impact of skin disease on the person. In *Dermatology in General Medicine,* Thomas Fitzpatrick, Ed. McGraw-Hill, New York, 1971, pp. 5–9.

18. Cohen, D. J., Shaywitz, B. A., Johnson, W. T., and Bowers, M. Biogenic amines in autistic, atypical, and epileptic children: CSF measures of HVA. 5HIAA. Submitted for publication, 1973.

19. Coppen, A. J., Whybrow, P. G., Noguera, R., Maggs, R., and Prange, A. J. Comparative antidepressant value of L-tryptophan and imipramine with and without attempted potentiation by triiodothyronine. *Arch. Gen. Psychiat.,* 26 (1972), 234–241.

20. de V. Cotten, M., Ed. Regulation of catecholamine metabolism in the sympathetic nervous system. *Pharmacol. Rev.* 24: 2 (1972), whole issue, 163–434.

21. Curzon, G. Brain amine metabolism in some neurological and psychiatric disorders, in *Biochemical Aspects of Nervous Disorders.* J. N. Cumings, Ed. Plenum Press, London, 1972, pp. 151–212.

22. Denenberg, V. H. The effects of early experience, in *The Behaviour of*

Domestic Animals, 2nd ed., E. S. E. Hafetz, Ed. Balliere, Tindall, and Cassell, London, 1969.

23. Dibble, E. *Fathers' and Mothers' Perceptions of Parenting Style in Relation to Children's Behavior.* The Catholic University of America Studies in Social Work No. 89. Washington, D.C., 1973.

24. Dibble, E. and Cohen, D. J. Companion instruments devised for measuring parental style in relation to children's behavior. *Arch. Gen. Psychiat.,* 1973, in press.

25. Emlen, W., Segal, D. S., and Mandell, A. J. Thyroid state: Effects on pre- and post-synaptic central noradrenergic mechanisms. *Science,* 175 (1972), 79–82.

26. Escalona, S. The study of individual differences and the problem of state. *J. Amer. Acad. Child Psychiat.,* 1: 1 (1962), 11–37.

27. Fish, B. The "one child, one drug" myth of stimulants in hyperkinesis. *Arch. Gen. Psychiat.,* 25 (1971), 193–203.

28. Fish, B. Visual-motor disorders in infants at risk for schizophrenia. *Arch. Gen. Psychiat.,* 28: 6 (1973), 900–904.

29. Freedman, D. X. and Giarman, N. Brain amines, electrical activity, and behavior. In Glaser, Gilbert *EEG and Behavior,* G. Glaser, Ed. Basic Books, New York, 1963.

30. Freud, A. *The Ego and the Mechanisms of Defense.* International Universities Press, New York, 1946.

31. Freud, S. Letter to Le Disque Vert. *Standard Edition of the Complete Psychological Works,* Vol. 19. Hogarth Press, London, 1961, p. 290.

32. Frohman, L. Clinical neuropharmacology of hypothalamic releasing factors. *New England J. Med.,* 286: 26 (1972), 1391–1397.

33. Goldberg, A. and Welch, B. Adaptation of the adrenal medulla: Sustained increase in choline acetyltransferase by psychosocial stimulation. *Science,* 178: 4058 (1972), 319–20.

34. Gottesman, I. and Shields, J. *Schizophrenia and Genetics.* Academic Press, New York, 1972.

35. Goy, R. Organizing effect of androgen on the behaviour of rhesus monkeys. In *Endocrinology and Human Behavior,* R. Michael, Ed. Oxford University Press, London, 1968, pp. 12–31.

36. Graham, F. K. and Jackson, J. C. Arousal systems and infant heart rate responses. *Adv. Child Devel.,* 5 (1970), 59–117.

37. Hartmann, H. *Essays on Ego Psychology: Selected Problems in Psychoanalytic Theory.* International Universities Press, New York, 1964.

38. Henley, E., Moisset, B., and Welch, B. Catecholamine uptake in cerebral cortex: Adaptive change induced by fighting. *Science,* 180: 4090 (1973), 1050–1052.

39. Hill, L. W. *The Treatment of Eczema in Infants and Children.* Mosby, St. Louis, 1956.

40. Hingtgen, J. N. and Bryson, C. Q. Recent developments in the study of early childhood psychoses: Infantile autism, childhood schizophrenia, and related disorders. *Schizophrenia Bull.,* No. 5 (Spring 1972), 8–54.

41. Hirsch, J. Behavior genetics and individuality understood. *Science,* 142 (1963), 1437–1442.

42. Hutt, S. J., Hutt, C., Lee, D., and Ounsted, C. A behavioural and electro-

encephalographic study of autistic children. *J. Psychiat.* Res., 3 (1965), 181–197.

43. Hutt, S. J., Lenard, H. G., and Prechtl, H. F. R. Psychophysiological studies in newborn infants. *Adv. Child Devel.*, 4 (1969), 127–172.

44. Janowsky, D. S., El-Yousef, M. K., Davis, J. M., and Sekerke, H. J. Provocation of schizophrenic symptoms by intravenous administration of methylphenidate. *Arch. Gen. Psychiat.*, 28: 2 (1973), 185–191.

45. Joffe, J. M., Rawson, R. A., and Mulick, J. A. Control of their environment reduces emotionality in rats. *Science,* 180: 4093 (1973), 1383–1384.

46. Juel-Nielsen, N. Individual and environment. A psychiatric-pschological investigation of monozygotic twins reared apart. *Acta Psychiat. Scand.*, 40 (1964), Suppl. 183. Munksgaard, Copenhagen, 1965.

47. Kaye, H. Infant sucking behavior and its modification. *Adv. Child Devel.*, 3 (1967), 2–52.

48. Kessen, W. and Mandler, G. Anxiety, pain, and the inhibition of distress. *Psychol. Rev.*, 68 (1961), 396–404.

49. Kuhlin, H. E. and Reiter, E. Gonadotrophins during childhood and adolescence: A review. *Pediatrics*, 51: 2 (1973), 260–271.

50. Landsberg, L. and Axelrod, J. Influence of pituitary, thyroid, and adrenal hormones on norepinephrine turnover and metabolism in the rat heart. *Circulation Res.*, 22 (1968), 559–571.

51. Lobitz, W. C. and Campbell, C. J. Physiologic studies in atopic dermatitis (disseminated neurodermatitis). I. The local cutaneous response to intradermally injected acetylcholine and epinephrine. *Arch. Derm. Syph.*, 67 (1953), 575.

52. MacLean, P. *A Triune Concept of Brain and Behavior.* The Hincks Memorial Lectures, T. Boag, Ed. Toronto University Press, Toronto, 1972.

53. Martin, J. Neural regulation of growth hormone secretion. *New England J. Med.*, 288: 26 (1973), 1384–1393.

54. Mason, J. Organization of psychoendocrine mechanisms. *Psychosom. Med.*, 30: 2 (1968), 565–570, 576–607, 631–653, 666–681.

55. Miller, N. *Selected Papers.* Aldine, Chicago, 1971.

56. Mohr, G., Tausend, H., Selesnick, S., and Augenbraun, B. Studies of eczema and asthma in the preschool child. *J. Amer. Acad. Child Psychiat.*, 2: 2 (1963), 271–291.

57. Money, J. and Ehrhardt, A. A. *Man and Woman, Boy and Girl.* Johns Hopkins University Press, Baltimore, 1973.

58. Money, J. and Ehrhardt, A. A. Prenatal hormonal exposure: Possible effects on behaviour in man. In *Endocrinology and Human Behaviour.* R. Michael, Ed. Oxford University Press, London, 1968, pp. 32–48.

59. Mosher, L., Pollin, W., and Stabenau, J. Families with identical twins discordant for schizophrenia: Some relationships between identification, psychopathology, and dominance-submissiveness. *Brit. J. Psychiat.*, 118 (1971), 29–42.

60. Murphy, D. L. and Wyatt, R. *Nature,* 238 (1972), 225.

61. Newman, H. H., Freeman, F. N., and Holzinger, K. J. *Twins: A Study of Heredity and Environment.* University of Chicago Press, Chicago, 1937.

62. Offer, D. and Freedman, D. X. *Modern Psychiatry and Clinical Research.* Basic Books, New York, 1972.

63. Olds, J. Hypothalamic substrates of rewards. *Physiol. Rev.*, 42 (1962), 554–604.

64. Olds, J. Hypothalamic substrates of rewards. *Physiol. Rev.*, 42 (1962), *Psychopathology in Childhood*, L. Jessner and E. Pavenstedt, Eds. Grune & Stratton, New York, 1959.

65. Ornitz, E. M. and Ritvo, E. Perceptual inconstancy in early infantile autism. *Arch. Gen. Psychiat.*, 18 (1968), 76–98.

66. Pollin, W. A possible genetic factor related to psychosis. *Amer. J. Psychiat.*, 128:3 (1971), 311–317.

67. Pollin, W. and Stabenau, J. Biological, psychological, and historical differences in a series of monozygotic twins discordant for schizophrenia, in *Transmission of Schizophrenia*, S. Kety and D. Rosenthal, Eds. Pergamon Press, London, 1968, pp. 317–332.

68. Pollin, W., Stabenau, J., Mosher, L., and Tupin, J. Life history differences in identical twins discordant for schizophrenia. *Amer. J. Orthopsychiat.*, 36: 3 (1966), 492–509.

69. Pollin, W., Stabenau, J., and Tupin, J. Family studies with identical twins discordant for schizophrenia. *Psychiat.*, 28 (1965), 60–78.

70. Prange, A., Wilson, I., Knox, A., McClane, T., Breese, G., Martin, B., Alltop, L., and Lipton, M. Thyroid-imipramine clinical and chemical interaction: Evidence for a receptor deficit in depression. *J. Psychiat. Res.*, 9: 3 ((1972), 187–205.

71. Prunty, F. T. G. and Gardiner-Hill, H., *Modern Trends in Endocrinology*, Vol. 4. Appleton-Century-Crofts, New York, 1972.

72. Rhyne, M. B. Genetic aspects of eczema. Conference on Infantile Eczema. *J. Pediat.*, 66: 1: Part 2 (1965), 168–170.

73. Richmond, J. B. and Lipton, E. L. Some aspects of the neurophysiology of the newborn and their implications for child development. In *Dynamic Psychopathology in Childhood*, L. Jessner and E. Pavenstedt, Eds. Grune & Stratton, New York, 1959.

74. Richmond, J. B., Lipton, E. L., and Steinschneider, A. Autonomic function in the neonate: V. Individual homeostatic capacity in cardiac response. *Psychosom. Med.*, 24 (1962), 66–74.

75. Richmond, J. B., Lipton, E. L., and Steinschneider, A. Observations on differences in autonomic nervous system function between and within individuals during early infancy. *J. Amer. Acad. Child Psychiat.*, 1 (1962), 83–91.

76. Rosenthal, D. *Genetics of Psychopathology*. McGraw-Hill, New York, 1971.

77. Rutter, M. *Infantile Autism: Concepts, Characteristics, and Treatment*. Churchill-Livingstone, Edinburgh and London, 1971.

78. Sachs, B., Pollak, E., Krieger, M., and Barfield, R. Sexual behavior: Normal male patterning in androgenized female rats. *Science*, 181: 4101 (1973), 770–771.

79. Schildkraut, J. J. *Neuropsychopharmacology and the Affective Disorders*. Little, Brown, Boston, 1970.

80. Schildkraut, J. J. and Kety, S. S. Biogenic amines and emotion. *Science*, 156 (1967), 21–30.

81. Sedlis, E. Natural history of infantile eczema: Its incidence and course. Conference on Infantile Eczema. *J. Pediat.*, 66: 1: Part 2 (1965), 158–163.

82. Shaywitz, B. A., Cohen, D. J., and Bowers, B. Brain monamine turnover in children: Preliminary results in epilepsy, minimal brain dysfunction, and movement disorders. *Neurology*, 1973.

83. Stabenau, J. and Pollin, W. Early characteristics of monozygotic twins discordant for psychopathology. *Arch. Gen. Psychiat.* 17 (1967), 723–734.
84. Stein, L. Neurochemistry of reward and punishment: Some implications for the etiology of schizophrenia. *J. Psychiat. Res.*, 8 (1971), 345–361.
85. Stevens, J. R. An anatomy of schizophrenia? *Arch. Gen. Psychiat.*, 29: 2, (1973), 177–189.
86. Sulzberger, M. Atopic dermatitis, in *Dermatology in General Medicine*, T. Fitzpatrick, Ed. McGraw-Hill, New York, 1971, pp. 680–684, 687–697.
87. Thomas, A., Chess, S., and Birch, H. G. *Temperament and Behavior Disorders in Children.* New York University Press, New York, 1968.
88. Vandenberg, S. G. Hereditary factors in psychological variables in man, with a special emphasis on cognition, in *Genetic Diversity and Human Behavior*, J. N. Spuhler, Ed. Aldine, Chicago, 1967.
89. Weil, A. P. The basic core. *The Psychoanalytic Study of the Child*, Vol. 25, International Universities Press, New York, 1970, pp. 442–460.
90. Weinshilboum, R., Raymond, F. A., Elveback, L., and Weidman, W. Serum dopamine-beta-hydroxylase activity: Sibling-sibling correlation. *Science*, 181 (1973), 943–945.
91. Winnicott, D. W. *Collected Papers: Through Paediatrics to Psychoanalysis.* Tavistock, London, 1958.
92. Wise, C. D. and Stein, L. Dopamine-B-hydroxylase deficits in the brains of schizophrenic patients. *Science*, 181: 4097 (1973), 344–347.
93. Wolff, G. and Money, J. Relationship between sleep and growth in patients with reversible somatropin deficiency. *Psychol. Med.*, 3: 1 (1973), 18–27.
94. Wolff, P. and White, B. Visual pursuit and attention in newborn infants. *J. Amer. Acad. Child Psychiat.*, 4 (1965), 473–484.
95. Wolff, P. H. The causes, controls, and organization of behavior in the neonate. *Psychol. Iss.*, 5: 17 (1966).
96. Wolff, P. H. Natural history of sucking patterns in infant goats. *J. Comp. Physiol. Psychol.*, 84: 2 (1973), 252–257.
97. Wolff, P. H. The serial organization of sucking in the young infant. *Pediatrics*, 42 (1968), 943–956.
98. Wooten, G. F. and Cardon, P. V. Plasma dopamine-beta-hydroxylase activity. *Arch. Neurol.*, 28: 2 (1973), 103–106.
99. Wyatt, R. J., Murphy, D. L., Belmaker, R., Cohen, S., Donnelly, C. H., and Pollin, W. Reduced monoamine oxidase activity in platelets: A possible genetic marker for vulnerability to schizophrenia. *Science*, 179: 4076 (1973), 916–918.
100. Wyatt, R. J., Termini, B. A., and David, J. Biochemical and sleep studies of schizophrenia: A review of the literature—1960–1970. *Schizophrenia Bull.*, No. 4 (Fall 1971), 10–66.
101. Yalom, I. D., Green, R., and Fisk, N. Prenatal exposure to female hormones. *Arch. Gen. Psychiat.*, 28: 4 (1973), 554–561.
102. Zarcone, V. Narcolepsy. *New England J. Med.*, 288: 22 (1973), 1056–1166.

The Dakar Discussion: A Review

Cyrille Koupernik, M.D. (France)

The International Study Group discussed the presentations of *Lambo* and *Asuni* with great interest, since between them they spanned both the traditional and the emerging societies in Africa. *Lehmann* wanted to emphasize the role of plurality of beliefs, of models of interpretations, and of urges as a cause of insecurity in rapidly changing societies. The patients that he saw were a prey to contradictory wishes and cravings related to the conflicting demands made upon them. As a result, it was not always easy to understand their motivations. *Lambo* described the defense mechanisms of traditional society as flexible, but the flexibility was an adaptation within each type of society so that people leaving it would enter a rapidly changing society unprepared for the conditions of efficiency and competitiveness prevailing there.

Flexibility was found to be a useful device to help individuals through an acute psychotic regression to avoid more serious deterioration, but it only helped individuals return to the status quo, which is not enough help if one has to live in a Westernized setup. This was one reason for questioning the validity of occidental techniques of psychotherapy even in an urbanized African milieu. *Dores* also had doubts about flexibility. It was difficult for him to imagine that the ego of an individual, whatever his culture, could be more or less diffused than the ego of someone else. He was also doubtful about maternal surrogation within the extended family group and felt that the handing over of a child to a grandmother or maternal aunt had its own dynamic conflicts. The African child may react very much like his Western brother in similar circumstances: he will become frustrated, upset, and enuretic. In the African languages, the words for different members of the family may be the same, but the behavior expected of these various family members are quite distinct. The rivalry between co-wives of a polygamous family was similar to that between sisters (*wuoudiante dore ci domu mbey*).

Chilande wished to add a further criterion, essential for psychiatry, to *Hersov's* two criteria of normality: to live in conformity with one's ideals and within the average expectations of the culture. The third criterion referred to the optimal mental functioning that enabled the individual to experience to his fullest, to readjust flexibly to changes in his circumstances, and to enjoy a sense of well being.[1] Sometimes society can prevent these readjustments by excluding or confining individuals (with the help of the psychiatrists) before they have time to return to the expected range of functionings.

In response to *Leiderman's* presentation, *Marcus* reminded the group that different methods of infant rearing modified the rate of motor development. For instance, an urban infant, lacking physical closeness with his mother, may seem floppy until she goes back to her village and returns him to his traditional position on her back, whereupon the infant almost immediately braces up and demonstrates the same precocious motor development as the other infants in the village.

Senghar pointed out that prematurity needed to be carefully defined and that it was not enough for an infant to be born before term to be called premature. Strictly defined, the prematurity rate in Senegal was about 8 percent. It was *Senghar's* impression that pregnant women who worked long and hard in the field were liable to have premature births. The greatest risk to the developing fetus and to his central nervous system was malnutrition in the mother, part of the general malnutrition endemic in Africa. After birth and throughout his childhood, whether he lived in the rural or in the poor urban areas, he would be chronically undernourished.

Valantin, commenting on the urban population in Dakar, felt that the gains and losses in living conditions depended on how you looked

---

[1] The concept of normality is more fully discussed by Lebovici and Diatkine elsewhere in this volume.

at it. The urban child appeared to gain in language and social skills but, on the other hand, suffered degrees of maternal deprivation compared to children in the traditional society. Another observation of the urban child was the mastery that he displayed with regard to the functioning of his body and the good relationship that he established with the bodies of others. This left one wondering whether the physical aspects in changing communities tended to get eroticized. The mother in this setting could expect the child to become more rapidly autonomous and to fend for himself with regard to feeding. The behavior of any particular mother tended to be a compromise between individual and cultural demands, so that individual differences did exist and cultural differences did exist, and one could no more generalize about a particular district than about the African continent itself, where a high degree of diversity existed in all cultural matters. The one common denominator, it seemed to *Valantin*, was the lack of support for the developing child and his increasing vulnerability.

Sangaret said that the prematurity rate, the miscarriage rate, and the infant mortality rate were much higher than in Europe. The average birth weight of the newborn was about 20 percent lower (2900 grams). These obstetrical problems stemmed from three facts: the immaturity of the mothers, often pregnant by the age of 14 or 15; multiple exhausting pregnancies and consanguinous marriages heightening the risk of genetic recessive disease; and severe maternal anemia. Prostitution was often rife among school-age girls, but there was a resistance to sex education on the part of African families. Criminal abortion was also on the increase, a phenomenon previously unknown in Africa. *Sanokho* pointed out that in Africa the mother only and not the father would bring the child to the clinic, but this did not mean that fathers were segregated from their children. In the rural areas the contact was often very intimate and the fathers readily played with the children. *Leiderman*'s observations therefore were not conducted under typical conditions. *Sanokho* also had doubts about the validity of tests devised for European and American children. *Diallo* said that the prematurity rate in Senegal was 8.5 percent, but that only premature infants weighing under 1500 grams were in real danger. In his opinion the main problem was malnutrition, which was responsible for one-third of the deaths in childhood.

In response to the discussion *Leiderman* admitted that prematurity rates were different from those in the United States, but what he was stressing was the key role of the mother. In one respect it was perhaps not an advantage for the African infant to have rapid early development, since this would inevitably be associated with diminished maternal intervention. This was perhaps why some mothers in Africa even tried to delay this development. In lieu of birth control methods, the African woman attempted to lengthen the interval between pregnancies. For example, in some tribes, a woman may be forbidden sexual intercourse for four years following childbirth, a situation that was possible only in a polygamous setup. There is also a superstition in Africa that breast feeding by a pregnant woman can have harmful effects on the fetus, and in some places this has led to precocious weaning with harmful consequences of malnutrition and emotional deprivation. This was probably one of the etiological factors in kwashiorkor. With regard to infant testing, *Leiderman* pointed out that African children in the first year performed better on the classical infant tests, and therefore there seemed to be no valid reason for not using these tests. There were also time schedules of observation of the family.

Lebovici voiced the concern of the group for the distortions produced in normal family life by the intrusion of the observer teams. From his own experience in audiovisual work with families, he found that each member appeared to have his own reasons for participating and his own reactions to participation. *Lebovici* himself had some difficulty in equating the family he knew in real life to the family that appeared on the screen. Time sampling had obvious limitations. He recalled one observational study in which the mother is preparing to go to the hospital to have a baby, and she asks her two children to help her with the packing, which they do very willingly. She then leaves the room for a brief period, and the two children wilt into a state of marked depression. Had the session been terminated at the leaving of the mother, an important part of the dynamics of family life would have been missed. Incidentally, this young mother was quite uninhibited for all the time she was in front of the camera, except when she had her first glimpse of her newborn baby. *Lebovici's* point was not in any way to underrate the importance of systematic observation of family life but simply to point to some of the complex and dynamic factors that could influence the procedures.

Diop said that in Senegal, as in other developing countries, the

parents and children often appeared to live in two different cultures
—traditional and modern—and due to the decay of traditional
culture, important traditions were no longer being transmitted. He
wondered to what extent parents, facing this rapid change, were at
risk and whether society might be able to devise methods for
preserving the treasures of traditional culture. *Diop* wondered, too,
under conditions of multiple fathering and mothering, as existed in
Senegal, whether the identifications of the child were with the group
or with the biological parents. He suspected that in traditional
societies the shared nucleus of beliefs was so powerfully effective
throughout the group that the deeper identifications were with this.

Makang Yaounde was of the opinion that it was impossible to
understand the development of the African child from a point of
observation between cultures. You needed to be inside a culture to
appreciate what was really taking place. The difference between the
two cultures was radical. In Europe and America the child achieved
autonomy by becoming independent from his family, whereas in
Africa maturity was reached without this separation. Furthermore,
the African family was much more a sociocultural institution than is
the small nuclear Western family. The whole environment of
development is differently perceived and conceived. Space and time
are not objective but profoundly loaded with emotional feeling. The
schedules are almost unknown. The African child eats when he is
hungry, not at any regular meal time. The Western observer might
well misunderstand the passivity of the parent in relation to the child,
not realizing that this ensures a greater freedom for the child from
living out the fantasies of his parents. The ancestral influence is
powerful in Africa but relatively minor in European or American
life. *Makang Yaounde* felt it was important for Africans to study
their own culture from within and not to place themselves on the
outside looking in. Finally, he thought that the idyllic picture
presented of the African child as absolutely devoid of aggressiveness
was also totally false.

In response to the discussion *Lambo* said that it seemed quite
obvious from the remarks that we were at the present time in Africa
at the crossroad, and badly in need of more knowledge. There also
appeared to be a discrepancy between theory and actuality. He was
optimistic that the future would lead to progression rather than
retrogression in spite of all the difficulties involved in emergent

societies. For example, it had been shown that children from middle-
class homes exhibited more psychopathology, more disengagement
and retreat than children from rural areas where they can disengage,
retreat, husband their resources, and remobilize for greater consolidation. For the purpose of clarification, it seemed to *Lambo* that the
Euro-American model was a straightjacket for the African and an
intolerable theoretical bind. He thought that women in general in
Africa needed to have their lives opened up and broadened if they
were really to become participant members in the advancement of
all Africa.

In response to *Asuni's* presentation, *M'Bodj* discussed the different
kinds of 4-year-olds in Senegal and the child living in the forest area,
in a residential district of Dakar, or in the poorest suburb of the
town. In traditional society the 4-year-old lived with his family with
a high degree of dependence on his mother. He joined the male clan
at the age of 7. In many respects the 4-year-old appeared to have a
special niche in the society and to be the very center of interest of the
family. There was a Wolof who said: "To give up one's 4-year-old
was to lose all that is pleasurable in life." In the urban and suburban
areas the situation was different. If the family was well-to-do, the
4-year-old went to kindergarten, and if the family was poor and the
home too small, he wandered in the streets.

Diallo made reference to the conflicts commonly occurring in the
latency child at school and manifesting themselves in psychosomatic
illness, learning problems, tension habits, and so on. In his opinion,
the traditional way of life was rapidly vanishing from the cities, and
it seemed obvious to him that the African mother in urban areas,
having to earn her living, was unable to give the children the affection
that they needed. Unfortunately, she still maintained the traditional
outlook that placed the greatest value in the greatest number of
children.

Rickards said that the elite obviously provided a high risk environment for their children, many of whom were becoming increasingly
vulnerable to its effects. He thought that the same problems occurred
in the elite environment of developed countries and that the
problems were aggravated for developing countries. *Thebaud* felt
that Africans were facing a brand-new situation for which traditional
culture had no answers. He reiterated that the risks were as great for
the adults as for the children. *Anthony* concluded that from what

they had heard it seemed that the physical risks were paramount for the young African child, but that in his traditional setting he seemed to be relatively immune psychologically or at least not to manifest classical psychiatric symptoms and syndromes. It was only with residential and social mobility that he appeared to become psychologically vulnerable and to develop the typical clinical picture, described by *Asuni*, that would take him to the child guidance clinic once the society was sufficiently developed to establish them.

Asuni, in answer to the discussion, emphasized that the problems of the children were actually the problems of the parents in failing to provide for the changes in circumstance. The schools, as in Europe and the United States, could serve as a port of entry into the family for the purpose of institutig the treatment. From a preventive point of view, it seemed important to provide buffers in this rapidly changing situation.

The next part of the discussion addressed itself to the presentations of *Comer* and *Cohen*. *Lambo* pointed out that the previous discussions centered on the cultural differences between Europe and the United States on the one side and Africa on the other. In *Comer's* presentation a third world was introduced, combining something of both, that of the black American. He briefly categorized the United States as a newly created country with a great amount of aggressiveness and competitiveness, and, what was especially interesting to the African, a large Black population that emerged out of Africa and out of slavery into a current situation that was partially segregated, unequal, and insecure. Comer referred to the importance of religion to the black American, and there was no doubt that the African was also deeply religious. As far as education was concerned, however, it was his opinion that the black African was much worse off than his American counterpart for the simple reason that the black American was a full citizen with the right and privilege to bring up his children as an American child with, at least theoretically, an equal opportunity for education. Until the last decade, this was quite different in Africa.

The colonial powers had entered Africa to exploit it, had failed to understand the African culture, and had tried to destroy it. All sensory and motor expressions of the African soul were regarded as primitive and erotic and to be deprecated. The British and French culture and outlook were superimposed, and the African culture was gradually attenuated. The African and his family were therefore in a state of conflict and confusion, and the African child was often confronted with the dramatic choice of remaining an African or becoming a quasi-Frenchman or quasi-Englishman. The confusion extended to education. Until recently, neither psychologists nor psychiatrists have had much influence on educational practice, and it has been left to teachers themselves to choose, somewhat randomly, from the two worlds open to them for their educational techniques. *Comer* was hopeful that help could be obtained from highly specialized individuals, who would apply themselves directly to the needs of the African in an African world and devise appropriate educational methods to fit in with the new demands of a changing world.

Asuni felt that the educational system in Africa tended to estrange a child from his family and from his natural environment. The school authorities generally did not take the rules and regulations of the traditional environment into consideration in dealing with a child from this environment. In many parts of Africa the village community was still responsible for meeting the fees of their children attending school, and this gave them a sense of responsibility for the child's education. In other parts of Africa the connection between the school and the community had been dissociated, and this had led to less cross-fertilization between school and community. Another problem was that the schools were training students for jobs which did not exist and preparing them for life in a modern world, and there was no room for them there. Furthermore, excessive emphasis was placed on the terminal examinations and on their significance, so that many of the students resort to drugs such as amphetamines to help them to pass. As a result, amphetamine psychoses are becoming much more frequent. Young people who left their safe rural communities to seek a life in the cities often ended up in delinquency, since the opportunities were very few. *Asuni* agreed with *Lambo* that the radical revision of the educational system was needed to preserve the spirit that was essentially African.

Thebaud wondered to what extent the plight of the black Americans was a financial one, and whether if this improved, the black American would be integrated completely into the American society. In reply, *Comer* said that even if environmental conditions were much improved for all groups in the United States, the main problems would remain. There was a risk entailed whenever an individual moved from a smaller to a larger community or from a poorer to a richer one, or from one lower down to one higher up on the social scale.

In the discussion of *Cohen's* presentation, *Asuni* mentioned that cases of infantile autism did exist in Nigeria, but because of the distances involved any follow-up study was extremely difficult. *Hersov* wondered to what extent personality traits observed during the neonatal period persisted when the child was reassessed at a later date, and in the case of the children who improved on testing, were there any indications of what factors influenced this development. *Rickards* reported a retrospective study of asthma and eczema which had found that parental depression was an important associated factor.

Anthony complimented *Cohen* on his model-making, which offered the conference a scientific basic for its deliberations. It was important for models to be used judiciously and parsimoniously and not to be overextended and overloaded. To understand a piece of work with a construct built into it, it was important to have some idea how the model came into being, what previous models had been constructed, and why this particular one had become the favorite of its inventor. He was in favor of model-making for the purpose of clarifying areas of research. They were easier to visualize and, in fact, easier to work with since they were more flexible than hypotheses. To be presented with a model fully fashioned and without a history, like the one given by *Cohen*, was unfair to the progenitor since we needed to know much more about the mode of construction and the reason for selection. The massive questionnaire method was one to which most clinicians were antipathetic, because one never knew what the questions meant to the respondents, what they understood by them, and what they misunderstood. The reliabilities appeared to be good, but this in itself did not help to obviate the built-in limitations of method. It surprised Anthony that sensitive clinicians still fell a prey to it because it seemed such an easy way of amassing a great deal of information in the shortest possible time. As in all research, a short-cut was often inadequate. In the psychophysiological responses of infants, the thresholds, the activities, and the sensitivities tended to have a normal distribution with the vulnerabilities polarized at both ends.

In response, *Cohen* thought it was a mistake to look for continuity of behavior traits from infancy to adulthood. This would be a very simplistic way to look at human development, and the picture is very much more complicated than that. Whether the response to stress took certain specific forms that persisted over time was another matter. *Cohen* agreed with *Anthony* that we needed to look at the extremes of the continuum for those at risk, and one certainly needed better population studies to know what the distributions were. With regard to the natural history of his research, *Cohen* felt that he might be able to rationalize and claim that it was in continuity with hypotheses generated by previous work. His use of questionnaires was in keeping with his resolve to remain open-minded in his methodology and to try techniques that seemed relevant and gave promise of good results. It was his hope that child researchers would show increased flexibility in exploring the clinical problems of childhood.

A Summing Up of the Dakar Conference

"Care for Your Children as You Wish Them to Care for Your Grandchildren"

Albert A. Solnit, M.D. (U.S.A.)

This summary begins with events of one year ago in Bled, Yugoslavia, when the International Study Group decided to meet in Africa. The decision was based on our wish to demonstrate and experience the international scope of our interests and commitments. We also decided to prepare ourselves by having two days of site visits before the conference to create a working mood that could be evoked by direct contact with children and their families where they live. We wished to sharpen our thinking about theoretical issues through observing directly the complexities of the child's life and development in a particular culture and society. Perhaps we should have arranged the site visits second rather than first because, as Serge Lebovici suggested, through a quotation from Lévi-Strauss, our observations would be more useful if they were directed by hypotheses and questions that our discussions would have provided.

In discussions of the site visits to Pikine, Medina, Sicap, Thies, Khombole, and magic carpet visits to Casamance, we realized we had been flooded by impressions and reactions. This reminded us to be modest about what we thought we observed and humble about the constraining, distorting tendencies in our observations, for example, in regard to children's toys and playful activities. In these new

settings, unfamiliar to most of us, the discomfort we experienced
tempted us to master our anxiety with a false sense of expertise.
Oh yes, we could understand and explain it. Then we settled down,
realizing the visits were a stimulus and an inspiration. And being in
Dakar reminded us how carefully we must weave together our
collaborative work if we were to be respectful of complexity, curious
about what we did not understand, available to the communications
of the Senegalese and our colleagues, observant of folkways that were
rich in their history and human feeling, and open to the questions
that could be asked if we were not too anxious, too guilty or too
ambitious.

We were repeatedly reminded that in the site visits, as with much
research, we usually contaminate the field which we are observing
through our entry into it. And yet certain observations may be
available only to the researcher in the field. In fact, the more useful
you are to those you are observing, the more likely they are to take
you into their community and let you in on their more personal,
more natural lives. It is doubtful that we were useful to those we
observed, hence we must be modest. In addition, we should not overlook the impact of being observed by those we came to see.

Professor Collomb has demonstrated this principle in a particularly
humane and scientific way and we are indebted to him for his
generosity in letting us see through his eyes. As clinicians and social
scientists, we continuously strive to be aware of how we contaminate
what we are observing and how to correct for it; how, in fact, blind
spots and tunnel vision in the observers are ubiquitous. It is necessary
to characterize these limitations in terms of the risk of distortions
and false generalizations, especially influenced by our own hypotheses,
biases, and tolerances.

I was reminded of an African saying about acculturation: When a
fool does not succeed in bleaching ebony, he tries to blacken ivory.
In this connection a Hausa saying may be helpful to us: Faults are
like a hill, you mount on your own and then see other people's. We
who are so aware of the needs and difficulties of self-understanding
can be aware of the importance of this folk wisdom.

Although we were not intending or presuming to become experts
on Africa though holding our meeting here, the warmth of the people
and our fascination with their customs and neighborhoods invited

us to learn and to return to our subject of vulnerability as preparation for clarifying our questions and moving slowly toward greater understanding. If we are to agree on a definition of vulnerability in childhood and what constitutes risk and mastery, we shall have to agree about what the child expects in his world and what the adults' expectations of the child are.

If conditions evoke the expectation of continuing wars or pestilence or starvation, then vulnerability under such conditions will not constitute the same characteristics as vulnerability under conditions of a peaceful, disease-free, safe environment with ample food for all. Similarly, if children are being reared in a technologically advanced or developing country, how will expectations and the impact of these expectations differ for these children compared to children growing up in an agrarian society? Finally, where the quality of life is characterized by one set of values it will have an influence that can be significant in shaping children as compared to the influence of a different set of values. For example, in those settings in which the community is in agreement that each family should have many children, as compared to the community in which each family limits itself to two or three children, the quality of life for children may be different, and the impact of economic and technological factors may be magnified and more difficult to cope with. Colin Turnbull has indicated this concern as well as many others.

And yet we do have criteria for healthy development that transcend variations of cultural settings and expectations. It appears that an affirmative answer can be supported when the criteria for sound mental health include the following:

1. Reasonably sound physical health.
2. The appearance of regularity in achieving maturational milestones indicating adequacy in locomotion, speech, and social responsiveness, and coordination that reflects a well-functioning neuromuscular system.
3. Capacity to move toward active mastery of situations that formerly required the care of an adult such as dressing and undressing, eating, and skills appropriate to the family and cultural setting.
4. Capacity to postpone impulsive behavior when it is unsuitable for the social setting.

5. A balance between adapting to the social environment and having an influence on modifying that environment in the service of the self and those to whom one is attached.
6. The resilient capacity to accept gratifications or experiences according to the family and cultural patterns which may be substitutes for those the child would seek or evoke for himself.
7. To have a reasonable sense of oneself as worthy of respect and affection according to the values of the family and community.
8. To be able to respond to the reasonable expectations of close adults, peers, and community institutions with satisfaction and without losing a sense of one's inner self and inclinations.
9. To undergo an exploratory, experimental phase in adolescence that leads to a new sense of self as an adult and that results in altered, more mature relations to parents.

The criterion of continuity in human relationships becomes a most important one in defining man's aims of caring for children, of protecting the community, and of dealing with the inevitability of death. Such a criterion may challenge the conviction of many here that one of the most favorable characteristics of African values and traditions is their focus on society rather than on the individual. Turnbull and others have amply formulated that point of view. However, can there be a focus on the one if there is not a balanced focus on the other? To be concerned with the well-being of the community assumes concern for the individual and his family. Our tendency, which I perceive as a risk, is to seek for an either-or solution.

Anthony's introduction provided a useful classification, a scaffold on which our observations and theories can be assembled in patterned ways. He suggested that various combinations of vulnerability and risk reflect not only the multiplicity of factors involved in determining vulnerability but also how the changes in maturation and in the environment will influence the dynamic states of vulnerability and invulnerability. He indicated that human beings have particular vulnerabilities at particular developmental periods.

Throughout the meeting there was strong agreement that the nations of Africa, like many other nations on other continents, are undergoing rapid change, especially with the advent of independence

from colonial status and technological advances. How does change
evoke strength? How does change evoke weakness?

Lambo's stimulating paper made it dramatically clear that just as
we say we cannot talk of a child without talking of his parents, we
should say we cannot talk of a mother without talking of her child or
children. Several provocative themes were evident in Lambo's paper
and throughout the meeting:

1. Are tensions, frustrations, and conflicts in the child in the first
    years of life undesirable and disadvantageous, regardless of the
    culture? Conversely, if it is possible, is it desirable to fully
    satisfy the child as soon as his need is expressed? What are the
    risks of arresting development by infantilizing the child?
2. How shall we talk to each other when we are using different
    magnifications? One of us wants to talk about the family and
    another about the community, society, and culture, and yet
    another wants to focus on the individual child. It is clear to me
    that we need all these magnifications, but it is most difficult to
    set them up simultaneously and to know how they fit together.
    I suspect we have tended to oppose these magnifications rather
    than to integrate them.
3. Under conditions of rapid urbanization, which traditions
    increase the family's capacity to make its way and to thrive, and
    which sap the family's strength under urban conditions of life?

The very thoughtful papers by Asuni and Leiderman reminded us
of two risks associated with improved family status and economic
conditions. We were confronted with the possibility that the parents,
by realizing their ambitions, are likely to loosen family ties, especially
as the child grows older. Should we speak of Europeanization and
urbanization of African families as a complicating force, one that
invites families to give up the old ways and buffeting resources for
new opportunities and alien traditions? Are we failing to recognize
the dissatisfactions with rural life that motivate families to move to
the city?

In Dr. Omololu's fine paper we are reminded that with the rapid
changes in Africa there is a widening discrepancy between what is
supposed to be the breast-feeding pattern and how it has been altered
in recent years in Nigeria and other parts of Africa. Malnutrition is

the inevitable destructive companion of low-income nations, of societies that have been unable to cope with rapid technological changes. Poor education about nutritional factors is a critical factor. Until Dr. Sanokho and Dr. Omololu called it to our attention, we tended not to give sufficient attention to the nutrition of mothers.

Throughout we were admonished to avoid overgeneralizing and to pay attention to individual differences as well as group similarities. Although it was not spelled out, the risk of idealizing the child's life and glossing over the child's difficulties was implied several times. Moreover, there was a hesitancy about looking at the disadvantages as well as the advantages of breast feeding until 18–24 months of age, of the child sleeping with the mother until 3 years of age, and other aspects of a "blissful" infancy without wondering if that is a sound preparation for the life that lies ahead. We are sorely lacking in the clinical observations that shed light on the child's inner life. This can be thought of as high-power magnification.

Our colleagues from Senegal, Nigeria, the Ivory Coast, the Cameroons, and Liberia reminded us tactfully and repeatedly about the children who suffer from asthma, behavior disorders, school learning difficulties, and other psychological problems. Dr. Diop in a searching analysis revealed to us how one cannot understand the development of the Wolof child without understanding his family, his cultural background, and the changes that are stressing what had been viewed as a stable and nurturing environment.

Dr. Comer's report required us to see differences and similarities that are disquieting. He challenged us to understand change and at the same time to see how many patterns are similar when a large population group is oppressed in different ways for a prolonged period of time. There is the important indication that being oppressed by outsiders in your own land is different. Subjects of such oppression may be less vulnerable, though not at less risk of such political, cultural, economic, psychological, and biological trauma and deprivation than those who were forcefully removed to an alien land and culture. American Blacks were subjected to over 400 years of slavery. This slavery was followed by a gradual trans-formation to a more subtle enslavement as second-class citizens. Comer focused on education and the responsibility and capacities of the schools to provide the child and his family with an appropriate and effective preparation for life and for moving into the mainstream of the life of a particular country and culture. He also called attention, as did many of our African colleagues, to the need to study how children express their strengths, their vulnerabilities, and their capacities for mastery. He reaffirmed what many others have emphasized, that is, the intimate, inextricable, and essential unity of the child with his family and the family with its community.

At yet another level of conceptualization is our need to join understanding from sociological and cultural studies to knowledge of psychic and biological dynamics that are so crucial for understanding individual behavior and development. Donald Cohen challenges us to accept multiple models to clarify the questions and to study the complexities of the child and his family at psychiatric risk. Is it true, as some have wondered, that the African child is less at psychiatric risk than at the risk of an unstable environment that threatens to deplete his emotional and cultural buffers and his individual resiliency?

In the study of individual children with kwashiorkor, as Dr. Collomb pointed out, the biological, psychological, and cultural contextual factors must be interwoven if we are to get a three-dimensional view of how this condition comes about for the individual child and how it appears epidemiologically. Both sources of understanding are necessary if we are to prevent this grave condition.

Donald Cohen developed a multifaceted model in which the investigation of endowment (genetic, biochemical, and neurophysiological) is combined with the study of personality and psychosomatic states that also reflect the impact of a particular environment. His report attempted to bridge these critical areas of knowledge and the techniques that uncover the data for such analysis. The study of sucking in newborns, of children with eczema, of the similarities and differences in twinships, and of children with psychotic development are related by a focus on sources of stress, individual differences, and the coping patterns evoked. Interventions can assist the child and clarify the miscroscopic and macroscopic mechanism (biological and psychological) that are elaborated in these states.

In these presentations there was a breathtaking scope of phenomena, methods of study, theories that clarify and are productive, and of multiple determinations involved in a balanced understanding of children at risk, the relative meaning of vulnerability, and the extraordinary resources children have available for mastery. Are we attempting too much for our limited capacities? At this time in our history we felt it would be less risky to try to keep in mind this complexity than to take advantage of restricting our vision to achieve a higher illumination of a narrower field. Both are necessary, but in recent decades we have emphasized the sharper focus and have sacrificed the effort to view more complex mosaics because it requires us to be less confident, more tentative, and to live with a greater amount of ambiguity. Ambiguity is less obvious, but it is still operational in the study of more restricted fields with higher illumination.

We also discussed the advantages of hypotheses that are testable as compared to model-building research. Our metaphors linked our science to the beauty of women and to the audacity of new automobiles.

Conclusions

In this conference we were fortunate to be challenged by presentations that represent a balance of naturalistic and experimental studies, of findings that embrace complexities and of findings that are derived from sharply focused, highly illuminated investigations. We ranged from anthropological theories of family function and structure and world views of urbanization to the biochemical cycles and linkages of the biogenic amines; from a consideration of the child's resiliency and resources to a focus on his vulnerabilities and risks and to an awareness of the influences of ever-changing societal and cultural forces and patterns.

Yes, we can think of the parable of the six blind men reporting on the elephant. Can we help each other see more clearly the different states of health and illness that are the reality of our times? We must have the patience and persistence of weavers concerned equally with beauty, usefulness, humanitarian values, and scientific explanation if we are to move ahead on the tasks outlined by this conference.

STUDIES IN RISK AND
VULNERABILITY

Enduring Disturbances in Behavior Following Acute Illness in Early Childhood: Consistencies in Four Independent Follow-Up Studies

John J. Sigal, Ph.D. (Canada)

There is a considerable literature dealing with the immediate psychological effects on the patient and his family of chronic or fatal illness in childhood. The common clinical observation that physical illness in early childhood may have psychological repercussions for the patient and his family long after the illness has disappeared has only infrequently been systematically explored. The results of those studies which have been done appear contradictory.

Stott [15] is the pioneer. He obtained teachers' ratings on the reading ability and on a standard measure of social adjustment of children 7 to 11½ years old who had been hospitalized for at least 2 weeks when less than 3 years old. Controls were matched for age and sex and attended the same schools as the former patients. The formerly ill children had more severe reading disabilities and were more inhibited or "unforthcoming," a term Stott used to describe children who were depressed, withdrawn, and excessively dependent, or lacking in normal assertiveness, but in no way affectless or hostile. Stott marshalls evidence to suggest that these defects are probably congenital, unrelated to environmental influences.

Green and Solnit [5] reported only on those aspects of their clinical investigations that dealt with children who are expected by their mothers to die prematurely. They found evidence to support the hypothesis that these mothers infantilize the children and that the children react with separation difficulties, hypochondriacal complaints, and school underachievement. Their sample of children ranged in age from newborn to 10 years when they had the illness or accident that triggered these maternal fears; the children were 17 months to 14 years at the time of the investigation.

Gibson [4] examined children who at least 4 years prior to the study, when they were less than 5 months old, underwent surgery for pyloric stenosis, atresia of the esophagus, or imperforate anus. He compared them with a group of children matched for age, sex, and intelligence from intact homes, who were deliberately selected to have no demonstrable psychological or social problems. On the basis of projective test findings with the children and structured personality tests of the mothers, he concluded that trauma in early infancy did not necessarily lead to later psychological disturbance. (The astresia group had an insignficant number of indices of disturbance). When there was a psychological disturbance it occurred in those children whose mothers were most disturbed or had the most negative attitudes to their children.

Costanza et al. [3] studied children who had been hospitalized when less than 1 year old from 4 to 7 years after hospitalization and compared them with all their siblings and with an age-matched subgroup of these siblings. They interviewed the mothers about each child, using a questionnaire consisting of some items dealing with normal behavior from the MacFarlane group's study [6] and other items dealing with personality, behavior at home and at school, and health. They found no differences between the formerly ill children and other control groups.

It is almost impossible to draw any logical conclusions from these studies. At the time of the illness or at the time of evaluation or both, the children in some studies were extremely heterogeneous by criteria of cognitive or dynamic development. As a result, negative findings (e.g., ref. 3) are open to serious question. Only those positive findings that occur in a significant proportion of the former patients (e.g., problems in impulse control in Green and Solnit's study) are suggestive of problems relatable to the earlier illness. Moreover, such studies as Gibson's apply measures which bear a tenuous relationship with actual behavior and make the results even more difficult to evaluate.

The studies conducted by my group [11–13], although having certain methodological defects, put some order into this chaotic state and provide some preliminary information on the question of long-term effects of early childhood illness. We examined three groups of children that were homogeneous by cognitive development criteria; they were ill between 2 and 5 years of age and were evaluated when they were 7 to 12 years. Furthermore, the same series of questionnaires and projective tests were administered to the children and parents in all groups, so intergroup comparisons are possible. We intended to evaluate separately by sex children within narrower age ranges who were ill at each of a number of dynamically meaningful ages. However, sample sizes precluded realization of this goal.

Because the ages at which the children were ill and at which they were followed up are within definite developmentally meaningful limits, our results can be compared with those of other studies that used defined age groups, enabling us to reach some conclusions concerning the interactional effect of the disease on the development and family transaction patterns.

Method

SAMPLES

In each sample of former inpatients all charts of the two major pediatric hospitals and of some general hospitals with pediatric wards in a large metropolitan area were examined. Attempts were made to contact all patients who met the following criteria: the patient had to be between the ages of 2 to 5 at the time of hospitalization and 7 to 12 years at the time of reading the charts; there was no evidence of mental deficiency, brain damage, or other physical or mental handicaps; the patient had at least one sibling who was 7 to 12 years old at the time of the study, who had not had a severe physical or mental illness at any time, and was not mentally retarded.

All the parents of these children who could be contacted by phone or by letter and who, after preliminary interviews, continued to meet the criteria outlined were included in the study. There was a very great attrition rate, primarily because the families could not be located.

Three independent groups of families were obtained in this way. In one group a child had suffered from nephrosis, in another from croup, and in the third from gastroenteritis. In all cases the illness had been severe enough to necessitate hospitalization, in some cases for extended periods of time or on several occasions. All cases were moderately to severely ill. Full details of the sample may be found in the original papers.

QUESTIONNAIRES

Only the objective questionnaire data will be discussed here, since we have not completed our analysis of the projective data. Peterson and Quay's Behaviour Problem Checklist (BPC) [7] was selected as one of the measures of disturbance in children's behavior for three reasons. First, repeated studies have suggested that the factors of behavior measured by the test are stable across the age ranges relevant to our studies. Second, the test was constructed to include the entire range of complaints for which children are brought to child guidance clinics. Third, one of the factors that emerges from the studies by the authors of the test is Conduct Problems (unsocialized, agression), which approximates the area in which we had noted behavioral disturbances in the clinical work that led to this series of studies. To verify the clinical observations further, and to measure functional strengths, a new scale, the Sigal-Chagoya Child Behavior Inventory (CBI), was developed as a second measuring device (see Sigal et al. [11, 12] for details. Both inventories were completed by the two parents jointly for each of their children included in the study.

Perceived parental attitudes and behavior were measured by Schaefer's Child Report of Parent Behaviour Inventory (CRPBI) [7]. This questionnaire was chosen because it has been shown to tap most parental attitudes explored by a wide variety of studies, and because its factorial structure is stable cross-culturally. The items were scored in two ways: once according to Schaefer's method, and again by grouping the same items under headings relating to our original clinical observations.

In addition, the parents of the croup children were asked a series of questions dealing with the nature and degree of their worry about their children's illness, about a number of other specific things, and about things in general. Their children were asked to rate the parents on similar questions.

Results and Discussion

What evidence is there from these studies for later psychological consequences of severe early childhood illness? The only factor in which the formerly ill children's behavior differed consistently from their siblings', although not always to a satisfactory level of statistical significance, was the Factor I of the BPC, Conduct Problems. On that factor the former patients scored higher than their siblings. Probabilities on a one-tailed t test were less than .10, .025, and .15 for the nephrotic, croup, and gastroenteritis groups, respectively. In addition, the croup group scored higher on Tests Limits ($p < .025$), Does Not Curb Aggression ($p < .10$), and the BPC Factor III, Inadequacy-Immaturity ($p < .20$). Their siblings scored higher on Curbs Aggression and Good Coping Behavior ($p < .05$ and $< .10$, respectively). The gastroenteritis group also scored higher than their siblings on the BPC Factor II, Neurotic Behaviour ($p. < .10$). Both croup and gastroenteritis patients scored higher than their siblings on Child Shows Excessive Dependence ($p < .10$ and $< .05$, respectively). The t tests for BPC Factors II and III were two-tailed, since no prediction had been made concerning the nature of the differences.

There were also consistencies in the children's ratings of their parents' attitudes. The three groups of former patients rated their parents higher than did their siblings on only one of the three CRPBI factors, Psychological Control. The variables in this factor—Control via Guilt, Hostile Control, and Instilling Persistent Anxiety—were responsible for this difference. In addition, there was a difference in the same direction for the croup and gastroenteritis groups in the area of Intrusiveness. On the CBI, patients more than their siblings, uniformly in the three disease groups, saw their parents as not fostering their independence, setting high standards, and setting limits. With a few minor exceptions, all differences were statistically significant for both parents in all groups on a two-tailed t test.

Since there is no way of knowing whether this sample obtained is truly representative of the parent population the results must be interpreted with caution. The most convincing results are those that are confirmed by other observers. Two of the studies previously mentioned do permit some comparisons. Unfortunately, the findings of one appear to agree with our results, whereas those of the other study are in complete disagreement. Green and Solnit's [5] data indicate that the symptoms most consistently mentioned might be grouped under the heading of impulse control, although they failed to note this when discussing their findings. This is consistent with the clinical observations that led us to initiate our series of studies and with our questionnaire findings. This support is weak, however, since Green and Solnit presumably wished to make a clinical point and reported only those cases that supported their hypotheses. They did not report on all cases that had been ill or injured, nor did they compare the incidence of the consequences they observed with the incidence of similar disorders in a control population. Furthermore, we have already mentioned their sample includes too wide a range of developmental levels.

We are incidentally able to confirm Green and Solnit's hypothesis about the parents' concern that the child might die. The children of parents who reported that they were concerned about the death of a child when he was ill had significantly higher Conduct Problem scores than those whose parents did not report concern about death at the time of the illness.

Stott's evidence [15] proves much more formidable and seems to directly contradict our findings. The "unforthcoming" children he describes seem to fit BPC Factor III, Inadequate-Immature, and to be the antithesis of our Factor I, Conduct Problem. The difference between the two groups is not likely to be due to the greater length of hospitalization of the children in his study, since he demonstrated that those who were hospitalized longest were least affected subsequently and Gibson [4] reported a similar finding.

It is in explaining the discrepant result of the two studies that the merits of the developmental-interactional approach proposed by Anthony [1] become clear. We and Stott both investigated children who were dynamically in latency and cognitively in Piaget's phase of concrete operations. The primary difference between the two sets of samples lies in the fact that Stott's group was ill at a younger age than was ours. Stott's sample was primarily at the age when object constancy develops, in the dynamic and cognitive sense, whereas the majority, if not all of ours had probably achieved object constancy before they were ill. The children in Stott's sample were much more dependent than ours on their mothers to mediate between their needs and the world, and their personality was much less structured. Stott's results suggest that the children remained in this state of dependence. He describes them as overaffectionate and dependent. For some reason they failed to achieve an independent existence. We might postulate that the illness interfered with the parents' ability to perform the normal task of facilitating ego growth to the stage of independent functioning with respect to the world. The dependent behavior then may be the consequence of a fixation that arises from interacting effects of mothers who were preoccupied and children whose egos were confronted with tasks which detracted from the normal developmental ones.

The data from our study of worries reported by the parents of children who had suffered from gastroenteritis suggests that it was primarily parental preoccupation that produced the type of behavior observed by Stott. We divided the group of parents into one group that reported a large number of worries not related to their children and a group that reported few such worries. The children of the general worriers scored significantly higher on BPC Factor III, Inadequacy-Dependency, the factor most descriptive of the type of disorder found by Stott.

Further supportive evidence for preoccupation as a causal variable derives from our studies of the families of survivors of the Nazi persecution [14]. We found that compared to appropriate clinic control patients, survivors' children who attended our clinics were rated higher on Conduct Problems when they were 8 to 12 years old and on Conduct Problems, Personality Problems, and Inadequacy-Immaturity when they were 15 to 17 years old. The preoccupation of the parent-survivors—not with the illness of their children, but with their own unending mourning and physicial debilitation—is well-known.

Ratings obtained from pediatricians of the likely duration of parental concern about each of the three illnesses studied adds further evidence to the hypothesized causal relationship between parental preoccupation and subsequent problems in impulse control in the children in our studies. Gastroenteritis was rated as the illness that evokes worry of the shortest duration, and it was children who were hospitalized for this illness who differed the least from the siblings in problems of impulse control.

Stott did not find the affectionless character described by Bowlby [2] or the problems of unsocialized aggression reported by Provence and Ritvo [8] because the children in his study had an interested, concerned mother, a significant object relationship in the dynamic sense of the term.

But why did we find problems in the area of impulse control? The children in our studies had already dealt with the discovery of the world. The parent-child interaction had been good enough to lay the groundwork for the child to come to terms with his existence as a separate entity. An essential aspect of this separation-individuation includes the appropriation of aggression. The task then was to lay the groundwork for coming to terms with himself and his impulses in relation to an outside world that had also acquired an independent existence. It was at this stage that the illness produced the failure in the parent-child interaction. The anxiety aroused by the concern that the child might die, as well as their general state of preoccupation prevented the parents from setting appropriate limits on the child. Since the controls are ineffectual, the child has no basis for an adequate internalization of them.

The data derived from the children's perception of their parents' behavior in our study, although current and not obtained over a period of years, and our clinical reconstruction of events [10, 11] are consistent with Solnit and Green's descriptions. The children in our studies rated their parents higher on the CRPBI variables, Instilling Persistent Anxiety, Control Through Guilt, and Hostile Control. This suggests the series of psychological events that are likely to occur in the parent when a child falls seriously ill. The thought that the child might die evokes anxiety and guilt, which the parent deals with in part by the mechanism of turning passive into active, that is, by making the child feel anxious and guilty too. The parent also feels angry with the child for inflicting this anxiety and guilt on him and for not responding to his attempts to control the child. The children perceived and reported all of these in the parents' interaction with them. The children's reporting (on our second sorting of the CRPBI items) that their parents set limits, set high standards, and do not foster independence reflects further interactional consequence of these parental attitudes and feelings.

It should be noted that although we have found consistencies in three independent studies and most of the differences are statistically significant, the overlap in the scores of patients and their siblings is so great that the results must be applied with caution. A severe illness in early childhood does not necessarily lead to disturbances in the parents, the child, or the parent-child interaction of later life. However, it occurs frequently enough to warrant alerting mental health professionals and pediatricians in this area of potential difficulty. Remedial measures may be indicated even if endowment is the primary basis for the vulnerability of some children, as Stott has postulated.

References

1. Anthony, E. J. A working model for family studies, in *The Child in His Family*, E. J. Anthony and C. Koupernik, Eds. John Wiley & Sons, New York, 1973.
2. Bowlby, J. *Maternal Care and Mental Health*, World Health Organization, Geneva, 1951.
3. Constanza, M., Lipsitch, I., and Charney, E. The vulnerable child revisited: A follow-up study of children three to six years after an acute illness in infancy. *Clin. Pediat.*, 7 (1968), 680–683.
4. Gibson, R. Trauma in early infancy and later personality development. *Psychosom. Med.*, 27 (1965), 229–237.
5. Green, M. and Solnit, A. Reactions to the threatened loss of a child: A vulnerable child syndrome. *Pediatrics*, 58 (1964), 58–66.
6. MacFarlane, J. W., Allen, L., and Honzik, M. P. *A Developmental Study of the Behavior Problems of Normal Children between Twenty-One Months and Fourteen Years*, University of California, Berkeley, 1962.
7. Peterson, D. Behavior problems in middle childhood. *J. Consult. Psychol.*, 25 (1961), 205–209.
8. Provence, S. and Ritvo, S. Effects of deprivation on institutionalized infants: Disturbance in development of relationship to inanimate objects. *The Psychoanalytic Study of the Child*, 16 (1961), 189–205.

9. Schaefer, E. S. Children's report of parental behavior: An inventory. *Child Develop.*, 36 (1965), 413–424.
10. Sigal, J. J. Familial consequences of parental preoccupation. Paper read at the Annual Meeting of the American Psychiatric Association, Dallas, May 1972.
11. Sigal, J. J., Chagoya, L., Villneuve, C., and Mayerovitch, J. Later psychological consequences of near-fatal illness (nephrosis) in early childhood: Some preliminary findings. *Laval Medical*, 42 (1971), 103–108.
12. Sigal, J. J., Chagoya, L., Villneuve, C., and Mayerovitch, J. Later psychosocial sequelae of early childhood illness (severe croup). *Amer. J. Psychiat.*, 130 (1973), 786–789.
13. Sigal, J. J. and Gagnon, P. Later psychosocial sequelae of early childhood illness (severe gastroenteritis). In preparation.
14. Sigal, J. J., Silver, D., Rakoff, V., and Ellin, B. Some second-generation effects of survival of the Nazi persecution. *Am. J. Orthopsychiat.*, 43 (1973), 320–327.
15. Stott, D. H. Infantile illness and subsequent mental and emotional development. *J. Genet. Psychol.*, 94 (1959), 233–251.

Long-Term Foster Care and Its Influence on Adjustment to Adult Life

Henry B. M. Murphy, M.D., Ph.D. (Canada)

When referring to children at risk, one's concern is implicitly with some danger yet to come, not with the damage that already exists. Children placed in boarding foster care and neither legally adopted nor able to be returned to their natural families within a short time have nearly always sustained some damage, whether it be from mistreatment, object loss, neglect, or an adverse inheritance. This damage and the abnormalities many foster children show have been the subject of much study, but the dangers that still lie in wait for them, either by reason of further mishandling or through a failure to mature properly, have received less attention. Studies of children still in foster care sometimes carry the gloomy implication that the prognosis must be bad [13, 19], but they do not go on to test that presumption. Follow-up surveys of former foster children are fewer and give a much more optimistic picture, but they scarcely look behind the personae which their respondents present to the world or discuss the probable state of those who refuse to give a reply [1, 8].

Since the foster child is often damaged even before the child protection authority learns about him, and because it is a general medical principle that prevention of further disease or damage

425

should take priority over the treatment of current symptoms, I believe that the organization and evaluation of foster care services for children should be based much more on the eventual production of healthy and adjusted adults than on their production of trouble-free children at shorter term. Prevention of the damage that usually makes the foster care necessary is still more preferable, of course, but it strikes me as a serious error to assess the foster home program itself on the basis of the foster family and child accepting each other [6] or on extrapolations from psychoanalytic theory [18].

The Former Foster Child Syndrome

In the 1960s two social work supervisors with exceptional memories and sources of information provided me with broad assessments of adult outcome for 316 Montreal children who had been at least five years in foster care during the period 1930–1959. The assessments were focused on social adjustment, and to provide both a check and a greater depth for these, 30 of the assessed subjects were traced and reassessed by research social workers and psychologists working with me. Of the 30, 10 had been thought by the social work supervisors to have made a satisfactory adjustment in the light of their backgrounds, 10 had been thought to have had poor adjustments, and the remainder were intermediate. They thus should have represented all degrees of outcome except the very worst, since we excluded persons who had recently been in trouble with the law or been in psychiatric care, so as to be assured of cooperation and to avoid disturbing the recent patients. (Persons who had left the region were also excluded.) For an idea of those worst outcomes, however, we also obtained abstracts from the records of every psychiatric patient at an English-speaking Montreal hospital who had been in foster care when young.

Despite the wide range of social outcomes and the exclusion of frankly psychiatric cases, a review of the 30 nonpatients revealed them to have certain personality traits in common, and since these traits are handicapping ones I am calling them a syndrome. Naturally the syndrome was much more handicapping in some than in others, but I believe that a search will reveal signs of it in many former foster children who appear well adjusted.

The first feature of the syndrome is a fear that society will hurt them, this fear masking a desire to hurt society. Neither the fear nor the hostility is likely to be admitted by the more adjusted subject and even some of the poorly adjusted deny the hostility, but the tendencies reveal themselves in many ways and are most easily demonstrated through the Rorschach Card IV whose commonest North American responses are "boots" or "feet" for adults and "animal skin" or "rug" for the college age [4]. Table I presents the abbreviated responses of the 14 former foster children who took this test; none give the "boots" response, only the most adjusted give the "skin" or "rug" response, two of the subjects are so disturbed by the card that they can give no responses at all, and the majority of the remainder project a frightening animal or monster. It is accepted that such responses on the Rorschach (found much more frequently in passive-aggressive delinquents than in other delinquents [17], for instance) represent hostility which the subject fears will be directed back at himself. Card IV is sometimes called the "father" card, but there is almost no correlation between what the former foster children report here and what we know about their actual fathers or their attitudes toward these fathers, and the interpretation of projected and feared aggression fits the rest of our data better.

Table 1   Rorschach Responses (condensed) Given by Former Foster Children to Card IV; By Adult Adjustment Rating and Rank on Mental Health Scale

Supervisors' Ratings of Adjustment	Mental Health Ranks	Sex	
Good	1	M	Bear rug; Général de Gaulle; goose necks
Good	2	M	Bear rug; standing animal; racoon skin
Doubtful	3	M	Bull's head; boar; fuzzy terrier
Doubtful	4	F	A big ape; a large tree root
Good	5	F	Cloud; trees; animal hide; rock
Good	6	M	Bird; gorilla; deerskin rug
Good	7	F	Hairy monster; seaweed; moth
Doubtful	8	M	Musk ox; savage man
Doubtful	9	M	Old castle tower; grotesque creature reclining
Poor	10	F	Gorilla carrying something wicked; pretty flower; waves falling over
Poor	11	F	Big gorilla in front of tree, going to charge any minute
Poor	12	F	(No response given)
Poor	13	M	(No response given)
Poor	14	F	Movie monster scaring me out of my wits

The second feature composing the syndrome is, not unexpectedly, an excessive concern with defenses against both the hurt and the hostile impulses. Perhaps this feature would have been less prominent if we had included subjects with a recent history of trouble with the police but I doubt it, since frank aggressiveness is rare in the subsequent histories of Montreal foster children. The researchers' reports on the 30 repeatedly mentioned guarding, constriction, execessive self-control, and an absence of freedom of expression, even though first impressions were often of an easygoing personality. A lack of ego strength, of intelligence, or of a coherent world view was *not* attributed to most of these subjects, and in some instances the presence of notable ego strength was remarked on, but it then was usually stated that this strength was being devoted to maintaining defenses. The less well-adjusted subjects were usually assessed to have little ego strength or self-control, and it was also observed that their activities were severely restricted, something which seems most likely to be due to the constant need to guard against impulse, a guarding that was not a luxury, judging from the histories of the psychiatric patients to be mentioned shortly.

The third feature in the hypothesized syndrome is a precipitate desire for marriage and home, combined with a low tolerance for the demands these can make. The marriage rate for the 30 was definitely higher than for the general Montreal population, age for age, and the rate of divorce or separation was many times higher than in the equivalent Montreal population, 5 of the 30 having been married and either divorced or legally separated by the age of 29[1] and 2 more having gone through a succession of common-law unions and separations. All 30 recognized that they had had, from the time they left their foster homes, a strong desire for their own home and children, although they often claimed to have been unusually sexually ignorant and unprepared. Several felt that their former foster parents or other adult counselors should have prevented them from marrying so young and one with a successful marriage was grateful that her first effort had been prevented.

The desire for children was genuine and the 26 ever-married subjects had 42 children, although their mean age was only 28, but

---

[1] These are 1965 data as related to the 1961 census. Divorce rates in the 1970s are substantially higher than in 1960s.

this seems to have represented an effort to experience vicariously a "normal" childhood rather than a desire for parenthood. Neither in their observed behavior with their own children nor in their psychological tests did most of them exhibit the easy, nurturant character of the effective parent. Sometimes they seemed to treat their children as rivals. It is possible that the difficulties experienced in many of their marriages were in part due to the difficulty of controlling hostility in so intimate a setting, but the main factor appears to be that the subjects had been looking for a nurturant partner, only to discover that their marriage-hungry partners had been looking for nurturance also, and neither had sufficient self-confidence to do the giving. Fortunately, where the marriages lasted both partners usually grew to learn how to give.

The syndrome just described was found, it must again be stressed, in persons who had not sought psychiatric care or broken down to an extent that such care had to be imposed on them. In the best adjusted of the 30 we could find only traces of it, just sufficient to make us regret that the effort at self-control was blocking so much of their potential talent. In the least adjusted there were many other symptoms present and there is a possibility that some of these also belong to the syndrome. However, these other symptoms might have been present without the foster experience, and it seems better not to cloud the issue by adding them.

What remains to be mentioned is what happens when this syndrome is associated with a frank mental breakdown, and for this one must turn to the 11 psychiatric patients with a history of long-term foster care. That number of patients is not excessive in relation to the relevant populaton at risk (those ill from childhood had been excluded), and the clinical syndromes spanned a wide range, but the factors which precipitated their breakdowns were often related to their foster experience and to a repressed aggression. Two became psychotic and attacked their natural mothers soon after rejoining them after a long separation, and a third attempted suicide under similar circumstances. Two broke down soon after the death of a foster parent, with symptoms of confusion or guilt rather than a simple loss reaction, and two more broke down after the birth of their first children, fearing to hurt the child or fearing to become a bad mother. I have no wish to argue that these breakdowns would have been avoided if the foster placement had not taken place, for in at least three instances there was a family history of psychosis, but it should be clear from these brief remarks that difficulties in handling aggression and in assuming the parental role were contributing factors.

"Natural Family" Influences

Before discussing what to do for such a syndrome it is normal to explore its possible causes, particularly if such exploration can provide a guide to prognosis and thus to the differentiation of the poorer risk from the better risk cases. For this exploration it is natural to start with the events that led to the placement, and since these events are often confused a more reliable prognosis source has proved to be what is recorded about the natural parents. The maximum impact of the latter's behavior may actually be later, or it may change character, but what one can learn about them at the time the placement is made provides a useful base from which to make a prognosis.

Coded abstracts were therefore made of the complete background data recorded on the 316 foster children whose later careers were sufficiently known to the agency supervisors for outcome assessments to be possible, and a search was made for correlates of these assessments. Since a rating of "poor adjustment" had to be based on solid evidence of some social or mental disturbance in adult life, whereas the difference between "good" and "doubtful" ratings was more subjective, and also because the rating of "poor adjustment" agreed very well with our own research ratings of poor mental health for a third of the 30 reassessed cases, it was decided to seek for indicators to a poor outcome rather than indicators to a good one, though the latter were not wholly ignored. Poor adult adjustments were assessed to have occurred in 14 percent of male and 26 percent of female subjects, and although my first inclination was to assume that the supervisors had given too much weight to sexual promiscuity or unmarried pregnancy for the girls, examination of the clinical pictures of the 30 more intensely investigated subjects, and of the patients, convinces me that the girls are more at risk, perhaps because they cannot assume a maternal role without "identifying with the aggressor."

After analyzing the percentages of "poor" adult adjustments made by foster children with different preplacement histories, the most significant prognostic indicator was clearly the structure of the natural family at the time the placement was initiated. This is shown in Figure 1 where one sees that over 50 percent of the girls whose parents were unmarried or casually separated adjusted poorly, whereas less than 5 percent of those coming from families broken by death or still unbroken turned out this way. With the boys it was not so much the normality of the family unit which was significant but the normality of the mother herself as judged by her record of heavy drinking, psychiatric treatment, and police arrests. If she had such a record and if she was unmarried or casually separated, then the boy she placed had only about a 60 percent chance of avoiding a poor adjustment. If she were unmarried or casually separated but had no other record of abnormality, then he had about 90 percent chance of avoiding that outcome, and if neither the mother nor the family were abnormal in the specified directions, he had a 93 percent chance. The actual percentages are not important, since they vary with one's criteria of outcome, one's criteria of parental abnormality, and the promptness with which the local courts and child-protection agencies intervene. What is important is that abnormal behavior on

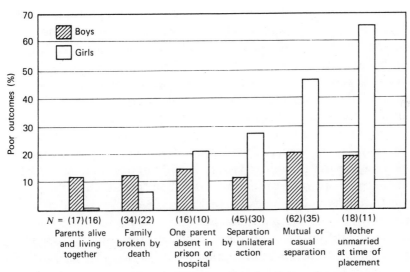

Figure 1 Percentage of poor outcomes as related to family structure at time of placement.

the part of the mother or on the part of the parents as a couple makes the prognosis for the placed child much worse than if the family has been more normal and the placement has been made necessary by death, sickness, or economic difficulties. The point is well known, but people sometimes do not appreciate how strong the difference is.

Abnormal behavior on the part of the father is of much less importance than such behavior on the part of the mother, and frank mental illness is of less importance than abnormal behavior due to alcoholism or psychopathic traits, judging from these data. This is not to say, of course, that schizophrenia in one or both parents can be disregarded, for we know from the work of Heston [5] and others that the offspring of such a marriage are at high risk even if they are transferred to another family at birth. But in most families requiring the foster placement of a child, schizophrenia (if strictly diagnosed) is rare in comparison to other types of mental disorder and the present data show that children of parents with some other type of mental disorder do not make poor adult adjustments unless that other disorder has been accompanied by alcohol abuse. (This conclusion is in harmony with one of Rutter's [15].)

Although the aforementioned prognostic indicators are present at time of placement, it must not be assumed that the adverse influence presumably underlying them has already come into operation and that preventive action is impossible. Even the child placed soon after birth has a poorer prognosis if the parents have been behaving abnormally than if they have not, though one can scarcely say that this behavior itself can already have had an impact. It is possible, of course, that such behavior derives from a genetic weakness which the child is liable to inherit, or that it induces perinatal brain damage, but it is also possible that the real trauma comes from the continuation of such behavior during later visits to the child, or simply from the absence of more normal behavior. For instance, if the natural parent is able to visit the child but does not, this very fact can be traumatic once the child knows about it and senses the rejection this implies. The idea that he is somehow rejected by a person who would normally accept him warmly is very important for all foster children, probably more important than object loss, and any apparent recurrence of rejection is dangerous, while any sign of acceptance by the natural parents can help.

When illegitimate children who are eligible for adoption are not adopted, then this is easily felt as a further rejection and such children show on their tests that they feel most of the world rejects them also. When a natural parent contributes financially to the child's upkeep, even without visiting, on the other hand, the percentage of poor outcomes is much lower than when the biological parent fails to contribute, even if visiting occurs in the latter case. When one considers adverse factors in the biological family background therefore, it is worth remembering that although these may have already operated before the child came into care, one may still be able to prevent worse damage if one prevents them from continuing to operate while the child is in foster care.

Heavy drinking or other disturbing behavior on the part of *both* parents carres a worse prognosis than on the part of only one, and the opposite-sexed parent appears more important than the same-sexed in this matter. Where the one supports while the other rejects the child, the social outcomes are better but some of our other evidence suggests that this may not reflect deeper mental health, since children with such a history exhibited a much greater tendency than other foster children to be manipulative, attention-seeking, poor at concrete problem solving, and lacking in true attachments. These data may be interpreted to mean that such children spent their energies in maintaining many contacts but avoiding intimate attachments that might later give them pain, and although we have no evidence that such behavor persists into adult life there must be a risk of this, a risk which could be overlooked if one paid attention to only what ex-foster children tell one.

Of course, when children are placed in foster homes soon after birth and then are neglected by their biological parents, one need not put the whole blame for their later difficulties on these parents. Failure of the agency to work with the biological parents, failure to make sufficient effort to achieve legal adoption, and failure by the foster parents to give the child a satisfactory picture of his status and of their devotion to his welfare can all contribute. Similarly, when newly placed foster children prove to have had an adverse family background, the prognoses suggested by Figure 1 do not immediately apply, for by no means all these children remain in long-term foster care. It cannot be said that if such children return soon to their natural parent(s), they thereby have a good prognosis, since to my knowledge no one has studied this; but what can be said is that the child protection agency cannot hold itself so responsible for the results.

The background variables associated with a high risk of remaining long in foster care prove, surprisingly, to be quite different from those associated with a high risk of a poor adult outcome. This time it is the age of the natural mother and whether she has ever been separated from the child before that are the strongest indicators, not the structure of the family or pathological behavior of either parent [12], at least as far as the Montreal cases are concerned. Before one attempts to use the outcome indicators for planning care, therefore, it is necessary to estimate whether the child is likely to remain long in care. If not, then probably the former foster child syndrome will not result, although other types of mental disturbance and distress may.

Foster Home Influences

Although the behavior of the natural parents before and after foster placement appears to be a major factor in the development of the former foster child syndrome, particularly if this behavior can be interpreted as rejection, it is not the only factor. The child-protection agency, the foster parents, society at large, and the lawmakers all can play their part. In Montreal the various options open to the agencies did not appear to make much difference, if one thinks of these in terms of number of children to a foster home, number of trial placements, type of home supervision, and similar matters. The character of the foster home, however, did prove to be important, and the government's policies concerning foster child support seemed to be.

Given the fact that the risk of later pathology in foster children is high and that one can with the foregoing indicators distinguish a minority with really high risk of poor outcome (52 percent in our sample) from a majority where that risk of social disturbance is much lower (7 percent) [10], some clinicians may be inclined to think that what should thereafter be important is not the character of the foster home but the character of the psychotherapy which the high risk cases should be receiving. In practice, however, the availability of psychotherapy for such children has always, up to the present, been too sparse, and when it is given it must usually be of brief duration. One's best chance of helping these children therefore is not through unrealistic plans for professional therapy but through a selection and manipulation of the foster homes open to them, with perhaps a sharpening of prognostic tools so that the little professional help that is available can be focused on the most needy cases.

For studying foster home influences two subsamples of the original 316 cases were chosen, one with 114 from adverse backgrounds and the other with 85 from the most favorable backgrounds. In each group preference was given to those cases where the information was clearest and the assessing supervisors most confident of their judgments. As before, we had to depend for our information about the earlier homes of the former foster children on the home records the agency had compiled, but to augment these sources approximately 50 current foster homes were also investigated, focusing on the foster mother and on one or more long-stay child,[2] and this provides depth to what might otherwise have been merely statistical associations. In both samples the children had been at least 2 years in their main foster home.

The first question raised in this phase of the research was: What foster home variable is most associated with poor adult adjustment on the part of the former foster child, after natural family background has been taken into account? The answer to this came as a surprise, for it was *suburban location*. Suburban homes did much less well than urban or rural ones, as Figure 2 shows. This association could not be explained on the basis of the agency having sent more difficult children there, nor on the basis of social class differences, the age of the foster parents, the social background of these parents, or the bad influence of one particular neighborhood. It was true that the difference between suburban and other outcomes was greatest when the home was a white-collar one and when the mother was over 45, but the poorer results from the suburbs were still in evidence when such homes were disregarded. Comparing children in the 50 current foster homes we found that the suburban-placed had a better identification with their foster homes than the urban-placed, were better accepted by the foster parents' relatives, showed more signs of personality integration, but on the other hand showed more signs of immaturity and neurosis and were much poorer at concrete problem solving. When mental health assessments were made of both child

---

[2] There were actually 61 children distributed over 50 homes for this phase of the research, but data were incomplete in two cases.

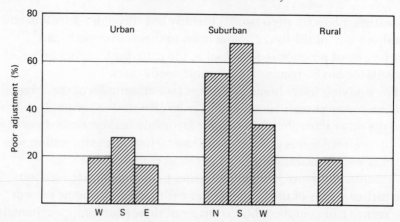

Figure 2 Percentages of former foster children who were rated to have made poor adult adjustments by type of background and location of main foster home. (Urban zone was divided into northern, southern, and western sectors. Rural homes were too few to subdivide in this fashion.)

and foster mother and these then compared, there was a correlation of .51 in the suburban group (significant at the .01 level) but of −.23 for urban pairs (not significant). Furthermore, when the contents of the children's Rorschachs were compared with those of their foster mothers there was significantly greater similarity between each suburban mother and child than between each urban pair.

These observations when taken by themselves or when related to the clinician's normal family practice are likely to leave one puzzled. The usual aim of foster placement is to have the child identify with the foster family, and since the suburban foster mothers were not less mentally healthy overall than the urban ones there would seem to be no harm in this. *Yet in that zone where one gets the best identification with the foster family one also gets the poorest results,* not just with the children from adverse backgrounds but with the children from favorable backgrounds as well. There is one major and at least one minor explanation for this paradox. The minor relates to the effect of suburban life on mental health. Although their general mental health was not worse, the suburban foster mothers were less confident about their maternal role and showed a greater tendency to depression, anxiety, and guilt. This harmonizes with the results obtained from other community surveys in the Montreal region [2], but its effects on the foster child are probably slight. Much more important is the effect of the stopping of state support for foster children at between the ages of 16 and 18 (the age has changed over the years).

Most foster parents depend to a slight extent on the income the child has brought in for them, many are affected by the same parent-adolescent frictions which affect ordinary families in North American society, and the child-protection agency often presses them to push the teenager out so that they have a place for one of the younger children that the agency must succor, younger children for whom the state will pay. Moreover, foster homes are discouraged from planning employment or a career for their charges since they are warned that the children may leave them before the end of official childhood, so that the idea of the adolescent going out to work and bringing some income into the foster home after official care has ended is often not broached. Of the 30 former foster children referred to earlier, 24 had left their main homes at the time state support ended, or earlier, and this percentage is probably lower than average for Montreal. Accordingly, those who had been rebellious and had resisted identification with the foster home were probably readier to make the jump and readier also to express resentment at this new rejection than those others, principally in the suburbs, who had identified strongly with the foster home and had been taught to repress their resentment and hostile impulses, particularly if the latter had also been encouraged to remain immature. The initial rejection trauma is likely to be reactivated by such treatment, but particularly so if dependency and identification have been encouraged.

The next foster home variable with a significant association to the children's outcomes brings out a similar point but then adds a twist to it. Foster mothers who express no particular preference regarding the ages and number of children to be given them achieve much better results with adverse background children than those that prefer only a single preschool child. The former type of mother is the more confident of her ability to handle children and is not looking for someone who will fill her own emotional needs, whereas the latter is thinking more of her own needs.[3] The former type

---

[3] A similar differentiation was obtained in a study of current foster children by Walker [18], who called his categories of foster mother "need-bestowing" and "need-appraising."

proves to be the more practical and puts less emphasis on affection, so that the children do not become so attached to her, are better at concrete problems, and hence probably are readier to make the jump into independence when the state support stops. However, whereas this type of foster mother seems to do better with the child from an adverse background, regardless of her location of residence, the pattern is almost exactly reversed when one looks at the children from favorable backgrounds, as Figure 3 shows. In adult life the latter type of child is the most likely to be rated as making a doubtful adjustment if he has been with a foster mother who had no preference or who preferred babies, and his chances of a good

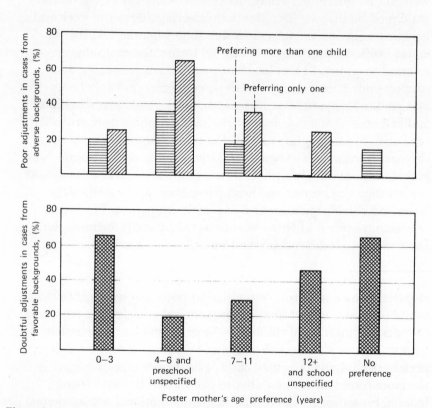

Figure 3 Percentages of former foster children showing respectively poor and doubtful adjustments to adult life, as related to their biological family backgrounds and to the age-preferences expressed by their main foster mothers. (For cases from favorable backgrounds the foster mother's preference respecting number of foster children made no difference.)

adjustment are best if she has expressed a preference for children between the ages of 4 and 11.

The explanation for this reversal leads us to another key feature of foster home handling, the provisions of roles. From quite a number of angles the analysis of our data makes it clear that *if children come from favorable backgrounds and hence are not too traumatized, then it benefits them to have some role or expectation that they can fulfill in the foster home, whereas if they come from adverse backgrounds and are more traumatized, the imposition of roles and expectations can harm them,* since they feel unable to respond and develop a still poorer self-image in consequence. If the foster mother has some emotional need that the child can respond to, if there is a younger sibling to take care of, or if the foster father is in skilled employment that the child can aspire to, then the child from a favorable background tends to make a better adult adjustment than if these are lacking, but the child from an adverse background tends to make a poorer adjustment in these circumstances.

Other foster home factors appear less important than these and hence do not demand elaboration in a summary paper such as this. The presence of the foster parents' own children within the home has a beneficial effect if they are older than the foster child but is of mixed significance if they are younger. The foster mother's assessed ability to set and maintain standards appears of more importance than her ability to provide affection. The foster father's characteristics are largely irrelevant if the children come from an adverse background, for then he tends to be ignored in favor of the foster mother (he is rarely mentioned in such children's Bene-Anthony tests and puppet play), but he becomes somewhat more important for the favorable-background children, particularly if there are no "own" children in the home.

Probably there are other foster home factors of more weight than those mentioned, but they are not measurable in this study, and we have had plenty of comments from the former foster children and indirectly from current children on what appears to be unsatisfactory. We cannot yet correlate these factors with adult outcome, however, or distinguish what the child has projected onto the situation from what actually occurs. Hence these must be ignored for the present. What seems undoubtedly to be of importance in the foster home is the provision of ego-building roles within the child's capacity and

the handling of separation at the end of official care. The latter type
of problem is something which therapists know well but which
governments and agencies apparently do not. The former is
something to which therapists and supervisors could give more
attention.

Sharpening Prognosis

Besides dividing foster children into high risk and low risk
according to their natural family backgrounds and then classifying
foster homes according to their suitability for each broad type, an
obvious step in improving the risk for these foster children would
be to identify more precisely the individual child's areas of
vulnerability and take special steps to strengthen him in these.
Whatever special services the child-protection agency had at its
disposal or could reach could then be directed at preparing the
future adult rather than at responding to petty crises. The great
problem here, however, is that although certain current weaknesses
in the children's characters are easily perceived, this is very different
from predicting which weaknesses are going to be most relevant
later. Follow-up studies of child guidance clinic populations such
as that by Robins [14] are presumably relevant here, but they are
not the same thing as a prospective study of children all sharing
the same major trauma.

A large proportion of the 316 Montreal foster children had
enuresis, truancy, theft, refusal to obey, and lying in their histories,
and these are characteristics which Robins found to be about the
best predictors, in combination, of a later sociopathic personality
[14, p. 157]. Yet only a few of these foster children developed into
sociopaths later. Moreover, it is not so much sociopathic behavior
which one should be seeking to avoid as the less obvious former
foster child syndrome, if my own observations are correct. I hope
in future to follow up the 61 foster children seen in the current
homes, but in the meantime we should consider what seem to be the
main additional prognostic indicators.

The worst indicator probably is a strong attachment to the foster
mother combined with a failure to really trust her or to identify
further with the foster family. This can be looked for only after the
child has been in the same foster home a reasonable time, of course,

and judging from what was said earlier about the suburban placements there could be a danger in identifying more widely with the foster family if that foster family later sent the child away as soon as government support for him stopped. Nevertheless, when one compares children from adverse backgrounds with those from favorable ones, these are the characteristics of the children whom we can assume to be the most damaged and who are in homes which seem least likely, for the reasons cited earlier, to succeed with children from adverse backgrounds. There is a strong association between rejection by both natural parents and affection being focused on the foster mother only ($p=.001$); the children from the most adverse backgrounds seem the least ready to ask for favors or to admit to mistakes ($p=.05$); children from adverse backgrounds with foster mothers who had preferred preschool placements less often name foster family members other than the mother in their own "Fairy Castle" test (a measure of identification devised for this research) and less often name adults for the Castles than do other foster children ($p=.01$).

After that broad indicator, those which our research next suggests are both derived from psychological tests that depend for their success on the clinician's skill and approach and therefore may not yield comparable results everywhere. Reference has been repeatedly made earlier to the children's ability to solve a concrete problem. This consisted of using everyday objects in unorthodox fashion, with failure usually being due either to too great rigidity of approach (inability to see the objects in other than their customary roles) or too uncontrolled fantasy, and results correlate highly both with the prognoses based on the biological family backgrounds and with those based on the foster homes.

The second measure that gave a good correlation with prognosis based on the biological family was the mental health rating developed on the basis of a sequential analysis of the Rorschach. This does not agree as well with the prognoses based on the foster home characteristics, since children placed with mothers preferring preschool children received better ratings than those placed with mothers preferring older children or having no preferences. However, there are possible explanations for this and the Rorschach still seems worth using, if in experienced hands. Should it be possible to obtain Rorschachs not just of the children but also of their foster

mothers, then a different approach to Rorschach interpretation can
be used which should also sharpen one's prognostic abilities, since
any similarity between the pathological signs of mother and those of
the foster child is definitely a warning. But it is not usual for foster
mothers to agree to take the Rorschach test.

Signs of a good prognosis can be as useful as signs of a bad one,
where one has isolated a group from adverse backgrounds and wishes
to know which children are *least* in need of special care. Here by far
the strongest indicator is identification with the adult world,
particularly the foster parents' world. Despite the fact that their
biological families had been more normal and hence supposedly
easier to identify with, it was the children from the most favorable
backgrounds that preferred the foster parents' names to their own
($p = .001$), gave the foster father the most mail on the Bene-Anthony
test ($p = .02$), and drew an adult for their first "free" drawing
($p = .005$). Children in presumably favorable current settings similarly
were most likely to name adults for their Fairy Castle and least
likely to exhibit fears of punishment and strangers. Nevertheless,
one has to look below the surface for these more favorable
signs, since global impressions tend to be wrong. It was the
children with the poorer prognoses that appeared more at ease
in their psychiatric interviews, and there was virtually no correlation
between the prognoses derived from the psychological tests or from
the prior research and the assessments given by the foster mothers,
teachers, and psychiatrists who had been in contact with the
children. Probably this is because currently disturbed behavior can
be a sign of attempts at self-repair.

Treatment Goals

Having by these means or others arrived at the group of children
that appear to be most in need of special treatment, what should one
do for them? I have no research data to provide on this point, no
results from a comparison of one approach versus another, and there
are many clinicians who would say that in any case the treatment
must be decidedly individually, not by categories. Nevertheless,
there are certain steps that appear logical in the light of this research.

The first step in many cases must be to assist the child in

recognizing his hostility and his fears (the children with the poorest prognoses could not admit to the fear that their foster parents might not keep them) and then to assist him in seeing that these might be justified yet unhelpful. This is a step well-known in child psychiatry and it is unnecessary to discuss the method. A second step may be to take the biological parent into therapy if she (and it is usually the mother) is either competing for the foster parents' affection against the child, something which one not infrequently detects if there is much visiting. A third step, though not for the same type of case, could be to assist the child in handling his fantasies regarding the biological parent, and to improve his reality testing. The adverse-background children who get too much visiting from the biological parent tend to be harmed by this, but the children who get no visiting are equally harmed (poor adjustment rates are about the same for each and much worse than for children that get infrequent visiting), particularly if the foster parents and agency have mistakenly screened the children from real knowledge about these parents.

Along with this better handling of fantasy should probably go training in reality testing of a broader nature, and modest encouragement of skepticism regarding the popular viewpoints. This last is necessary since the foster child who completely accepts popular opinions is going to acquire a poor opinion about foster children in general, including himself, and we found that the children with the better prognosis tended to give the fewer "populars" on the Rorschach, although one normally thinks of a paucity of "populars" as a danger sign. However, too much skepticism can also be dangerous. Regarding method here, I think an important element is helping the child to gather factual information about his biological parents and to get different viewpoints on them, but under guidance so that a tendency to fantasize on the basis of partial information is kept in check and so that he can be supported during the absorption of news that may be quite traumatic. Another element, however, could be training in concrete and social problem solving, a training that would involve looking at familiar situations in new lights.

These brief comments on treatment have related to what one customarily attempts in individual therapy, but how far such individual therapy can succeed against adverse environmental influences is highly questionable, as the Youth Consultation Service study in New York showed [9]. If governments, agencies, and foster parents could be persuaded to plan on the basis of the foster children remaining as attached to their last foster homes after finishing high school as other adolescents remain attached to their families, then I believe that cases with the former foster child syndrome would be many fewer, since it is the suggestion (or frank display) of rejection at this point which probably reawakens the earlier traumata, induces regression, and creates the syndrome as we observed it. In Scotland, where a much higher proportion of former foster children remain attached to their last foster homes, according to Ferguson [3], the rush into early marriage is much less and perhaps the other symptoms are less also. But if such further rejection seems likely, a major function of individual therapy should be to prepare the child for it.

Conclusions

To write a paper on the psychological damage created in foster children and former foster children without ever mentioning maternal deprivation probably seems surprising, and in any more theoretical approach to the question this concept would have to be returned to. The present paper has not been a theoretical one, however. It has described a clinically observed syndrome, has considered social maladjustment in a larger population with the same foster care background, and has attempted to explain with as little theory as possible the associations empirically observed between the syndrome, the maladjustment, and a variety of preceding variables. It so happens that the preceding variables which we could measure offered little information on whether maternal deprivation, in the strict sense of that term, had occurred or not. None of the children covered by the present research had suffered from the obvious lack of contact with a mothering figure which Spitz described in foundling homes [16] (as far as we are aware), and the more subtle types of deprivation were not detectable by our crude measures. Even if we had had the means of measuring such deprivation, however, there are good reasons for thinking that this concept is much less important than the simpler concept of rejection, as far as the present type of foster child is concerned. There is a big difference between our 30 former foster children and Bowlby's "44 juvenile thieves," and it is probable that the sense of being rejected, first in infancy and again later, is much commoner than the actual experience of maternal deprivation.

The prognostic indicators offered in this paper apply to the Montreal children under Montreal conditions, and they have not yet been validated by a follow-up of children for whom prognoses have already been established (although I hope that this will soon take place for the 61 children in the clinical study). Even if it is assumed that my interpretations are valid, it will still be necessary to take local conditions into consideration, conditions such as the greater readiness of Scottish foster parents to shelter their charges after the end of schooling or the greater difficulty which New York agencies have in finding adoptive homes for eligible Negro children. Nevertheless, I suggest that it is greatly preferable to plan care on the basis of attempting to prevent poor adult outcomes, rather than to plan it on the basis of current, possibly transitory symptoms and the vague opinions of social workers concerning what constitutes a "good" foster home.

References

1. Alten, I. *Oud-Pupillen Antwoorden.* Amsterdam, 1957.
2. Engelsmann, F. et al. Variations in responses to a symptom check-list by age, sex, income, residence and ethnicity. *Soc. Psychiat.*, 7: 3 (1972), 150–156.
3. Ferguson, T. *Children in Care—and After.* Oxford University Press, London, 1966.
4. Harrower-Erickson, M. R. and Steiner, M. E. *Large-Scale Rorschach Techniques.* Charles C Thomas, Springfield, Ill., 1945.
5. Heston, L. L. and Denney, D. Interactions between early life experience and biological factors in schizophrenia, in *The Transmission of Schizophrenia*, D. Rosenthal and S. Kety, Eds. Pergamon Press, London, 1968, pp. 363–376.
6. Kraus, J. Predicting success of foster-placements for school-age children. *Social Work*, 16 (1971), 63–73.
7. McCord, W. and McCord, J. *Origins of Crime.* Columbia University Press, New York, 1959.
8. Meier, E. G. *Former Foster Children as Adult Citizens.* D.S.W. Thesis, Columbia University, 1962.
9. Meyer, H. J., Borgatta, E. F., and Jones, W. C. *Girls at Vocational High.* The Russell Sage Foundation, New York, 1965.
10. Murphy, H. B. M. Foster-home variables and adult outcomes. *Mental Hygiene*, 48 (49), 587–599.
11. Murphy, H. B. M. Natural family pointers to foster care outcome. *Mental Hygiene*, 48 (1964), 380–395.

12. Murphy, H. B. M. Predicting duration of foster care. *Child Welfare*, 47 (1968), 76–84.
13. O'Reilly, C. T. *Foster Children; Profile and Problems*. M.S.W. Thesis, Loyola University, Chicago, 1961.
14. Robins, L. N. *Deviant Children Grown Up*. Williams and Wilkins, Baltimore, 1966.
15. Rutter, M. *Children of Sick Parents; an Environmental and Psychiatric Study*. Oxford University Press, London, 1966.
16. Spitz, R. A. Hospitalism. The *Psychoanalytic Study of the Child*, 1 (1945), 53–74.
17. Townsend, J. K. The relation between Rorschach signs of aggression and behavioral aggression in emotionally disturbed boys. *J. Projective Techniques*, 31 (1967), 13–21.
18. Walker, C. W. Persistence of mourning in the foster-child as related to the foster-mother's level of maturity. *Smith College Studies of Social Work*, 41 (1971), 173–246.
19. Williams, J. M. Children who break down in foster homes. *J. Child Psychiat. Psychol.*, 2 (1961), 5–30.

Antisocial Behavior Disturbances of Childhood: Prevalence, Prognosis, and Prospects*

Lee N. Robins, Ph.D. (U.S.A.)

Child psychiatric clinics were originally created in the United States to treat children with antisocial behavior disturbances. The child guidance movement began in response to the needs of juvenile courts in the early 1920s. Since that time most clinics treating children have found antisocial behavior disturbances to be a prominent part of their patient load. In 1964 Rosen et al. [23] surveyed psychiatric clinics throughout the United States and found that antisocial behavior disorders were still the most common problem seen in children's clinics. These disorders have always been particularly common among boys.

Although antisocial behavior may be the largest category of psychiatrically treated children, probably only a small fraction of all the children who would be diagnosed as having antisocial behavior disorders if they showed up in a child guidance clinic actually come to psychiatric attention. Many of these children land in the hands of the police and the courts rather than in psychiatric

* The work reported here has been supported by Research Scientist Award 36,598 and Research Grant MH-18864.

hands; many of them are diagnosed in school settings as underachievers because their academic performance does not match their
IQ scores, or as children with specific reading disabilities because
they somehow do not learn to read at the time that other children
do. Pediatricians and pediatric neurologists take care of many of
them under the diagnosis of hyperkinetic children.

Although children with antisocial behavior disorders do not
constitute the whole of any of these groups—neither of delinquents
nor of underachievers nor of children with reading disorders nor
of hyperkinetic children—the overlap between each such diagnosis
and antisocial behavior disturbance is striking. For example, the
average delinquent, although of normal IQ, is 2 to 3 years retarded
in his academic achievement and is thus an "underachiever." A
follow-up after 4 to 6 years of children originally diagnosed
hyperkinetic found a large proportion delinquent [29]. Cantwell
[4] found the same excess of sociopathy and alcoholism in the fathers
of hyperactive children that Robins [18] had found in children
referred to a psychiatric clinic for antisocial behavior, suggesting
that they are highly overlapping populations. Werry [30] points out
the impossibility of separating hyperkinetic children from children
with antisocial behavior disturbances.

Since childhood antisocial behavior disturbances are cared for in
a variety of settings, counting cases in psychiatric treatment gives
little idea of how common they are in the population. Recently,
however, Rutter, in an epidemiological study of psychiatric and
physical disability on the Isle of Wight, gave us our first approach
to an incidence rate [24]. His rate applies only to 10- to 12-year-olds,
since that is the group he studied. At this age level in England, the
incidence rate was 4 percent. Much more common in boys than
girls, antisocial behavior disturbance appeared in 6.4 percent of all
boys in this age bracket and in about 1.6 percent of girls. As Rosen
found these disorders the most common among treated children,
Rutter found them also the most common of all childhood
psychiatric problems, treated and untreated, accounting for 68
percent of psychiatrically disturbed boys and 32 percent of
psychiatrically disturbed girls. Although the great excess of boys over
girls is typical of findings in all studies of antisocial behavior
disturbance, the excess he found may be somewhat greater than
that he would have found if he had followed the children until they

were older, since this disorder appears to have its onset somewhat later in girls than in boys [18].

Since antisocial behavior disturbances are relatively common in childhood, it is important to know whether they have important prognostic significance. Are they just the extreme end of normal "childish" behavior, which will end with adulthood, or are these syndromes associated with adult disability? An answer requires comparing the adult outcomes of children with antisocial behavior disorders with outcomes of normal children and children with other disorders. Fortunately there have been studies following these children into adult life, beginning as far back as 1926 when Healy and Bronner did their classic follow-up study of delinquents in Boston [10]. We have located 23 studies which have followed children who were antisocial as evidenced either by a diagnosis in a child guidance clinic, by school difficulties, or by contacts with police and juvenile courts, and which obtained information about these children at least 10 years after the initial information was collected about them. Their outcomes have been compared with outcomes of normal children, of children suffering from neuroses, and of children suffering from psychoses. Whatever the outcome criteria and however the study was carried out, antisocial children were found to have worse adult outcomes than normals and than neurotic children. Their outcomes were not as dismal as those of psychotic children, a large proportion of whom spent much of their adult lives in mental institutions. Robins has reviewed the 23 studies tracing the outcomes of antisocial children for at least 10 years [19].

The prognosis for antisocial behavior disorders is better than that for childhood psychosis, yet the frequency of the antisocial disorders and their relatively poor prognosis should make them a very important concern of those interested in public mental health. They are followed by adult difficulties of much greater social consequence than are the later problems of psychotic or neurotic children. Psychotic children often need custodial care as adults. Neurotic children who do not recover (although most do) suffer internal misery. The antisocial child as an adult also is liable to suffer internal misery, contrary to the beliefs of those who see the adult "ne'er-do-well" as someone who enjoys life thoroughly, but he also contributes importantly to most of our major social problems.

It is from the population who show antisocial behavior disorders of childhood that apparently virtually all adult sociopaths derive. It is from this group that a very high proportion of the prisoner population comes as do many of our vagrants, our skid row inhabitants, those drug addicts who resort to crime to support their habits, and even substantial proportions of those psychotic adults who require restraint because of their aggressive and combative behavior. "Follow-back" studies of psychiatrically hospitalized adults who had been seen in psychiatric clinics as children have shown them to be more antisocial than the average clinic referral [17]. Also from this group come many of the parents whose children end on welfare rolls, as wards of the state, or as adopted children, because the parents simply do not provide sufficient financial or affectional care for them. These neglected, impoverished, or adopted offspring [11, 21] themselves have a very high risk of childhood antisocial behavior disorders, probably a consequence of an unfortunate mix of genes and harsh early environment. Thus the high frequency of antisocial disorders in the child population is preserved from one generation to another.

To get some impression of the frequency with which children with antisocial behavior disorders do grow up to have serious adult problems, we can look at the adult outcomes of children referred for antisocial behavior to a St. Louis child guidance clinic [18]. With a median age of 13 at the time of referral, by age 18 only 16 percent had permanently recovered. When interviewed at an average age of 43, more than 25 percent had had a sufficient variety and severity of antisocial behavior since 18 to warrant the diagnosis of sociopath. As adults, about 8 percent were alcoholic or drug addicts; about 11 percent were psychotic. This was in marked contrast both to children referred to the clinic for reasons other than antisocial behavior, who were more often well and rarely sociopathic as adults, and to a comparison group of normal school children, 60 percent of whom were well and only 2 percent sociopathic.

When we put aside diagnostic labels and look at adult social adjustment, we find extraordinary rates of adult difficulties. Children seen for antisocial behavior had as adults a high frequency of criminal activity, of divorce, great geographic mobility, much unemployment, excessive drinking, and social isolation.

Perhaps more important than the finding that antisocial behavior disorders in children were frequently continued into adulthood is the finding that serious antisocial behavior virtually *never* began in adulthood in patients or control subjects free of it before age 18. This observation, made first in white child guidance clinic patients and normal white schoolchildren from lower-class homes [18], was confirmed in the follow-up study into their thirties of urban black schoolboys [22]. Thus even in a population with the provocation to acting out that discrimination and economic disadvantage must produce, gross chronic antisocial behavior did not develop de nouveau after the age of 18. The possible implications of these findings for public policy are impressive. They suggest that if one could interrupt the antisocial patterns so readily discernible by children's parents, teachers, and peers, one might greatly reduce the scope of the world's social problems.

There are those who do not approve interrupting antisocial disorders of childhood because they interpret them as "normal" or even desirable reactions to the inequalities and oppressions faced by the children of the poor and minority groups in an affluent society. They believe that the solution is to change societies so that such reactions are not evoked. This is a viewpoint that cannot be categorically dismissed, since there does seem to be an association of antisocial behavior disorders with lower class and with some minority ethnic groups, but there are also findings that argue against this interpretation. First, these disorders are not exclusively in disadvantaged children, and when they do occur in majority group, middle-class children, they are indistinguishable in symptom patterns from the antisocial disorders of poor children. Second, prognosis is no better or worse in terms of adult adjustment when these disorders occur in middle-class children than when they occur in lower-class children. Third, there is no evidence that the ending of disadvantage by improving schools, incomes, or affection leads to a marked diminishing of the disorder. Finally, even for children who do suffer serious disadvantage in our society, this reaction is atypical and is not functional for them either in terms of improving their chances in the society or of making them leaders of groups who might achieve social reforms. With the problem behavior go subjective symptoms of alienation and hostility that make children with antisocial behavior unpopular not only with their teachers and parents but with their peers. Unable to engage in successful interpersonal relations, these children do not become leaders. Thus successfully treating aggressive behavior in childhood would not seem to mean stamping out potential creative rebellion. Rather it should save the affected children from what will turn out for a substantial proportion of them to be a future of poverty, lovelessness, and isolation.

Efforts at Prevention and Treatment of Antisocial Behavior Disorders

Although the need to prevent or treat antisocial behavior disorders in children is great in terms of their social and personal cost, there are not yet available methods of treatment or of prevention which have been demonstrated to be effective [20]. Most of the efforts that have been labeled prevention of antisocial behavior disorder or delinquency might better be seen as efforts to forestall the full display of the disorder in children who are already showing the early warning signs discussed above. Perhaps the only example of primary prevention has been the Craig and Furst effort [8], which chose first-grade children to treat entirely on the basis of their coming from high risk families, not on the basis of their own behavior. In general, the distinction between other studies that have been labeled prevention and those that have been labeled treatment is almost entirely based on who decides it is time to do something about the child—the researcher or the authorities. When the researcher selects the child for special programs on the basis of teacher nominations as troublesome, before he has been referred to psychiatric services or dropped out of school or been declared officially delinquent, the program is usually labeled prevention. If the child has already been referred for help or is in official trouble, it is labeled treatment.

Programs aimed at preventing the emergence of antisocial behavior or of more serious antisocial behavior than the child has yet shown have been uniformly disappointing [1, 8, 15, 16, 27]. All these studies have, however, strongly confirmed the predictive value of family patterns, underachievement in the early school years, and teacher selection of potential delinquents and dropouts, since a large proportion of the children selected for preventive programs because they were considered at high risk have indeed shown serious antisocial behavior in adolescence. Failure to prevent has met not only the traditional social casework tried in most of these studies but also efforts to modify the school experience by providing work-study programs along with tutoring in the Ahlstrom and Havighurst study [1].

Treatment regimens aimed at reducing the present level of behavior problems in children already referred for psychiatric care or delinquent have shown some short-term success, but there have been few adequate long-term evaluations against control groups receiving either no treatment or traditional treatments. On a short-term basis the stimulant drugs in double-blind studies have been able to improve classroom behavior and behavior at home in children labeled hyperactive, but controlled long-term follow-ups have not been conducted. Clearly the stimulant drugs are no panacea, however, since children treated with these drugs show much more school failure and delinquency at follow-up than do normal children [12, 29].

Behavior modification techniques have also shown dramatic short-term results in diminishing disruptive classroom behavior and improving academic performance of schoolchildren and reducing disciplinary problems among incarcerated delinquents [5, 26]. But again there has been no long-term follow-up to learn whether these improved behaviors can be maintained after the behavior modification therapy is terminated.

Less structured therapeutic programs, including admission to conventional child guidance clinics [25] and residential educational settings [28], have shown little or no advantage over no treatment even on a short-term basis. Techniques recently used, such as contingency contracting, television feedback, and aversive conditioning, look promising but have not yet been investigated over long enough periods and with adequately matched control groups to provide answers.

Some forms of treatment have been shown to be worse than no treatment at all. Children who had committed offenses that could require appearance in juvenile court were less likely to be recidivists if they somehow avoided contact with the courts, and particularly if they avoided being sent to a "reformatory" [18], although carefully controlled studies of the effect of diversion of delinquents from the juvenile court system have not yet been done. Delinquents assigned to Synanon-like "therapeutic communities" in California, instead of typical youth programs, showed significantly *more* recidivism than controls [3]. These findings suggest that the juvenile court system may achieve the opposite of the purposes for which it was designed.

Future Directions for Research

IMPROVING PREDICTION

As the Gluecks [9] discovered late in their research with delinquents, whereas families of delinquents differed from families of nondelinquents, differences between the two groups' own early behavior patterns were even greater. The Gluecks found the predelinquent history to be that of risk-taking, antipathy for school, associating with children older than themselves, and persistent truancy. Although these observations were retrospective, later studies showed teachers, parents, and fellow students able to predict prospectively on the basis of early behavior which children will have serious deviant behavior later [e.g., 6]. However, we still know very little about what the best behavioral clues are for such selection of high risk children and at what ages the indices become sufficiently stable to allow confident prediction. Studies of normal children are contradictory about whether stable patterns can be discerned before the age of 6 [14, 31]. Comparison of the detailed natural history of the age of occurrence of deviant behaviors in normal children with antisocial child patients should be useful in discovering the earliest meaningful signs of threatening antisocial behavior disturbance.

At the present time when professionals are asked to select children likely to have serious problems later on, they tend to select too many [13]. Natural history studies of the progression and age of onset of specific symptoms associated with antisocial behavior disorders should enable us to distinguish behavior that is truly ominous from that likely to be transient. We could thus reduce the number of cases nominated for treatment. Being able to reduce the number of predicted deviants to a figure closer to their actual number has obvious advantages in terms of allocating manpower and funds for prevention. In addition, it reduces the number of children labeled as deviant and protects more of those who do not need treatment from any possible risk from the treatment itself. Once an efficient set of early indicators is found, we can proceed to study, perhaps more successfully than heretofore, methods of prevention and treatment.

PREVENTION AND TREATMENT

There are clues in existing research that suggest profitable methods of prevention and treatment. It is well-known, for instance, that children with antisocial behavior are usually seriously retarded in academic performance. We do not know at this point whether academic failure usually preceded or followed the onset of the antisocial behavior. If experiencing academic failure contributes to the occurrence of antisocial behavior disorders, then it is clear that preventive efforts should include efforts to forestall failure through programs such as those currently endeavoring to improve the IQ's and academic success of disadvantaged children either by educating their parents to stimulate them as infants or through a variety of educationally oriented day care and preschool programs. No one has yet measured the effect of these programs on behavior disorders. It should be relatively easy to include evaluation of the frequency of serious deviant behavior along with the IQ testing and standardized achievement tests now used to compare children in these programs with children from the same socioeconomic groups who have not been exposed to these programs.

Among the treatment techniques that warrant further investigation are not only those that have already been shown to be effective on a short-term basis, for example, behavior modification and stimulant drugs, but also those that have been reported successful by clinicians but never evaluated in a standardized way. For instance, some physicians believe that the primary defect in antisocial behavior disorders is too high a threshold for anxiety. They train parents to increase the child's anxiety level, by catching him in minor lies, for instance. Another hypothesis around which treatment has been designed is the idea that antisocial children's recklessness and aggressiveness stem from a low responsiveness to external stimuli. This makes them seek excitement and risks that would be uncomfortably overstimulating for "normal" children. Based on this hypothesis plus the hypothesis that conformity requires a positive self-image are programs which teach survival in the wilderness, where an antisocial child can successfully pit himself against truly exciting external hazards. Again there has been no long-term follow-up of the success of these programs, although delinquents are supposed to respond well to them.

A third hypothesis is that antisocial behavior results from association with other antisocial individuals. The therapeutic inference from this hypothesis is that if one could flood the child's environment with conforming individuals, he would accept them as models rather than the antisocial models from whom he has learned his problem behavior. This is the view which has prompted the assignment of children to conventional foster homes rather than to institutions where they are exposed to other delinquents. In some parts of the United States it is now public policy to close down institutions for antisocial children and replace them with foster home placements. This seems to present a superb opportunity to compare unselected cases in areas where these innovations have been made with cases treated traditionally to learn whether such treatments do have an effect on recovery rates. Research into these various methods of treatment would not only increase the armamentarium of effective treatments available to the therapist if some are found to be useful, but it might also answer some of the questions about possible underlying causal mechanisms.

EXPERIMENTS IN TREATMENT DELIVERY

Assuming that evaluation of treatment shows some of these methods to be effective, there will be important research to be done in how to involve children in treatment. Antisocial disorders are common in children with negligent, inadequate parents. Such parents seldom are aware that their child needs help and may resent interference from authorities who point out the need; even if they accept the fact that the child needs help, they may themselves be too undisciplined to keep appointments regularly. When Rutter attempted to interview parents about their children on the Isle of Wight, he found he had the highest refusal rate among the parents of antisocial children.

Since parents often are neither ready nor willing to seek treatment for their antisocial children, alternative routes to treatment need to be explored, with due regard for the necessity for obtaining parental permission. Since treatment results may be better if the parents themselves are also involved in treatment, methods of involving reluctant parents should be explored. The failure of Ahlstrom and Havighurst's experiment in providing a work-learning program for boys predicted to drop out of school and become delinquent was attributed by them partly to the fact that selection for treatment was itself a stigmatizing experience for the boys. The problem of how to make treatment available to antisocial children without stigmatizing them is one deserving of considerable exploration.

An Overview of the Current State of Knowledge About Antisocial Behavior Disorders in Children

Previous research on antisocial behavior disturbance in children has shown great convergence. Almost every study has confirmed the high prevalence rate of these disorders, their early onset, their association with maleness and severe school retardation, their persistence into adulthood, the facts that they come to treatment only under duress, that they run in families, and that they do not yield to conventional psychotherapeutic treatment techniques. These findings have already led to important changes in the field of child psychiatry. Mental health professionals have recognized that they cannot indulge in their traditional role of sitting back and waiting for these children to seek treatment and then offering them psychotherapy while the parent gets traditional social service. When the child does appear for treatment, it is typically after many years of behavior problems when he is deeply committed to delinquency and has already suffered what may be irreversible educational deficits. Having found that conventional treatment methods are not effective, mental health professionals have been going into the community to offer help early and have been devising innovative and original methods that appear more effective than psychotherapy. Unfortunately, none of these new techniques has yet been shown effective in the long haul, nor have they been shown ineffective. They simply have not been sufficiently tested to know whether they will work or not.

Another result of research in these disorders is an alteration in some of our stereotypes about antisocial children. It now seems clear that antisocial behavior in boys is *not* simply normal masculine behavior unacceptable to middle-class female schoolteachers. It has now been shown that there are no striking differences in terms of acceptability of such behavior according to the sex of the teacher. It is also known that for many children these are not transient phenomena that will disappear as soon as the child is out of the classroom. Indeed many of these children grow up to adult lives that are subjectively unrewarding and threatening to the community. Another stereotype that seems to be dispelled by research already done is that the behavior of antisocial children is functional and reasonable in the light of their location in socially deprived minority settings. The idea that most delinquents are well adapted to their environments has simply turned out to be false. There are indeed street urchins who are "rational" delinquents because their survival depends on their illegal activities. But the typical antisocial child in our culture gets along well with *no one*, neither his middle-class critics nor his lower-class peer group. His high rate of subjective psychiatric symptoms reveals his discomfort with himself as well.

Despite the consensus among studies, we have not learned nearly as much as one might have hoped from research that began back in the 1920s with Burt [2] and Healy and Bronner [10]. One of the reasons that progress has not come faster may be the failure of the various disciplines that deal with the antisocial child to pool their knowledge about these children. In addition, their diagnostic labels such as "underachievers" and "hyperkinetic" have had etiological implications which have led each discipline to focus on the treatment method consonant with that hypothesis. For instance, the school system has offered remedial education to "underachievers" without trying to improve peer group relationships, school attendance, relationships to teachers. Similarly, physicians have often treated hyperkinetic children with drugs without simultaneously treating the social and psychological contributors to antisocial behavior.

Probably the most urgent area of further research in antisocial behavior disturbances of childhood is in treatment methods. Antisocial behavior disturbances in childhood are so common and have such lasting effects that the need for effective treatment is great. Yet so few scientifically satisfactory evaluations of treatment for children have been done [20] that guidelines for how to tackle this large and urgent problem are absent. The scarcity of adequate treatment evaluations grows out of the failure to provide training for researchers in evaluation methods, the rather primitive state of development of these methods, and a scarcity of grant funds of sufficient magnitude and duration to complete reasonable studies. Since children with antisocial behavior disorders grow up not only to contribute heavily to the major social problems of crime and dependency but also to become the parents of a new generation of children at high risk of these disorders, it is in our self-interest to make every effort to prevent and treat them, quite aside from our responsibility to prevent and relieve their subjective distress.

References

1. Ahlstrom, W. M. and Havighurst, R. J. *400 Losers.* Jossey-Bass, San Francisco, 1971.
2. Burt, C. *The Young Delinquent.* Appleton, New York, 1925.
3. California Youth Authority. The Marshall Program—Assessment of a short-term institutional treatment program. Part II: Amenability to confrontive peer-group treatment. Research Report No. 59, August 1970.
4. Cantwell, D. P. Psychiatric illness in the families of hyperactive children. *Arch. Gen. Psychiat.,* 27 (1972), 414–417.
5. Cohen, H. L., Filepczak, J. A., Bis, J. S., Cohen, J., and Larkin, P. Establishing motivationally oriented educational environments for institutionalized adolescents, in *The Psychopathology of Adolescence,* J. Zubin and A. M. Freedman, Eds. Grune & Stratton, New York, 1970.
6. Conger, J. J. and Miller, W. C. *Personality, Social Class, and Delinquency.* John Wiley & Sons, New York, 1966.
7. Conners, C. K., Eisenberg, L., and Barcai, A. Effect of dextroamphetamine on children: Studies on subjects with learning disabilities and school behavior problems. *Arch. Gen. Psychiat.,* 17 (1967), 478–485.
8. Craig, M. M. and Furst, P. W. What happens after treatment? A study of potentially delinquent boys. *Social Service Rev.,* 39: 2 (1965), 165–171.
9. Glueck, E. T. Distinguishing delinquents from pseudodelinquents. *Harvard Educ. Rev.,* 36: 2 (1966), 119 130.
10. Healy, W. and Bronner, A. F. *Delinquents and Criminals: Their Making and Unmaking.* Macmillan, New York, 1926.
11. Hutchings, B. and Mednick, S. A. Registered criminality in the adoptive and biological parents of registered male criminal adoptees, in *Genetics and and Psychopathology,* R. Fieve and D. Rosenthal, Eds. Johns Hopkins University Press, Baltimore, in press.
12. Laufer, M. W. Long-term management and some follow-up findings on the use of drugs with minimal cerebral syndromes. *J. Learning Disabilities,* (1971), 519–522.
13. Macfarlane, J. W. From infancy to adulthood. *Childhood Education,* March 1963.
14. Macfarlane, J. W., Allen, L., and Honzik, M. P. *A Developmental Study of the Behavior Problems of Normal Children Between 21 Months and 14 Years.* University of California Press, Berkeley and Los Angeles, 1954.
15. Meyer, H. J., Borgatta, E. F., and Jones, W. C. *Girls at Vocational High.* Russell Sage Foundation, New York, 1965.
16. Powers, E. and Witmer, H. *An Experiment in the Prevention of Delinquency.* Columbia University Press, New York, 1951.
17. Ricks, D. F. and Berry, J. C. Family and symptom patterns that precede schizophrenia, in *Life History Research in Psychopathology,* M. Roff and D. F. Ricks, Eds. University of Minnesota Press, Minneapolis, 1970,

18. Robins, L. N. *Deviant Children Grown Up: A Sociological and Psychiatric Study of Sociopathic Personality.* Williams and Wilkins, Baltimore, 1966. pp. 31–50.
19. Robins, L. N. The adult development of the antisocial child. *Seminars in Psychiatry,* 2 (1970), 420–434.
20. Robins, L. N. The evaluation of psychiatric services for children in the U.S.A. Proceedings of the World Psychiatric Association Second Symposium on Psychiatric Epidemiology, in press.
21. Robins, L. N. and Lewis, R. G. The role of the antisocial family in school completion and delinquency: A three-generation study. *Sociol. Quarterly,* 7: 4 (1966), 500–514.
22. Robins, L. N., Murphy, G. E., Woodruff, R. A., Jr., and King, L. J. Adult psychiatric status of black schoolboys. *Arch. Gen. Psychiat.* 24 (1971), 338–345.
23. Rosen, B. M., Bahn, A. K., and Kramer, M. Demographic and diagnostic characteristics of psychiatric clinic outpatients in the U.S.A., 1961. *Amer. J. Orthopsychiat.,* 34: 3 (1964), 455–468.
24. Rutter, M., Tizard, J., and Whitmore, K. *Education, Health and Behaviour.* Longmans, London, 1970.
25. Shepherd, M., Oppenheim, B., and Mitchell, S. *Childhood Behaviour and Mental Health.* Grune & Stratton, New York, 1971.
26. Staats, A. W., Minke, K. A., and Butts, P. A token-reinforcement remedial reading program administered by black therapy-technicians to problem black children *Behav. Ther.* 1 (1970), 331–353.
27. Tait, C. D., Jr., and Hodges, E. F., Jr. *Delinquents, Their Families, and the Community.* Charles C. Thomas, Springfield, Ill., 1962.
28. Weinstein, L. Project re-ed schools for emotionally disturbed children: Effectiveness as viewed by referring agencies, parents and teachers. *Exceptional Child,* 35: 9 (1969), 703–711.
29. Weiss, G. Minde, K., Werry, J. S., Douglas, V., and Nemeth, E. Studies on the hyperactive child: VIII. Five-year follow-up. *Arch. Gen. Psychiat.,* 24 (1971), 409–414.
30. Werry, J. S. Organic factors in childhood psychopathology, in *Psychopathological Disorders of Childhood,* H. C. Quay and J. S. Werry, Eds. John Wiley & Sons, New York, 1972.
31. Westman, J. C., Rice, D. I., and Bermann, E. Nursery school behaviour and later school adjustment. *Am. J. Orthopsychiat.,* 37 (1967), 725–731.

Children at Risk from Divorce: A Review

E. James Anthony, M.D. (U.S.A.)

Introduction

In the field of preventive psychiatry at the present time there is a growing concentration of interest and research on children who are likely to become, for constitutional or environmental reasons, psychiatric casualties. This high risk group constitutes one of the major clinical challenges currently confronting us, and the extent to which we become able, as clinicians, to diagnose the prospect of disorder before it occurs could prove a revolution in the management of human affairs. Up to this point our clinical efforts have been dedicated to the detection and amelioration of existing illness and maladjustment, and we have given little time in our busy therapeutic lives to anticipate possible but still nonexistent developments. In the absence of systematic investigation we are, however, still operating largely in the dark in our attempts to ascribe vulnerability to specific causes and to prescribe logical and effective steps of intervention.

Thus we have progressed very little beyond the realization that vulnerability to psychological stress is relative to the situation and circumstances. (This has been found to be equally true of physical stresses; for example, it has been found that animals in isolation succumb to lower doses of poison than animals living in groups.) The degree of resilience in the human individual varies with the age and stage of development, with the sex, with the quality of the early

461

environment, with the amount of stress already experienced, and with the umbrella of security and protection raised over development by the significant caring figures in the environment. Vulnerability has been shown to vary not only from individual to individual within the same family group or same community, but it fluctuates within the same individual at different times, in different places, and with different stresses.

Divorce can be regarded as a traumatic experience in the life of a child, and its occurrence places him in the category of individuals at psychiatric risk. An attempt will be made here to explore the clinical liabilities for the children of divorce and the extent to which these can be modified by appropriate interventions. Before embarking on this, we will consider the size of the problem and its current rate of growth, although it should be remembered that the figures presented are rapidly being outdated.

The Facts of Divorce in the United States

The facts of divorce, as they relate to children, are impressive in their enormity. The United States has the highest divorce rate among Western nations, and the figures are increasing. Almost 70 percent of divorcing couples have minor children, and almost 9 million children (or one in seven) are children of divorce. About 25 percent of marriages end in divorce, and this is even higher in certain sections of the country. This does not take into account the number of permanent separations or desertions (the poor man's divorce), which are believed to equal the number of legal divorces. If we combine divorce and desertion, about 18 million children in the United States will have experienced a disruption of the parental relationship during the period of their childhood. Since about 85 percent of divorced persons eventually remarry, and of these 40 percent again divorce, a large percentage of children have endured the trauma of divorce more than once; many have endured this more than twice, since 80 percent of third marriages are likely to end in divorce.

What then are the possible risks for this large group of children and how many are vulnerable? The first risk is that the child may become psychiatrically disturbed during the period of childhood, either acutely, as in a traumatic neurosis, or chronically maladjusted and malfunctioning at home or at school. The second risk is that the child will turn away from marriage as an unsatisfactory mode of human relationship or repeat his parents' pattern of unsuccessful marriage ending in divorce. The third risk is that the children of divorce will subsequently develop psychiatric disorders in adult life. Before examining the details of these three eventualities, a closer look will be taken at the nature of the stress involved.

The Stress of Divorce

It is difficult to gauge how much of a stressful situation registers with any particular child. One must take into account his perceptiveness, his general sensitivity, his age and intelligence, and his level of emotional participation within the home. Many children of latency age are already beginning to preoccupy themselves, both emotionally and socially, with situations and people outside of the family, and they may even use this extramural preoccupation as a defense against closer involvement in the parental relationship. The trauma of a pathological situation correlates with the degree of perceptiveness, and it is the subjective rather than the objective appreciation of a given reality that governs the individual's response to it. Every child in a family therefore has his own reality to contend with in the context of divorce, and what is perceived and felt by him may not be perceived and felt by another child. This by itself makes for some perplexing variations in reaction.

When the clinician is examining the intimate side of peoples' lives, he has to bear in mind the so-called *Rashomon* principle, postulating that every member of the family has his own peculiar perspective on a shared problem. The individual systems of pathological defenses and coping mechanisms also ensure an idiosyncrasy of response, although family members do share a certain number of these. Wish fulfillment and denial can powerfully distort the perception of reality, which is why surveys of happy marriages must be regarded with a certain amount of skepticism. The ratings of "very happy," "moderately happy," and "somewhat unhappy" may make a lot of sense to the statistician but little to the clinician. One has only to recall the essayist William Hazlitt, whose years were filled with domestic discord, unrequited love, financial trouble, and chronic ill health, stating, as he lay dying: "Well, I've had a happy life." If that statement were to become part of a statistic, we could be completely misled in a way not possible by a careful, clinical examination of Hazlitt's life.

A number of discrepancies are possible between the actual and perceived reality of a relationship. There is the reality as seen by the world, the reality as seen by the parents, and the reality as perceived by each one of the children. First, there is a discrepancy between what the world outside knows of a marriage and what is actually happening in it. In one of his novels, John O'Hara writes: "A married couple always presents an absurdly untruthful picture to the world, but it is a picture that the world finds convenient and a comfort . . . what goes on between a man and woman, the world never knows, and could not possibly know."

Divorce comes as a moment of truth, and the convention of eternal monogamy is then debunked as a piece of culturally determined fiction. Children are taught to believe in this permanence as a necessary part of their security, and it is gradually incorporated into their psyches as a sustaining fantasy that is often strong enough to withstand all the bickering that they witness and the unconscious death wishes stemming from the need to disrupt the parental union so they can have the preferred parent to themselves. The breaking up and reconstructing impulses are constantly canceling each other out as the child fluctuates between wish and fear. But little of this enters consciousness undisguised since the powerful defense of denial forbids the close consideration of birth, copulation, disruption, or death. At times it almost looks as if everyone is actively conspiring from childhood onward to preserve the sacramental institution of marriage. For all these reasons divorce tends to come as a surprise not only to the world at large, or to the children in the home, but often to the conflicted marital partners themselves, who may have been hovering over it for decades without reaching a decision. It may take a long time coming, but those in contact with it often seem in no way prepared for its arrival.

To understand the stressfulness of divorce, one must abandon the view of it as a relatively short-term legal event and envision it instead as an almost indefinite process of stages with each stage having its own psychological impact conducing to its own set of disorders.

The Predivorce Stresses

These may be operative from the beginning of the marriage, and the children of the union may represent a series of therapeutic

attempts to heal a sick relationship. Around 1960 the child
psychiatrist Despert [1] had the impression, shared by most people,
that children of divorce numbered largely in any group of disturbed
children. When she went to her files, she found to her astonishment
that there were proportionately fewer children of divorce, a fact that
led her to postulate that it was not divorce but a bad marital
situation, with or without divorce, that determined a child's
adjustment. She found that a child was very disturbed when the
relationship between his parents was very disturbed, and she referred
to this parental relationship as "emotional divorce." Emotional
divorce always preceded legal divorce but was not always followed by
legal divorce. Despert concluded that divorce itself was not automatically destructive to children and that the marriage which the
divorce brought to an end might have been much more so.
"Emotional divorce" often begins a long time before actual divorce,
and it makes more sense to consider as a failure the whole experience
of marriage rather than the proceeding itself, which may not be so
destructive.

This clinical hunch has been tested more systematically and found
to be valid: Children from unhappy, intact homes are often more
disturbed than children of divorce. One can conclude that it is hardly
worth saving a bad marriage for the sake of the children, if the
children are made worse by the marriage. In fact, although divorce
is always a major upheaval in the child's life, it should not be
regarded as automatically synonymous with disaster, since on occasion
it can lead to actual improvement in the child's clinical condition.
With good management the child may even come to accept and
understand the total failure of a parent who has been rendered unfit
for parenting as a result of mental illness.

One of the problems that retrospective studies pose for outcome
studies relates to the idealizing tendency of the child. The majority
of grown-up children (almost 80 percent) recall the predivorce period
as one in which their families were closely united, happy, free from
conflict, and mutually secure. Only a minority (22 percent) report
any constant, open warfare between the parents. This could, of
course, represent an authentic middle-class reaction where husband
and wife strive desperately to keep their differences sequestered to
the bedroom and present a fake united front to the children, but
there is also no doubt that children under heavy emotional stress do

develop inordinate capacities for not seeing the obvious. In some middle-class homes, however, and in many lower-class homes, the parental conflict is often open and tempestuous, and the children can become frightened witnesses of dreadful scenes [3].

In still another type of marriage the relationship becomes gradually devitalized; there is nothing to complain about, but there is also nothing to enjoy. A sense of void is predominant, and family life is characterized by tediousness and boredom. There are authorities who believe that this dreary development is "natural" to the middle years of life and represents an expectable stage in the evolution of the nuclear family.

Whereas the children from conflicted marriages are inclined to be irritable, restless, aggressive, and difficult, the children from devitalized marriages generally react with flatness and lack of zest. For the family as a whole, the home becomes a "habit cage," and continuation is ensured by the absence of any alternatives. When divorce intervenes, it almost looks as if the marriage has faded away to nothingness, and the postdivorce phase is equally characterized by an absence of reaction. The children grow up knowing nothing of the ecstasies that belong to warm and compelling human relationships.

Abnormal, in the sense of clinical, marital relationships, where one of the parents is psychiatrically ill, are especially prone to give rise to pathological disturbances in the children, particularly if prolonged into the latter part of childhood and adolescence. In a neurotic marriage the children may be caught up in hysterical coalitions with either partner and exploited emotionally, aggressively, and even sexually. In obsessional relationships the children are often participant observers of seemingly fierce sadomasochistic transactions that run the gamut of petty cruelties. In many of these it is what Freud referred to as "the narcissism of small differences"—the squabbling over the issue of butter or margarine—that eventually wrecks the marriage and devastates the family rather than any major disagreement or incompatibility. The children can serve as pawns, scapegoats, go-betweens, spies, informers, manipulaters and allies in the underground battles that are constantly waged, and they may be confidants to all the bitter secrets of an unsuccessful marriage.

A parent who functions psychopathically can destroy any hope of happiness for the children since the degree of violence generated can completely undermine all sense of safety. A psychotic parent, on the

other hand, can confuse and mystify the child, subjecting him to a
constant bombardment of irrationalities and incongruities. As a
general rule pathological marriages exert such a potent influence on
the development of children that divorce can hardly save them from
the prospect of becoming, in some way, psychiatrically disordered.
However, one must again emphasize that vulnerabilities vary
surprisingly from child to child in the same family, and prognosti-
cation is still a very inexact science in the area of risk.

The quality of the marriage prior to divorce therefore has a close
relationship to the quality of the disturbance engendered in the
child. Conflicted marriages make for conflicted children, *"emotional
divorce"* breeds affectionless children, *skewed marriages* lead to
dominant or dependent children, and *neurotic marriages* may so load
the child with unconsciously transferred feelings, reactivated from
liked or disliked parental siblings, that nothing the child can do in
reality makes any difference to the way he is treated.

The Crisis of Divorce

We come next to the crisis of divorce itself, which the child,
however prepared, is never ready for and is rarely able to accept.
The final act of disruption, even in the worst marriages, can tax his
coping capacities to their limit. Divorce and desertion are in many
ways different from bereavement in that they alter the form of family
relationship rather than cut it short. The major affect during the
crisis of divorce is grief associated with guilt, and the major affect in
the period after divorce is shame coupled with strong resentment.
Since the divorce rate is highest in the first few years of marriage,
the affected children tend to be young, and so the major disturbances
focus around separation anxiety. When the young child first learns
about an incipient divorce, his characteristic response often is denial
to such an extent that the parents may seriously question his affection
and involvement. Even when he has been repeatedly and painstakingly told about the impending separation, he may still quietly
go on asking when the missing parent will return and why he has not
yet come back. The middle-class parents who refrain from expressing
feeling in front of the children may actively foster such mechanisms
of denial and repression.

The immediate reactions to divorce will depend on the emotional loading carried over from the predivorce period and will therefore vary with the configurations of conflict, adultery, cruelty, desertion, drunkenness, criminality, drug addiction, or mental illness. If the predivorce marital relationship has been within the normal range, the children predictably manifest certain common reactions that can be diagnosed, within the nomenclature, as transient situational disorders. These include some degree of clamming up, a certain amount of regression, especially in the younger children, and a host of somatic disturbances such as overactivity, tachycardia, anorexia, nausea, vomiting and diarrhea, urinary frequency, and disturbed sleep with nightmares. The child may run away from home, run to the lost parent, grieve openly or covertly for him, display hostile feelings toward the remaining parent, and at times seem confused and disoriented about himself and his surroundings.

These symptoms generally can be regarded as crisis reactions rather than psychiatric symptoms, unless they persist or worsen. The danger signals are the same as for any other crisis situation and include the persistence of silence, panic, guilt and hostility within the home, an increase in somatic symptoms, learning disabilities or a refusal to attend at school, an outbreak of various forms of delinquency, and withdrawal from all relationships outside the home. As the condition gets worse, characterological obsessive-compulsive reactions may appear together with tics and habit spasms, dissociability, mutism, and disturbed sexual behavior (transvestism, homosexuality, etc.).

A controversy has been raging for some time as to whether so called "good" or "bad" divorces are more potent in causing psychiatric disturbances. The "good" divorce is defined as one that transforms the marital relationship into a friendly relationship with an absence of accusation, recrimination, and court battles over custody, alimony, and maintenance. The children preserve a good relationship with the absent parent with the full cooperation of the parent with custody. The reverse of this is true with the "bad" divorce. The divorced couple seem to have even more to fight over than when they were married, and visitation rights especially provoke endless animosity in which children are constantly pulled in two directions. Generally speaking, bad marriages produce bad divorces and badly disturbed children.

Recently the "good" divorce has come under suspicion as leading to internalizing disorders. This has been attributed to the fact that the child finds it more difficult to make sense out of the situation. In his own thinking, when people fight they part, and when they're friends they stay together. In the "good" divorce the child is confronted by two people who speak well of each other, relate well together, and apportion no blame, and it may be hard for the small child especially to understand this curious double communication which says in effect: We like each other and want to remain friends, but at the same time we do not get on and have decided to separate. It may be difficult for children to interpret this in terms other than hypocritical.[1]

The period of divorce is undoubtedly a difficult period of adjustment even for nondisturbed children. As a general human response, they will attempt to reconstitute the fragments of their lives, maintain continuities with happy experiences in the past, idealize the absent parent, preoccupy themselves with a vast number of activities, find substitute love relationships (although somewhat warily at first), plan for their custodian's reunion with the old parent or possible remarriage with a new one. (In this last situation they may characteristically do everything to promote a new marriage and everything to sabotage it.) The sense of abandonment always exists, even in the best managed divorces, and grieving may persist for some time. The child should not be dissuaded from mourning for what he has lost, and he may even need to be helped to mourn.

The Postdivorce Stresses

These, like the proverbial snowball, gather accumulations from the predivorce and divorce periods. In about half the cases, divorce does not end the marital relationship. The interaction continues relatively unchanged. The partners may become obsessed with ideas of punishing or remarrying each other. In the other half of the cases indifference toward the former spouse sets in and grows until after a while the one can scarcely believe that he was ever married to the other.

Westman [5] has used a crude index of good or bad divorces

---

[1] "Psychological death" is no answer to this problem since it raises new difficulties in understanding. Even in the universe of children people do not disappear mysteriously without leaving a trace behind. It is like trying to explain the disappearance of his biological parents to an adopted child. In 40 percent of cases the children become clinically disturbed.

derived from the absence or presence of postdivorce legal contests. About half the divorces involving children are followed by legal contests, and about a third of these showed evidence of repeated and intensive interaction between the divorced couple for a two-year period following the decree. Issues focused on money or children about equally. Postdivorce turbulence persisted because the couples remained embroiled in their predivorce conflicts, attempting to harass and punish their former spouses, using the children as pawns in the continued conflict, and in some cases even continuing to maintain amorous relations. Westman has described four types of turbulence to be seen in this period: a parent-centered turbulence in which the children manipulate the parents to continue their discredit each other with the children; a child-centered turbulence in which the children manipulte the parents to continue their conflicts, these being the children who have generally driven their parents to divorce; a parent-child type of turbulence where a parent and child gang up against the other parent; and a type of turbulence generated by relatives, especially meddling in-laws.

The children of divorce seen in a child guidance clinic (about 15 percent of all cases) are generally disturbed, and the disturbance is usually associated with some form of postdivorce turbulence, a third of which is parent-centered turbulence.

These disturbed children of divorce tended in general to distort the explanations of the divorce, particularly maximizing their own contribution to it and wishing hopelessly for a reunion of their parents even when remarriage had occurred. The exaggerated fantasies entertained by these children regarding their part in bringing about the divorce are reinforced by the postdivorce financial bickering which leads the children to assume it was the cost of their upkeep that caused the father's departure, and that they are therefore responsible.

McDermott [4] found several symptom clusters in this disturbed group centering around running away from home, delinquency, and poor home and school behavior. Depression, of clinical intensity, occurred in about a third of the children, sometimes overtly and sometimes in the form of depressive equivalents, such as accident-prone behavior and absconding. The latter symptom could well represent an appeal to people to take note of the child's growing fear of abandonment. The overall syndrome of the postdivorce period is what Odier labeled the neurosis of abandonment, characterized by alternations between inner depression and outer aggressiveness, a grieving for the lost family unit, and feelings of being small, weak, and intensely vulnerable. The child is often too ready to interpret divorce as an expression of hostility on the part of the parents and to assume that this is provoked by the child's wrongdoing, which the parent is punishing deservedly by means of hostile rejection, even if this entails a certain amount of circular reasoning. For example, a child who began to steal after divorce as a symptom of deprivation explained that his stealing was the reason for his parents' divorce. In many cases, the child is actually right in his belief that he is the major cause of the divorce, but he may frequently be led to assume this when the struggle over child support becomes acute.

In addition to feeling himself a causal agent in the divorce, the child may also experience the feeling of being a pawn in the conflict between his parents and is often close to the truth in this matter as well. "My mother wants me to stay with her so that my father can't have me."

The reactions of the parents may also create difficulties for the children. What is destructive for a child's development in a divorce is not so much the absence of a parental figure with whom to identify, but the way in which the remaining parent is manipulated by the child into the role of the absent parent. Furthermore, there is sometimes an unconscious collusion between the parent and child to recreate the lost parent through the child's identification with parental traits.[2] This can then lead to a parent-child struggle that often bears a striking resemblance to the previous mother-father struggle. The projection of the father image onto a son by the mother giving him a pseudo-identity is fraught with danger. It is not surprising that after a while the child begins uncannily to live up to the mother's picture of the bad father in becoming delinquent, lazy, stupid, bad, and immoral. In the predicament in which these children sometimes find themselves, a fantasy of the rescuing father coming to take them away and save them is not infrequent. At other times, the grief-stricken and angry mother may attempt to force the child to identify with her, making him an extension of herself,

[2] The remaining parent puts the child into the role of the absent parent—the child puts the remaining parent into the role of the absent parent and the situation is charged with all the potential disturbances of the predivorce marital relationship.

possibly neat, clean, and feminine. The son may then act tough to avoid assuming the passive, helpless, and nonmasculine position, or balk at occupying the male role in the family not only because of the vulnerability that has become associated with it but also because of his anger and helplessness at being deserted by the father.

The developmental stage of the child, of course, has an influence on the symptomatic picture that he presents. At the critical point when the son turns to the father as the personificaion of his ideals to hear him devalued or described as oversexed and promiscuous can provoke a lot of resentment and resentful behavior. The son may even try to desert the mother in the manner of his father. The orderly development of conscience was often interfered with when the divorce took place at this critical stage. The child experienced his parents as sadists and masochists, exploiters, and scandalmongers. It is not surprising that children exposed to such perversions of human relationships and corruption of spirit should develop ideas that this is a "dog-eat-dog" world in which anything is acceptable. These were children who developed "superego lacunae" and fantasies of violence that were sometimes acted out.

The neurosis of abandonment occasions such separation anxiety that the child may insist on staying constantly with the remaining parent and of even refusing to go to school. In terms of his infantile logic, his insecurity may be intensified by the thought that if one parent can leave him, there is nothing to stop the second from doing the same. If his mother can get rid of his father so easily, she can also rid herself of him with equal impunity. He may become overcompliant and ingratiating to avoid being deserted a second time. The parent with whom the child is living may also attempt to make the child a companion and overtax his maturity considerably, a fact that may increase his insecurity as he sees himself incapable of meeting the demands made upon him. In addition, if the parent places any of her hostility and resentment on him, it can intensify his sense of worthlessness and badness. In this predicament the child needs to be reassured that his bad wishes have not been realized and that he is not responsible for extruding his father. The hostilities within him may also give rise to anxiety and eventually to the formation of phobias.

The loss complex is radically different in the case of death and divorce. After death the absent parent is usually idealized, but after divorce he is often devalued. In either case, however, the image is distorted, and therefore healthy identification is impaired. In the conflictual postdivorce world there may be few opportunities for the child to use reality testing to correct his misconceptions about the absent parent. The intensification of the child's difficulties may be brought about by a seductive parent encouraging him to take over the role of the lost spouse and then treating him punitively for being like the bad father. In the case of a daughter, the child may sense her mother's continued attachment to the absent father and may assume a male identity to ensure the mother's interest in her. In both instances homosexual developments may take place. The remote divorce developments therefore include the dangers of one-parent development, step-parentage (what Jones referred to as the "Hamlet complex"), the reconstitution of two broken families into one whole family (unfortunately, they tend psychologically to remain two broken families living together), and the development in the child of blatantly manipulative and exploitative tendencies.

In some communities the children of divorced parents may be stigmatized, and even in highly tolerant settings the child may feel different and become ashamed to bring children home and may even conceal the facts of divorce from friends. This duplicity adds to the child's feelings of low self-esteem. It sometimes happens that the children of divorce are rejected by children from intact homes who may feel threatened by their presence. On the other hand, they may resort to excessive questioning of the child, eliciting details of the divorce as a means of alleviating their own anxieties.

If the divorced parents remain in conflict, the child may take advantage of their discord and play one against the other for his own ends. He may foment the conflict, assuming that a bad relationship is better than no relationship at all. They may also waste a lot of waking time obsessing with ideas of reconciliation even after many years. This generally reflects a failure on the part of the child to obtain satisfactory substitute relationships to compensate for the loss of the parent. In the extreme form the child may even make use of peers as surrogate parents and may undergo traumatic experiences as a result.

In rare instances a child's postdivorce reactions may be so severe that he exhibits extreme decompensation, manifested by vague wanderings, severe regressions, detachment, and impairment of reality sense. The child who reacts like this, however, has probably suffered from significant psychopathology before the separation, the divorce acting as no more than a precipitating factor.

In the postdivorce phase visitation may bring its own complications. The father becomes a nice guy who provides entertainment, and the mother is regarded as mean because she imposes the restrictions and discipline. Because the child has been already traumatized and the parents feel guilty, they may hesitate to apply reasonable controls. At other times visitations may become a chore for both father and child, each feeling compelled to live up the full allowance of time stipulated by the divorce contract, and all the time resenting it.

When the mother starts to work, the child may exhibit anger and depression, experiencing it as further loss. The mother may come to resent this. Still later, her dating may arouse in the child reactions of confusion, jealousy, anger, or denial. The child may attempt to get rid of each new date for fear his position with the parent will be jeopardized. A common reaction is that of displacing the hostility the child feels toward the absent parent onto the date.

One of the major ultimate dangers that divorce holds for the child is that he may generalize from his childhood experience and eschew marriage because of its unreliability and traumatic significance. A second danger is that he will reproduce in his own marriage the same pathological interactions his parents have exhibited. Thus the most damaging thing for the child to contend with is the vilification of the parents of each other—their diatribes, their rages, their distorted criticisms, their recriminations, their vengeances, and their use of the child as a spy or tattletale.

The Vulnerable Child in Divorce

The vulnerability of the child to divorce stems from a number of different factors. It may be his age at the time of the divorce, his sex in relation to the departing parent, his general hypersensitivity as a constitutional factor, his level of nervousness as an acquired trait from earlier experiences, a history of exposure to previous separation, for example, through hospitalization, and the existence of some handicap, disability, or chronic illness.

The psychodynamic indices include an intense attachment to the parent of one or other sex, a high degree of dependency and tendency to regression, manifestations of separation and phobic anxiety, an inability to be alone, an early preoccupation with death and disease, a failure in the development as a separate person, a low self-esteem, and an undue propensity toward guilt, shame, anxiety, and depression.

With certain groups of children, such as handicapped, adopted, and children with chronic illness such as asthma, epilepsy, and diabetes, the divorce process may bring about a psychosomatic crisis demanding hospitalization.

Crisis Intervention with Children in Divorce

Most children whose parents divorce are not in need of psychiatric treatment, but all of them are in need of some form of support which they may gain from an extended family group, from friends, or from practitioners. Sensible and commonsense management of the children at this time may be sufficient, which means an understanding of the child's situation in relation to the divorce and his particular perception of it, and support during the difficult period after the divorce.

The vulnerable child, on the other hand, needs to be convoyed very carefully during the whole process. This requires dealing with the complex of affects in the predivorce period, the use of surrogation and transitional objects during the period of change, the establishment of continuity between the predivorce and postdivorce self-conception, the maintenance of good relationships with the absent parent, the stimulation of mourning processes and the working through of attendant guilt. In the younger child one is dealing with the problem of how to substitute for loss, and in the older child how to grieve adequately for the loss.

In the therapeutic process with the disturbed child of a divorce, it is often possible to work with a central fantasy, a special restitutive kind of "family romance" with which the child attempts to repair the fragmentation of his inner life. In this utopian fantasy the child will often recreate a world signifying his needs, his dissatisfactions, his conflicts, and the ways in which all these can be resolved. In one case a child after prolonged and pregnant silence in his first interview gradually evolved his idea of a perfect city model which he proceeded

to describe in great detail. The city was in two parts, but each of the
streets ran through both parts so there was easy communication.
In the middle was a monument to peace. At the four corners of the
square city there were places that dispensed food, medicine, books,
and information so that all basic needs were catered for. The
university offered courses in being happy and in knowing how to care
for children. Nothing was left to chance in the city, so that there was
no place for misunderstandings, misconceptions, or conflicts; and the
ruling family was together for "a very long time and possibly
forever."

Using this utopian fantasy as a healing device, we explored the
child's inner feeling of being split into two, of becoming incomplete,
and his need to bring things together if he were to stay one person.
At one point he said, "I feel as if both my mother and father are
inside me and are fighting, and then they are walking away from
each other, breaking up my body so that I would go with them both,
but if I did that, of course I would die. I would be all broken up.
I can only be a real live person if they join together again." We faced
the unreality of this, the fact that he was a person in his own right,
and the ways in which we could bring the pieces together inside him
without necessarily having them come together in the outside world.

In Retrospect

A retrospective study of children of divorce brought up a number
of interesting findings [2]. The children from unhappy homes
reported in later life that they now believed that their parents'
marriage was a mistake in the first place and should never have
occurred. They also felt that they were "used" during and after the
divorce and that divorce increased the emotional distance that
already lay between them and their fathers. Their own attitude
toward marriage was also seriously affected by the divorce, and they
exuded much less confidence in their ability to have a successful
marriage.

It is interesting that although the experience of divorce in
childhood leads to divorce in adult life and although the expectations
of happiness and success in marriage are reduced by the experience
of divorce in childhood, there is a "family romance," a utopian
union, that survives even the most disturbing, depressing, and

devastating experiences of human relationships. It is this unconscious fantasy that can be used in the service of therapy. In the treatment of divorce one is concerned not only with the treatment of psychiatric disturbances caused by unhappy family relationships or disruption but also with the nurturing of the inner fantasy that might help to make future divorce less inevitable.

The concept of marriage as a desirable thing for human beings has managed to survive the ease with which divorce is now becoming available. As Linton pointed out, divorce statistics are no guide to the number of really successful marriages in a community, and he feels that probably there are as many happy marriages today as there ever have been, the only difference being that unhappy partners are now in a better position to do something about it. Linton feels that a congenial marriage can provide more contentment and emotional security than any other human relationship and that in a world in flux these are becoming increasingly important to individual happiness. He points out that the ancient trinity of father, mother, and child has survived more vicissitudes than any other human relationship and is the bedrock underlying all other family structures. Even under conditions of collapse or disruption, somehow the rock remains. He has this last portentous thing to say: "In the Götterdämmerung which overwise science and overfoolish statesmanship are preparing for us, the last man will spend his last hours searching for his wife and child."

References

1. Despert, J. L. *Children of Divorce*. Doubleday, Garden City, N. Y., 1962.
2. Landis, J. T. The trauma of children when parents divorce. *Marriage and Family Living*. 1950.
3. Le Masters, E. E. Holy deadlock: A study of unsuccessful marriages. *Sociol. Quarterly*, 21 (1959), 86–91.
4. McDermott, J. F., Jr. Divorce and its psychiatric sequelae in children. *Arch. Gen. Psychiat.*, 23 (1970), 421–427.
5. Westman, J. D., Cline, D. W., Swift, W. J., and Kramer, D. A. The role of child psychiatry in divorce. *Arch. Gen. Psychiat.*, 23 (1970), 416–420.

The Effects of Parental Divorce: The Adolescent Experience

Judith S. Wallerstein, M.S.W. and
Joan Berlin Kelly, Ph.D. (U.S.A.)

This essay, which discusses the effects of parental divorce upon the adolescent, is the first report from a three-year study[1] designed to observe and record the impact of divorce on children and on their families as discerned at the time of the divorce decision and again approximately one year thereafter. These research goals were combined with efforts to develop counseling models and specific techniques of psychological guidance for the participating families. Of the 131 children in our total sample, 21 were 13 years old or older at the time of the divorce decision. Although this represents a relatively small group, the findings are nonetheless notable, partly because they are at some variance with generally held conceptions regarding the response of adolescents to family disruption and partly because there have been no systematic studies reported in the literature regarding the phase-specific impact of parental divorce at this developmental period.

[1] The Children of Divorce Project was supported by a grant from the Zellerbach Family Fund of San Francisco at the Community Mental Health Center of Marin County, California. The project staff comprised Judith S. Wallerstein, M.S.W., principal investigator; Joan B. Kelly, Ph.D., co-principal investigator; Angela Homme, Ph.D.; Doris Juvinall, M.S.W.; Susannah Roy, M.S.W.; Janet West, M.S.W.

Marin County, stretching northward from San Francisco, contains some 206,000 people and is considered one of the most beautiful as well as most affluent areas in the United States. It has at the same time one of the highest marriage and divorce rates in the country and in the world.[2] The population is young, relatively well educated, racially nearly homogeneous, and generally vigorous. Because of these considerations it was reasoned that the phenomenon of divorce might in this milieu be more susceptible of highlighted systematic study than in settings where divorce is accompanied by high crime and poverty rates, crowding, and other disorders of urban living which contribute to the strain of family life. In effect it was hoped that a relatively stable setting would better enable the divorce themes themselves to emerge over time with greater clarity.

Accordingly, in 1970 the project reported here was begun at the Community Mental Health Center of Marin County, directed to the general divorcing population. People who had taken the decisive step of legal filing for family dissolution were advised of the availability of our free counseling service for themselves and their children. The counseling was explained as child focused, primarily preventive in nature, and including an individual evaluation of each child and counseling sessions with the parents. Help was offered to parents in interpreting the family dissolution to the children, in planning postdivorce arrangements, and in discussion with each parent of ways of easing the effects on the children. In effect we threw a wide net into the general divorce population pool, and we brought in 60 families with 131 children between the ages of 3 and 19 who were seen by five experienced clinicians trained in work with children and parents. The subjects were seen during a 6-week initial counseling period and invited to return for further follow-up interviews, again individually for each family member, at 12 to 18

[2] In 1970 the divorce rate in the United States was 3.5 per 1000 population, in California 4.2 per 1000, and in Marin County 5.7 per 1000. The highest divorce rate outside of the United States in 1970 was in the USSR (2.6 per 1000). In other European countries where divorce is legal, the divorce rate was considerably lower.

Between 1962 and 1972 in the United States the rate of divorce has increased 81 percent while the marriage rate has risen only 27 percent. A comparable analysis for California indicates a 96 percent increase in the divorce rate with a 26 percent rise in the marriage rate. The number of children under the age of 18 involved in divorce is also greater in California (16.6 per 1000 children in 1969) than in the United States as a whole (10.3 per 1000 children in 1969).

months postcounseling. Thus our data derives from these subjects seen initially at the height of the divorce decision or crisis, and subsequently when relationships had presumably had a chance to achieve a more stable equilibrium. A subgroup encountered serendipitously in the course of this study was those parents who, as children, had experienced the divorce of their own parents. Their revived memories and feelings provided an additional, although retrospective, source of data.

Although marital crisis and divorce have received considerable professional and community attention in the post-World War II United States, the effects of divorce on children have been very little scrutinized. At the time that this study was launched only McDermott had collected direct observations on a nonclinical population at the time of parental divorce, and his sample was limited to 22 children of nursery school age [19]. Subsequently, Hetherington reported an experimental study of the behavioral responses to male interviewers of adolescent girls who had lost their fathers through earlier divorce as compared with girls who had lost their fathers through death and girls from still intact families [13]. Hetherington found intensified seductive and somewhat maladroit behaviors in her experimental sample. In these instances the divorces also were not recent but predated the girls' adolescences. There have been some social science survey studies [5, 12, 14–16, 21] attempting through retrospective questionnaire data to establish correlations between parental divorce and certain emotional and behavioral sequences such as alteration in self-esteem regulation, dating patterns, and deviant or delinquent behavior patterns. As with Hetherington's findings the divorce in most instances had been in earlier periods. Finally there are reports of studies of court and clinical populations [18, 28] trying to ascertain common psychological or social characteristics of the divorcing families and their children, and accumulated experience and extrapolations from clinical practice [7, 23, 27]. None of these were addressed specifically to the youngster who had reached adolescence at the time of the parental divorce.

In our project we attempted to study parental divorce as an individual psychological experience to be followed over time for its impact on and consequences for each of the participants in the family drama, the children individually and in interaction across

generations with their divorcing parents. In doing so we have been
guided by a number of general theoretical considerations and
conceptualizations which set the framework for our study.

First we have taken for granted the complex interplay of adaptive
and defensive strategies that determine each child's capacity to
maneuver the divorce stress, each with his idiosyncratic distribution
of areas of achieved mastery and growth alongside emotional
difficulties and compromise formation. This interplay is represented
by the following example. The child of divorcing parents who
expresses guiltily his responsibility for having caused the divorce
may indeed be doing so to ward off the more terrifying feeling that
he has no control or indeed no influence whatsoever on the course
of events in his environment. This particular conflict resolution with
anxiety and guilt generated may actually be in the service of the most
effective coping with an otherwise overwhelming situation.
Therapeutic work directed solely to the exposure and resolution of
the conflict over neurotic guilt can thus concurrently undermine the
most effective coping strategy available to that child at that time.
Similarly, Anna Freud stressed the role of psychological regression
and of denial as significant and necessary parts of normal childhood
and adolescent development. Clinical judgment regarding the
efficacies of these maneuvers must take into account the specific
adaptive as well as defensive purposes and value of each in
formulating an overall judgment regarding the child's psychic state
in relation to the event or phenomenon being coped with.

A second guiding generalization was that judgments of pathology
in coping could be made confidently only over time, because we
have no established, understood, or agreed upon normative behavior
models for effective response to the kind of life crisis represented by
divorce. Do we know anything, for example, about expectable
response or spectrum of response to family disruption that can
differentially portend ultimate mastery or failure to master? Can
the capacity to maintain development as the central criterion for
mental health be assessed clinically at the time of divorce or indeed
only when viewed within the perspective of time, and if so at what
appropriate time or distance from the event? Further, can theoretical
and clinical models for assessing normal and pathological response
to family disruption, comparable to stages of mourning or object
loss, be constructed and how can these be assessed except over time,

and if so over what time? It is because of these considerations—this desire to study evolution over time—that while making full use of clinical formulations at the initial study we have tried to reserve overall clinical judgments until we have had the fullest advantage of the maximum time perspective afforded by the follow-up inquiry. In consequence, as much as possible we suspended final judgment on the need for intervention at the time of the initial counseling and moved to intervene therapeutically at this time only where the suffering of the child seemed acutely to require it.

Third, we were interested in the age-specific normal developmental tasks of the children caught up in the divorce. In this part of the study being presented here our concern is with the adolescent subgroup and the impact of the divorce on the process of resolution of their phase-specific tasks. As developed by Anna Freud [11], Erikson [9], Blos [3], Laufer [17], and others, the appropriate mastery of these adolescent tasks is the necessary prologue to adulthood and true heterosexual identity formation. Blos has summarized this as follows: "The adolescent process proceeds from a progressive decathexis of primary love objects to increased narcissim and autoeroticism to heterosexual object finding and involves a detachment of psychic institutions from the parental influence . . . this process of detachment is accompanied by a profound sense of loss and isolation equivalent to mourning" [3, p. 125].

Our own formulation here, consistent with our study data and clinical observations, is that the family disruption by virtue of the particular interplay between the divorcing adults and the interplay between each of the parents and the adolescent poses a very specific hazard to this normal adolescent process of progressive decathecting of the primary love objects. As such it carries the potential for severely overburdening the adolescent ego in its maturational, time-appointed tasks. At the same time, the very same situation of hazard carries with it a concomitant potential for the stimulation of a developmental spurt and of accelerated growth toward adulthood which, *if it does not come prematurely* (i.e., before the normal detachment has begun to take place), may indeed even facilitate the road to independence and maturity.

Related to this formulation is our additional emphasis on the other side of the interaction—the psychological position of the parents—and the powerful reverberations in the adolescent of the impact of the divorce on the parent. Thus the adolescents and their parents were conjoined within the vicissitudes of the parent-adolescent relationship as set within the divorce frame of reference. The young people were facing parents who were responding to the combination of stresses and promises in the current family disruption, sometimes with frenetic, regressive, even disorganized behaviors.[3] At the same time their relationships to the parents were shaped by their personal versions of the complex phase-specific and usually conflicted interactions of the parent-child relationship and by the history and style of this relationship at earlier stages in the family life as well as its forerunners in the childhood and adolescent experiences of the parent himself.

Pushed by regressive forces, the parents often reverted to their own preadult or adolescent behavioral life-stages or patterns in identification with or in competition with their own children and or their own past.[4] Many parents of both sexes driven by vulnerabilities, threatened by a loss of self-esteem with depressions, rages, and sexual impulses set free characteristically turned to their adolescent children for support, comfort, battle alliances, and moral vindication. Or sometimes the same parents manifest a desperate need to use the adolescent as an unconscious or conscious extension of themselves in the conflicted relationship with the spouse, creating difficulty in maintaining proper distance and separateness from developing youngsters despite intellectual recognition that the child's burgeoning autonomy needs protection. Thus Mrs. Y., a divorcing mother of four, protested that she was unable to forbid the 15- and 13-year-old-daughters from having continuing sexual relationships with their boyfriends, because "they had just lost their father." Both girls were engaged in considerable sexual activity when seen at counseling.

Some parents for a time preceding the divorce live out sexual impulses with much younger partners or move into a marketplace of available partners patterned after adolescent or young adult behavior. The adolescent child may then be experienced by the parent as a peer or competitor in these liaisons. For example, Mrs.

---

[3] A recent study [4] points to a higher incidence of serious psychiatric illness among divorced people.

[4] A related set of observations by Elson [8] suggests that some parents embark on abrupt life changes including divorce in response to the adolescents' departure for college.

B., age 33, who became depressed and anxious when she was without a date began to bring home a succession of young men in their twenties. She wore her skirts very short, her clothes very tight, her hair loose in the manner of a teenager. Her manner was flippant, bright, and hard. She complained to us that her 13-year-old daughter was chronically peevish and disobedient. "Probably" she said smilingly, "because she is jealous."

Sometimes hostile and destructive impulses were released at the time preceding and during the divorce in people who had been able to bind such impulses previously in obsessive-compulsive defenses and had functioned previously with apparent intactness in their responsible adult roles. Mr. C. at the time of the divorce explained to his adolescent son that his mother had developed a postpartum psychosis after her delivery requiring both hospitalization and electric shock, and that subsequently he needed to be cared for by somebody else during his infancy, emphasizing his scientific conviction that mental illness is inherited. His son, age 13, was clinically depressed and suicidal when seen by us. And still other parents tried to prevent independent relationships between their youngster and the separating parent. Mrs. L. appealed with repeated tears to her adolescent daughters for support against their sinful father. She endured their visits with the father with great tension, cross-examining them after each visit, making them voyeurs regarding the detail of the father's relationship with his girlfriend.

Shared Responses to the Divorce Experience

Certain experiences and responses to the divorce appeared in our data with sufficient frequency to be considered as common or characteristic of the adolescent group as a whole. The commonality of response undoubtedly has its roots in the developmental psychology of the adolescent and for the most part represents that aspect of the adolescent's functioning devoted to active mastery of, and adaptive coping with, the disorganizing impact of the divorce.

DIVORCE AS A PAINFUL EXPERIENCE

The 21 adolescents in our sample almost without exception experienced the divorce process as an extraordinarily painful event. Painful feelings were legion, and at times seemed too intense for the young people to deal with. These feelings we suggest reflected the precipitousness with which psychological processes and changing perceptions that usually unfold developmentally over time often had to be telescoped into excessively brief time spans under pressure of the divorce happenings. Predominant affects generated were those of great anger at the parents for breaking up the family at a point critical to the adolescent, considerable sadness and sense of loss, and a sense of betrayal by the parents if not both. Intensely strong feelings of shame and embarrassment prevented some from sharing any of their misery, and several adolescents had not even told closest friends of their parents' divorce. The helpless immobilization implied in "I just *couldn't*" suggests that to talk of their pain and embarrassment would somehow reveal *them* as failures, rather than their parents. Other youth caught in loyalty conflicts experienced much guilt when in fantasy or reality they aligned themselves with one parent, with resentment at both parents the inevitable result. The extent of unhappiness in all forms was initially of considerable surprise to us all, since the general expectation of both the professional and lay communities was that the more vulnerable, dependent preschool and latency aged children would experience more overt distress. Despite the expectation that the adolescent process of decathecting the parents in the psychological move out of the house would lessen their pain, the acute distress repeatedly and forcefully conveyed to us was inescapably real.

Openly expressing resentment at her mother for bringing her to the counseling service, D. burst into angry tears. "God! This *would* have to happen just when things were settling down . . . (more tears) . . . this really *upsets* me! I could have used your help a long time ago, but I've *already* talked this out. (Did it help?) Yes! And now I want to forget about it!!!" Alternately laughing at and apologizing for being so emotional at 15 years, she tearfully continued to demonstrate her inability to "forget about it," unleashing a torrent of anger, sadness, confusion, and helpless feelings.

A 14-year-old confided "the rug was pulled out from under me" when he learned his parents would divorce. Surprised and shocked, G. cried for some time, then undertook heroic efforts to effect a reconciliation. "I begged and begged . . . I tried to talk sense to my mother until I was almost *mute*," he even emphasized that a reconciliation would save lots of money. At counseling he sadly admitted his helplessness in this hopeless endeavor, but nevertheless asked the therapist to try once more for a reconciliation on his behalf.

Occasionally an adolescent insisted the divorce was not a particularly painful or disrupting experience, assuming a detached stance of "That's their problem . . . it doesn't really affect me." Only a year later were such adolescents able to reveal their pain. Thus a 17-year-old, asked at the follow-up session what advice he would give to parents contemplating divorce, quickly replied, "Don't divorce!!!" Because he had been cool and detached 1½ years earlier, the therapist replied that it sounded as if the divorce had been more painful than he had previously admitted. He emphatically agreed.

The pain of divorce for adolescents did not appear consequent to any feeling of responsibility for the parents' divorce. This is in contrast to the preschool and latency aged children studied, who assumed in their thinking varying degrees of responsibility for causing the divorce, which then increased their anguish and guilt. It is unclear why these adolescents did not feel this sense of responsibility. It may be that any assumption of responsibility would too gravely accentuate the revivified oedipal pressures, in part phase-specific and in part heightened under the impact of the divorce. Additionally we can say of the pain of parental divorce at adolescence that it may remain a persistent and unresolved aspect of the psychic life of the individual; at least it was so from the reports of the parents in our group who had themselves sustained a parental divorce when they were adolescents (as distinct from those to whom this had occurred at earlier ages). This fresh and unremitting psychic pain was often stated to be responsible for the sometimes lengthy delays in obtaining the current divorce.

ANXIETY ABOUT FUTURE MARRIAGE

Another significant finding was an enormous concern, shared by the more intact adolescents, about their future as marital partners. Whereas for some this was a painful problem expressed at the time of the initial counseling, for others it appeared to crystallize only during the year that followed. Because the breakdown of the parents' marriage comes at a time when the adolescent is expending considerable thought and psychological energy in the service of his heterosexual object-finding, the divorce experience interjects itself into his thinking in several relevant ways. It confronts the adolescent with the inescapable concern that divorce may also occur in *his* future adult life. For our adolescents, two different reactions occur in response to this salient anxiety about future divorces. The first is a decision that he or she will *never* marry, heard commonly at the time of the initial counseling. Some who initially asserted their doubt about future marriage modified their position somewhat by the time of follow-up.

One attractive 15-year-old expressed firmly her doubt she would ever marry. L. would "travel a great deal and live with a man." "If we had a child then I suppose we would have to take some appropriate action . . . but I just don't know about getting married." A year later, L.'s stance was essentially unchanged, and in fact may have been consolidated by the newly discovered, disturbing information that her mother had been married twice before.

For those who had not ruled out marriage, much thought was given to marrying later than their parents had, with an attendant conscious intent to be quite selective, and wiser than their parents, in the choice of marital partners.

G., 16 by follow-up, said he "would be more careful than my parents were." "Actually, I'm not sure I'll ever marry . . . certainly not until I'm in my thirties." He expressed many questions about marriage—"it seemed to ruin so many lives." Further, D. emphatically stated, "I never would have children . . . unless I got to be a millionaire and needed an heir."

Early in the divorce process, one 16-year-old had already given considerable thought to her future marriage. "I won't marry young . . . I want to develop *my* interests and skills first. Love and respect are necessary . . . but companionship is the most important thing in a marriage. Each person has to have separate interests and respect the other person's interests, but it's really important to have common interests and goals, too. My parents didn't respect each other at all, and the only common interest they had was us kids."

Unfortunately, there is not much evidence that such conscious intent to select a mate more carefully actually eventuates in a more compatible marriage, although one would hope that such might be the case for these adolescents painfully thinking through their futures. In analyzing the 60 families in the sample we were repeatedly struck by the absence of love, compassion, and intimacy among the parents of these children, even in their descriptions of the earlier history of their marriages. These young people have hardly experienced and internalized any concept of marriage as characterized by giving, caring, and loving. Thus, although their caution is admirable, their experience with alternatives is sadly

limited, and it is hard to predict whether their caution will be in the
service of better choices.

Related to the concern about being or finding an adequate
marital partner was evidence in some of our adolescents of
considerable anxiety about adequacy as a sexual partner, either in
their current dating or future married life. Although this coincides
with normative adolescent anxieties about developing sexuality, the
identification with the parent as a sexual failure enhanced these
anxieties. Some adolescents had been told in explicit detail of the
sexual inadequacies or peculiarities of one parent by the other angry
or self-justifying one. Two older adolescent girls dramatically accused
their mothers of "making" them frigid because of the divorce action.
Despite their ability to later relinquish this stance, the self-esteem
of both girls as sexual beings in their own heterosexual relationships
was threatened, demonstrating again how divorce can painfully
collide with adolescent development.

WORRY ABOUT MONEY

One interesting observation was the often unrealistic concern
about finances seen predominantly in those adolescents functioning
reasonably well. Because money was one of the most common
battlegrounds between divorcing parents, many of the children and
adolescents became "money-wise" somewhat prematurely. For
latency-age children anxiety about money was diffuse and related
to overall feelings of deprivation, whereas for adolescents the anxiety
about finances became focused around their future needs. Some
adolescents were sure that neither parent would finance their college
education, despite the obvious fact that sufficient funds were indeed
available. Further, they were disinclined to settle the matter by
definitively discussing the matter with the parents separately for
fear of starting new arguments and bitterness. Other adolescents
were told by their mothers that no money would be available at the
same time that their fathers were insisting that college support was
part of the final settlement given to the mother.

By the time of follow-up, even those adolescents most accustomed
to affluence had adopted a more realistic stance toward the
availability of money and tended to be less demanding in terms
of personal luxuries. This did not necessarily mean they had forever
given up the notion of personal affluence. Rather, there was

evidence of an increased capacity for delay of gratification, a more
realistic understanding of financial priorities, and a certain
gratefulness for getting what they could. In general, the divorce
appeared to create a more mature attitude toward financial matters
in the long range, despite the initial anxiety and anger about being
deprived. Being more realistic generally seemed to be one of the
benefits of divorce for those adolescents able to actively master the
divorce experience in a reasonably healthy manner.

PRECIPITOUSLY CHANGED PERCEPTIONS
OF THE PARENTS

Adolescent development involves the disengagement from the
primary love objects and the accompanying move toward heterosexual
object choice. Normally this process is a gradual one. One significant
finding of our study was the fact that divorce shortens the normally
available time span for the gradual accomplishment of these tasks,
instead plunging the child abruptly into the process of having to
disengage from and shift his perceptions of his parents. Because
these teenagers had little opportunity to establish their own tempo
in this regard, feelings of loss, emptiness, and loneliness were much
exacerbated.

In our adolescent sample, for example, the divorce process forced
a *precipitous* deidealization of the parent. The previously overvalued
parent, considered unrealistically and with awe, becomes abruptly
undervalued, a painfully fallen idol. Typically, the adolescent at
this time feels personally betrayed by his parents' divorce, and often
vigorously defends against such feelings of loss by expressing
considerable rage. In the process, he overzealously undervalues and
derogates at least one of these fallen parents. Because of the
continuing tie with the parent, and those internalized aspects of the
ego ideal derived from the parent, there is the risk that such
precipitous deidealization may interfere with the consolidation of
the adolescent's own consolidating self-esteem.

Angry at her mother for seeking a divorce, D. described her mother as
"weak, artificial, inadequate, and *totally* dependent upon her therapist," while
insisting that her father, previously very rejecting of her, was brilliant, good,
"a fine person." Viewing both assessments as unrealistic, the therapist was
concerned about this girl's future feminine identification and self-esteem if
such unbalanced assessments were to persist. With gentle persistence the

16-year-old's rage collapsed to reveal a profound sadness related to both parents' weaknesses so dramatically revealed in the divorce conflict. "They *should* be more mature . . . I feel like *I* have to be the adult," she said wistfully.

For one 13-year-old the abrupt deidealization of her father did not occur until a year following the divorce when she accidentally encountered her rather proper father with a young woman at a local art fair. This coalesced with the recent discovery of other pertinent information about her father which had been withheld. Both events led to a sense of moral indignation, a tumbling of her father in her esteem, a new feeling that he was not a man of moral integrity. Her sense of disappointment, of loss, was as painful as her anger as she mourned the father of her childhood fantasy and her preadolescence.

ACCELERATED INDIVIDUATION OF PARENTS

Divorce also appears to force the adolescent to separate out each parent as an individual, to formulate differential views of his parents qua individuals earlier than would be developmentally required. One factor precipitating this earlier scrutiny and differentiation is the active process of working through the stated and unstated reasons for the divorce. The explanations provided by the parents initiate the process, providing powerful impetus to differentiating the parents into people with incompatible needs, interests, and goals. When a parent states that "we never really loved each other"; "she wants a different kind of life style"; "we just weren't interested in the same things"; or "he won't stop drinking . . . he needs more help than I can give him" the adolescent is forced to think beyond the parental unit to very distinct individuals. The individuation process is increasingly consolidated as each parent is seen functioning in geographical and psychological separation.

This process of differentiation may proceed in several directions, depending upon the capacity of the adolescent to integrate the observations about his parents and make constructive inferences that will influence his maturing personality. For those capable of such inferences, and whose parents permit this to occur by allowing the adolescent to make some of his own independent assessments, the result seems to be an earlier, more realistic acceptance of personality differences, a greater sense of closure about the divorce, and a

smoother process of their identity formation. For some this
contributes to a more mature look at the hazards and potentialities of
marital interactions. The abrupt individuation of the parents forced
by the divorce may at the same time serve a defensive function by
transforming feelings of helplessness into a sense of control via
active mastery.

Poised and responsive, J., a 17-year-old, indicated at the following session
she had taken a much more objective stance toward both parents. Previously
furious at both, with attendant feelings of helplessness at her vulnerable
position, J. viewed her relationship with each as considerably improved.
Much to her relief, her father "doesn't get upset as much these days." "I
guess I'm also seeing him more as a person than as my important daddy." Her
mother's newly found happiness also pleases her, and she enjoys being close to
her in a new and more mature way.

Just 15 at follow-up, S. indicated in a variety of ways that his relationship with
his mother had deteriorated. "She does strange things . . . unreasonable things
. . . like she has this plan to keep changing our rooms around, and when she's
finished we won't be able to go back to our old rooms, even if we like them."
"My mom told me she didn't hate my dad, but now I know she does. She does
things just to punish him . . . like she waited until my dad drove all the way
out to our house before telling him we couldn't go on the camping trip. Lots of
times she gives reasons for things that aren't the real reasons." S. accurately
perceived his mother's behavior as frequently irrational, yet seemed to have
come to grips with it.

HEIGHTENED AWARENESS OF PARENTS
AS SEXUAL OBJECTS

One further aspect of the abruptly changed perception of the
parent attendant upon the divorce was seeing the parent as a sexual
object. A certain number of adolescents became overtly anxious
about their parents' sexuality, suddenly now visible where before it
could be more readily denied. Having a mistress, frequent dates,
or a boyfriend sleep overnight inescapably presented the adolescent
with more evidence than he cared to see that his parent was indeed
a sexual being and now very much in the same marketplace as the
adolescent in terms of heterosexual object-finding. Undoubtedly the
anxiety was due to increased sexual and reawakened incestuous
fantasies: the parent was no longer a "safe" object. This was
complicated by the fact that quite a few fathers had found girlfriends
close in age to their adolescent daughters. Several adolescent girls

handled their anxiety and dismay by significantly but quietly curtailing the number of visits with their father. Others were scornful or morally indignant, primarily as a defense against their own incestuous fantasies, yet did not share these feelings with the parent.

LOYALTY CONFLICTS: THE NEED TO CHOOSE

In many of the divorcing families in our sample, one or both parents consciously or unconsciously required that the child align with him in the continuing struggle. This demand on the adolescent frequently resulted in feelings of despair, anger, guilt, and depression. At the time of the initial counseling, early in the divorce proceedings, more than half of our adolescents were profoundly conflicted by issues of allegiance and loyalty, and angrily protested the role they felt was being forced upon them.

After some initial resistance to becoming involved in divorce counseling, W. settled back and said, "Okay, mother and I hassle." When asked what about, she replied, "my mother tries to get me to say critical things about my dad and I don't want to!" When the therapist supported her stance, the 14-year-old warmed up and continued, "mother demands that I take her side . . . she expects that I will share her anger toward dad for leaving her for another woman . . . and if I just stay silent, then it means that I agree with her!" W. described how she actively fought back against her mother. Later in the session, when the therapist shared her feelings that it was unfair for anyone to be caught between parents, W. cried, "But I *am* in the middle . . . I *am* in the middle . . . it *is* my struggle! I'm loyal to my father and I love my mother. I want to help my mother and I know that she needs it . . . but she keeps going about it in the wrong way!!

It is significant that by the follow-up a year later, virtually all of these adolescents had been able to disengage themselves from such active loyalty conflicts. This is in striking contrast to the latency age children seen in this study, many of whom were unable to detach themselves from this destructive process by virtue of their age and dependence on the parent for continued support and nurturance. The normal adolescent process of decathecting the parental figures combined with the early abrupt differentiation of parents as separate individuals functioned as an invaluable assist to the adolescent caught in divorce. Instead of feeling forced to align oneself with one parent and reject the other, the adolescent was able to detach himself from both parents, including the parent making the demand for the allegiance.

At follow-up a year later, W.'s anger at her mother remained, but she could now openly discuss her feelings and was very much in control of herself. She said that "things are just the same . . . my mother is just as angry, just as bitter, and just as jealous of my father's girlfriend." The intensity was the same, but the expression of the mother's feelings was perhaps a bit muted now. What had changed was that they, the children, had learned to talk less of their father, and when the mother asked if the girlfriend was present during their visits, they lied to the mother now, and solved the problem that way.

This adolescent had learned to deal adaptively with her difficult mother. She no longer felt pulled by either parent, and in fact gained self-esteem in the move away from both of them. What was necessary, however, was a compromise of the high moral sense of the adolescent, that is, the need to lie to keep the peace. Whereas a year earlier such a need to compromise created moral outrage and angry outbursts against the mother, this was now accepted as a necessary adaptive solution. In those adolescents, not few in number, who were forced to compromise their integrity in such ways, there was no evidence that their moral sense was compromised in other areas.

Related to this was the observation that our adolescents were forced to grapple openly with issues of morality raised uniquely by the divorce. Less universal in scope than the traditional moral searching of adolescence, these concerns centered around which parent was right or wrong in those attitudes and actions causing the marital conflict and eventuating in divorce. Most adolescents struggled with such moral questions not only in the service of making judgments about the parents, but more importantly in the service of consolidating their own conscience and moral development, particularly in determining appropriate ethical and sexual conduct for themselves now and for the future. For some it was a question of which parent represented the appropriate moral attitude to be identified with, while others determined that both parents' moral and ethical behavior was found wanting.

E. talked at counseling of changes over the past few years in her life, stating, "even though my mother and father were dishonest, and I used to be, I've suddenly stopped. I don't know why . . . I just decided I didn't want to be like them." A year later at follow-up, E. indicated she'd thought a lot about her parents "cheating on each other" (sexual affairs) . . . "I think it's terrible!"

This is especially significant for this adolescence because, lacking adults of high moral conduct available as role models, her move toward higher ethical standards came from within as she increased the distance between herself and her parents after the divorce.

STRATEGIC WITHDRAWAL

All of the adolescents in this study tried with varying degrees of success to make use of distancing and withdrawal as a defense against experiencing the pain of the family disruption. Sometimes this distancing took the active form of much accelerated social activity or staying away from home, which was especially threatening to some parents, particularly those parents who had been apprehensive initially about acting out of their adolescent children, and whose apprehensiveness may have increased by virtue of their own newfound sexual freedom. Some youngsters declared vehemently their lack of involvement with parental problems despite behavior and many tears to the contrary.

A certain percentage of adolescents in our study held steadfastly to detachment and distance verging on aloofness. Some of these were indeed young people for whom the divorce essentially legalized and consolidated a family life style and relationship pattern between the parents which had preexisted for many years. These young people had already set a particular course.

Thus P., age 16½, an essentially intact youngster, who continued to do well at school and elsewhere, said of his father (whose combined job and mistress had previously kept him absent from the home), "Dad was never around before. We learned to get along without him. The divorce won't make any real difference." P. volunteered that he had felt sad at times, because he never had a real father; he missed this when he was a "growing child." He hoped that the divorce would bring some relief for his mother's anger and chronic unhappiness.

P.'s older brother, who was into serious, rebellious acting out, drunkenness, drug abuse, car accidents, and violent outbursts in the family said the divorce would change nothing for him. His social behavior and relationship patterns within the family continued essentially on the same hurricane course, perhaps somewhat accelerated. At age 18, within a year of the divorce, he became involved in a drunken accident during which he demolished a friend's car.

The group that particularly interested us were young people in their early or mid-adolescence who before the divorce had not led lives essentially detached from their families. Rather it seemed to be primarily in response to the divorce decision that their behavior veered away from the parental figures. Their "cool" manner was in fact a source of some initial concern to us as to whether the central developmental impact of the divorce might indeed be an increase in narcissistic investment and a diminution in empathic response. Thus R., a very bright 15-year-old, stoutly maintained that his parents divorced only because they had undertaken to build a new home and could not agree on the number or placement of the bathrooms. He held to this position concretely and not meta- phorically throughout the entire counseling sessions. I., when initally seen, delivered herself of some very strong opinions with surprisingly mild affect. Her dispassionate recounting of her parents' marital failures and their personal faults and her clear interest only in her own life was striking and troublesome in this 13-year-old girl.

It is therefore of central importance to report that these particular adolescents looked the best to us in our entire sample at follow-up not only in terms of their having matured considerably during the intervening year but primarily in terms of their now demonstrated capacity for empathy, warmth, and compassion toward at least one parent. Moreover, this sometimes took a form well beyond verbal support and extended to considerable help in the home. Thus L., in contrast to her previous cool stance and self-centered behavior, had willingly assumed responsibility for helping her mother with the younger siblings and expressed genuine concern about her mother's welfare.

When seen at follow-up, R. no longer maintained his previous superficial explanation of his parents' divorce. He seemed much more outgoing and poised and considerably less preoccupied with his own needs. This time he said that he thinks his parents behaved foolishly, that he feels his mother's needs for support, help, and intimacy, but that he feels that he can be of no help to her, and it would not benefit him or them for him to enter into the difficulty between his mother and his father. He was willing at this follow-up to admit how painful the divorce had been in the past year.

A., who had been spending most of her time out of the house at the initial counseling, also seemed to have mellowed considerably. She was less defensive and less angry. Whereas previously she said, "I don't care about him or her" in relation to her parents. A. now said that her dad had problems, but she was not going to let his problems upset her, and "bother my activities and my life." When reminded of her statements the year before, and her fighting with her siblings and feelings of injustice on the part of her parents, A. laughed freely, and said, "Was I like that? Wow, I really was a brat then."

It would appear that for those adolescents the emotional detachment at the time of the parental divorce represents a strategic withdrawal in the service of maintaining the integrity of adolescent development. It seems clear that the distancing at the time of the height of the struggle saves the adolescent from anguish, humiliation, and emotional depletion, and enables him at a later date—at a time appropriate to his own timetable and needs, and when the external turmoil has subsided somewhat—to be supportive, empathic, and sensitive. Nor is there any reason to assume that such capacities for empathy, compassion, and protectiveness will not endure into adulthood. These findings would be very much in accord with our understanding of the significant place of withdrawal and denial in the normal development of children and adolescents.

Major Psychopathological Formations

Finally we must consider these subgroups among our youngsters in whom the divorce triggered or consolidated serious psychopathological response as assessed within the time perspective of initial counselling and subsequent follow-up. We consider these the young people *at risk* and needful of psychotherapeutic intervention. One case illustrative of each such subgroup is presented here.

PROLONGED INTERFERENCE WITH ENTRY INTO ADOLESCENCE

For several young people in our study the primary impact of the parental divorce experience can be considered as a developmental interference in which the entry into adolescence and the mastery of the normative tasks of adolescence seemed delayed or held back indefinitely by the particular conflict configuration and parent-child interaction which obtained at that time.

T. is an early adolescent whose aggressive, driving father was often caustic and verbally abusive with his wife and three children. At other times the father was passionately and demonstrably affectionate with his son, but rarely with any other members of the family. T.'s mother suffered with a severe

hysterical illness with disabling psychosomatic symptoms of many years standing
for which she had recently entered psychotherapy. She was chronically
depressed, and had made several suicide attempts, which were known to the
children. T.'s mother was close to her three children and attempted consciously
within the limits of her own low self-esteem to shield them from the husband's
depreciation. To compensate for her husband's disinterest, she had always been
especially close to T., and he in turn worried about her illness, her depression,
and her suicide attempts.

When T. was told by his parents of their divorce decision, he ran from the
livingroom screaming, "You're trying to kill us all." Following his father's
moving out of the household, T. began increasingly to assume a protective role
with his mother. He checked her social activities, monitored her telephone
calls, requested the check at restaurants, sat in his father's place at the dinner
table, and lay down on the sofa with her on occasion. Some of the impetus for
this behavior doubtless derived from the mother's gratification with T.'s
attention, which was supportive of her at a time when she felt intensely
deprived, rejected not only by her husband but also by the maternal grandparents, who strongly opposed the divorce.

When seen a year thereafter the boy's preoccupation with his mother's health
had intensified. His jealousy of her other relationships and particularly of her
intimacy with her psychotherapist was undiminished. He flew into jealous
rages when she dated, was indeed sleepless when she went out on a date, and
worried about her continually, especially about her possible death from cancer.
His own attachment to his friends had lessened, as he had become more
preoccupied with his mother, although he continued to do well academically.

T., at 14, is clinically at risk, manifesting a delayed entry into
adolescence and is in active need of psychotherapeutic intervention.
A year following the divorce he is still suffering with increasingly
intolerable conflict which binds him into a conflicted, overly
eroticized oedipal attachment to his mother, an attachment which
has been given real and fantasy impetus by the father's departure and
the mother's divorce-intensified needs. T's panic at the announcement
of the divorce decision by the parents presaged the difficulties which
he did indeed encounter. A year following the parental separation
he is further away from his own autonomy and independence.

TEMPORARY INTERFERENCE WITH
ENTRY INTO ADOLESCENCE

H., age 13, an adopted child of a marriage which came to divorce after 1½
years of no conversation, no sex, and no meals between the parents, who
communicated entirely by written notes during all of this time, had an intense
relationship with her father, who had held her on his lap until she was 11 years

old. He was a violent, abusive, and authoritarian figure to his wife and two sons, but never to his daughter. The mother was a petulant, long-suffering woman who seemed helpless for many years to resist the father's tantrums, moodiness, and beatings. After the mother filed for divorce, the father refused to leave the house and returned nightly in a towering rage. When the divorce was granted he disappeared, leaving no forwarding address, although he continued to send child support money from a post office box.

When H. was seen, she was apprehensive, depressed, and inarticulate. Her sadness, her sense of loss, her worry about her father, her forlorn hope that he still loved her despite his desertion and her tattered self-esteem came out gradually, but without relief or diminution of her depression. H. gained 20 pounds in the three months following the mother's decision to file for divorce. During this period she began to drop contact with her friends, to engage in doll play with younger children, and to sleep in her mother's bed.

At follow-up, approximately two years later, H. was in the process of reconstituting her predivorce state of functioning. She was gradually regaining an appropriate age level performance at school, although still having difficulty. She had, however, resumed friends in her age group and was succeeding in losing much of her excess weight gain. Although still somewhat subdued and stolid in her responses, she seemed to have moved into age-appropriate adolescent development. Her recovery from the regression and resumption of age-appropriate behavior coincided with the mother's remarriage and H.'s good relationship with the stepfather.

This case represents a delay rather than a full blocking of the youngster's entry into adolescent development. We note in passing that sleeping with her mother following the divorce is not a common occurrence among adolescents, but was more common following parental divorce where there are latency or younger children in the family. There are many such instances in our sample in which the parent is apprehensive about sleeping alone at this time. In this case it is important to point out that B. was not able to resume her own developmenal agenda until she was set free from the regressive interaction with the mother and the multifaceted impact of the father's desertion by the mother's remarriage and her good relationship with her stepfather.

PSEUDO-ADOLESCENCE IN RESPONSE
TO PARENTAL DIVORCE

One danger specific to adolescence is entry into heterosexual activity, prematurely, before having acquired the preconditions for true heterosexual love relationships. To the extent that the sexual activity occurs under the dominance of an incestuous tie to the parents or as an extension of the parents' unconscious or conscious needs and impulses the adolescent can be said to be living out a pseudo-adolescence rather than a true emancipating adolescent experience.

C., age 15 at counseling, began her sexual activity at age 14 at the time that her father began a sexual affair with a neighbor. C. was full of rage at her father, whom she considered an adulterer, and freely admitted throwing rocks at the windows of his mistress and similar harassments. She described in obscene language her fantasies of her father's sexual performance with his mistress and shared these and other confidences regarding her father's sexual activity with her mother in what appeared to be an ongoing relationship in which mother and daughter developed strategies together regarding the father and his mistress. These consultations seemed at times to reach bizarre limits, as for instance when the mother found an unsigned note addressed to no one in particular, saying, "I want to love you," and called a family conference to ascertain what strategies should be undertaken.

C.'s father, a mild-mannered, gentle, chronically depressed professional man, referred to his marriage as a "blur," made increasing use of pot, which seemed to be affecting his judgment especially at work, and seemed unable to see any connection between his behavior and consequences either for his wife or for his children. C.'s mother, a teacher who had been relatively organized in her functioning prior to the divorce, suffered a severe regression at the time of the divorce decision. She began to show increasingly poor judgment and seemed to be warding off a disorganizing depression through a variety of disjunctive behaviors including inviting numbers of young men to live in the household, probably in a desperate effort to deny her intolerable perception of the husband's departure and absence. In various ways it seemed clear that the mother in her regressed state seemed unable except in a verbal way to differentiate her needs from those of her daughter.

C. continued on a course of sexual activity with a succession of young men in the year following the divorce. At school her performance was poor. She seemed unmotivated, educationally and vocationally, and primarily interested in the male teachers. At follow-up both mother and daughter seemed essentially unchanged. The family had gone from crisis to crisis, and the house had become almost a boarding home in which a variety of young men lived, some of whom were sleeping with the daughter.

C. is a severely disturbed adolescent whose symptoms included drinking, drug abuse, promiscuity, and poor impulse control. She is much at risk, and in urgent need of both psychotherapy and environmental controls.

REGRESSION FOLLOWING LOSS OF EXTERNAL
VALUES AND CONTROLS

Another subgroup of young people at risk were those for whom
the parental divorce signified primarily the loss of external
behavioral constraints and models which still provided a necessary
part of their psychic economy. Specifically the external presence
of the parent, usually the father, served to reinforce and organize
still insufficiently consolidated inner-control mechanisms. Therefore
for these youngsters the disruption of the family structure, the loss of
the father's physical presence, the discovery of sexual, aggressive, and
"amoral" behaviors in parents with the consequent sense of
disappointment and betrayal triggered acute anxiety and intense
conflict. It seemed clear that the controls and tenuous identification
and ego ideals of these young people were unable to contain
heightened sexual and aggressive impulses in the absence of the
familiar external reinforcement and threats.

B., a junior college student, discovered accidentally that his father was having
a sexual liaison with a young woman before this information became known to
his mother and before the divorce decision. This discovery caused B. intense
and unremitting anguish. "I began to feel a lot of anxiety. What should I do;
what shouldn't I do? Should I do it now, should I do it later?" With the
father's decision to request the divorce B. was enormously shocked and felt
that his father had betrayed his major philosophy of life, namely, never to
quit. "It was rare that you could go to my dad with any kind of a problem
and not have him say, "You have to stay with it." In this case my dad was
chucking away what was the basis of my philosophy that he had taught me. It
meant to me that maybe my point of view was wrong since my dad threw it
away. It felt like I was taking a creaky ship into the storm" (referring to his
own future ventures into adulthood and particularly to his plans to become
engaged to a young woman).

B. developed a series of somatic symptoms, including dizzy spells, sleepless-
ness, and fears of being alone. These culminated in an emergency episode when
while driving a car across a bridge B. felt unable to proceed. He became acutely
fearful that he was going to die, began to sob uncontrollably, and pulled his
legs up into a fetal position. He was taken to a hospital by the police. Shortly
thereafter B. was admitted to a psychiatric hospital where he remained for 10
days as an inpatient, and eventually, successfully began to work out the conflicts
triggered by the divorce and in particular his feelings that he was "incapacitated
by my father's desertion."

B.'s father, an aggressive and somewhat blustering businessman, had indeed ventured into what appeared to be an adolescent fling at middle-age. B.'s mother was a dependent, somewhat unrealistic woman who lived in B.'s view "in that upper-middle class world that exists for women who drive station wagons and work hard on charities." Central in B.'s breakdown was his statement "I think that the beliefs which gave me the ability to deal effectively with life were blown apart for me."

DIVORCE AS A SUPERIMPOSED TRAUMA

Finally there were in our study youngsters at serious risk whose life experience had been unhappy and fraught with conflict and insecurities for many years. For these adolescents the divorce itself represented one more link in a long chain of experiences out of which they drew the same lesson: the reasonable needs and wishes of the children had little or no priority within the family. These adolescents find themselves without role models, prodded by the wish to achieve independence from the unhappiness and rejection they have known, but without the inner integrations needed to face the complex and exacting demands of adolescence. In a true sense they are in flight *from* rather than to, and there was no doubt that without intense psychological help over the long term they would not be able to make headway toward adulthood. In addition, the parents of these youngsters burdened themselves and their children with their own unresolved or unmodified need for immediate gratifications, with frantic efforts to ward off psychotic disorganization and profound depressions which threatened to engulf them, and in direct competition with, and depreciation of, the capacities and physical appearance of their children.

E., age 13, came from a family in which both her father and mother had struggled throughout the marriage to maintain adulthood, but had little sense of the dimensions of the parental roles except as economic providers. Each had had throughout a succession of open love affairs often with the other's friends. The father, a handsome, narcissistic man with an explosive temper, had precipitated the divorce, because he wished to marry an older woman "who would be good for me." The mother, a tense, pretty, young woman, had warded off a profound chronic depression by a variety of maneuvers including staying out of the home, and needing the constant company of a man. At the time of the divorce decision both parents were preoccupied with their own needs: the father with his wish to move out as easily as possible; the mother with the acquisition of a new man to cover her loneliness, rage, and threatened depression.

At counseling, E. explained that she had no use for any adults, particularly her parents, that she wished only to live alone, because she finds adults deceitful, selfish, irresponsible, and without morality. The parents' divorce confirmed and underscored this view. Her affective life centered around an encapsulated fantasy of horses who led an erotic, wild, and beautiful life, mating endlessly and producing in polygamous society happy children whom they treat with love and compassion. E. said, "Whenever things get tough I go into my room, and I talk to my horses, and my horses talk back to me." E. had few friends and was doing poorly at school.

At follow-up E. said there was one adult in the world that she trusted. That was the matron in the local school who permitted her to smoke. E. was smoking excessively with some mild drug use, a great deal of loneliness, and a desperate yearning for affection, friends, and interest from any quarter where it might be forthcoming. She had established herself in those high school groups identified with antisocial behavior. Although she had mostly relinquished her preadolescent fantasy of horses, she had hardly replaced it and was feeling empty, restless, and hungry for stimuli.

E. is suffering with a serious depression of long standing, is predelinquent, with a lifelong history of emotional deprivation and erratic parenting. She is very much in need of long-term psychotherapeutic help and environmental supports.

Conclusions

It appears that following parental divorce many young people live through an acutely painful experience which, although time limited for most, is marked by a rapid acceleration and telescoping of normative adolescent perceptions, conflicts, preoccupations, and responses. Some of the distress may indeed be related to the rapidity with which the changes occur under the press of the divorce impact and the diminished ability of the adolescent to exercise control over the tempo of change. Nevertheless, most of the young people whom we studied were able within a year following parental separation to take up their individual agendas and proceed toward adulthood at a more measured pace. Moreover, it seemed that except where the response to divorce caused delays or ruptured development, they were able to continue at a level equivalent to their previous achievement or enhanced even by their mastery of the inner and outer events of the preceding year.

Those youngsters who entered adolescence and encountered the parental divorce with a history of long-standing difficulties seemed to follow a more troubled course. These difficulties in many instances were intensely exacerbated by the difficulties of the parents at the time of the divorce. Of particular relevance to the experience of the adolscent was the degree of the parental regression, particularly to preadult or adolescent modes of behavior, and the tendency of some parents to cross generational boundaries out of the intensity of their own needs and conflicts. Many youngsters caught up in this interacting web were severely limited in their capacity to address complex adolescent tasks.

Finally, it seemed that the adolescents who appeared to do best were frequently those who were able at the outset to establish and maintain some distance from the parental crisis and whose parents, whether willingly or reluctantly, permitted them to do so. As noted, these young people at first impressed us as seeming somewhat self-centered and perhaps insensitive. We discovered over time that these were the youngsters who were able at the end of the year to develop that remarkable combination of realistic assessment of their parents along with compassion, which augurs well for their future.

Repeatedly, throughout this study, our attention was drawn to the central importance of the particular patterning of the parent-child relationship obtaining both at the time of the divorce and previously, and to the particular unconscious and conscious dissonances and congruities which are present in the interacting needs, impulses, conflicts, and defensive configurations. All of these seem centrally related to the capacities of each family member to hold to the separation of generations and to his individual growth potential.

References

1. Anthony, E. J. *Parenthood, Its Psychology and Psychopathology*. Little, Brown, Boston, 1970.
2. Blos., P. The concept of acting out in relation to the adolescent process. *J. Amer. Child Psych.*, 2 (1963), 118–143.
3. Blos, P. *On Adolescence*. The Free Press, New York, 1962.
4. Briscoe, C. W., Smith, J. B., Robins, E. Marten, S., and Gasking, F. *Divorce and psychiatric disease. Arch. Gen. Psychiat.*, 29 (1973), 119–125.
5. Burchinal, L. G. Characteristics of adolescents from unbroken, broken, and reconstituted families. *Marriage and Family*, 26 (1964), 44–51.
6. *California Statistical Abstract, 1971*. State of California, Department of Public Health, Sacramento, Ca.

7. Despert, J. L. *Children of Divorce.* Doubleday, Garden City, N.Y., 1962.
8. Elson, M. The reactive impact of adolescent and family upon each other in separation. *J. Amer. Acad. Child Psych.*, 3 (1964), 697–707.
9. Erikson, E. H. The problem of ego identity. *Psychol. Iss.*, 1 (1959) 101–164.
10. Freud, A. *Normality and Pathology in Childhood: Assessments of Development.* International Universities Press, New York, 1965.
11. Freud, A. Adolescence. *The Psychoanalytic Study of the Child*, 13 (1958), 255–275.
12. Goode, W. J. *Women in Divorce,* The Free Press, New York, 1965.
13. Hetherington, E. M. Girls without fathers. *Psychology Today*, 6 (1973), 47–52.
14. Landis, J. T. A comparison of children from divorced and nondivorced unhappy marriages. *The Family Life Co-ordinator*, 11 (1962), 61–65.
15 Landis, J. T. Social correlates of divorce or nondivorce among the unhappy married. *Marriage and Family Living*, 25 (1963), 178–180.
16. Landis, J. T. The trauma of children when parents divorce. *Marriage and Family Living*, 22 (1960), 7–13.
17. Laufer, M. Object loss and mourning during adolescence. *The Psychoanalytic Study of the Child*, 21 (1966), 269–289.
18. McDermott, J. F., Jr. Divorce and its psychiatric sequelae in children. *Arch. Gen. Psychiat.*, 23 (1970), 421–427.
19. McDermott, J. F., Jr. Parental divorce in early childhood. *Amer. Psychiat.*, 124 (1968), 1424–1432.
20. Murphy, L. B. The stronghold of norms on the individual child. *Childhood Education*, 4 (1973), 344–349.
21. Nye, F. I. Child adjustment in broken and in unhappy unbroken homes. *Marriage and Family Living*, 19 (1957), 356–361.
22. *Statistical Abstract of the U.S., 1972.* U.S. Department of Commerce Publications, Social and Economic Statistics Administration, Bureau of the Census, Washington, D.C.
23. Steinzor, B. *When Parents Divorce.* Pantheon, New York, 1969.
24. *United Nations Statistical Yearbook, 1971.* Statistical Yearbook, 1971. Statistical Office of the United Nations. Department of Economic and Social Affairs, New York, 1972.
25. *Vital Statistics of California, 1962–1971.* State Department of Public Health, Sacramento, Ca.
26. *Vital Statistics of the United States, 1969.* Volume III, U.S. Department of Health, Education and Welfare, Health Services and Mental Health Administration, National Center for Health Statistics, Washington, D.C.
27. Westman, J. C. Effect of divorce on a child's personality development. *Med. Aspects Human Sexuality*, 6 (1972), 38–55.
28. Westman, J. D., Cline, D. W., Swift, W. J., and Kramer, D. A. The role of child psychiatry in divorce. *Arch. Gen. Psychiat.*, 23 (1970), 416–420.

A Reasearch Strategy for Studying Risk for Schizophrenia during Adolescence and Early Adulthood*

Eliot H. Rodnick, Ph.D. and
Michael J. Goldstein, Ph.D. (U.S.A.)

Various strategies are possible in selecting for intensive study a population of children or adolescents who may have a higher than random likelihood of developing schizophrenia. We have chosen one particular route since it involved reasonable parsimony in assumptions regarding the possible etiology of schizophrenia. It was consistent with current knowledge regarding precursors of schizophrenia and provided access to a subject sample that could be studied intensively while meeting enough of the needs of our subjects to ensure their active cooperation during a period of intensive study.

Our overall strategy had several components. First we attempted to identify conditions which current evidence suggests may contribute to the onset and course of development of schizophrenic behavior. Second we studied a cohort of adolescents intensively to isolate those who might possess the kind of attributes considered likely as precursors of adult schizophrenia. Third the adolescent

[1] The research reported here has been supported by NIMH grants MH-08744 and MH-13512. An earlier version of this paper was written for the Dorado Beach Conference on Risk Research in Schizophrenia, Puerto Rico, October 18-22, 1972.

cohort is followed into adulthood to assess the extent to which the precursors indeed predicted adult psychopathology. Fourth specific retrospective studies with a new sample of acute, young adult schizophrenics then provide the opportunity to cross-validate the predictive significance of those precursors identified in the prospective study.

We can best describe the particular strategy we used by considering our research design, the assumptions underlying our choice of variables to be investigated, and their relevance to the issue of identifying those who are potential high risks for schizophrenia by discussing the issues in terms of the four stages of research strategy presented in Figure 1.

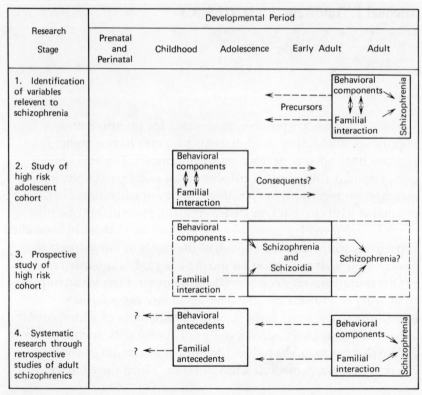

Figure 1   A strategy for sequential research on cohorts with high risk for schizophrenia.

Stage 1. Delineation of Relevant Precursor Variables Related to the Occurrence of Schizophrenia

From the whole array of possible precursor variables we selected those that could be identified objectively, and to which we might have access in a research study. After examining and then rejecting a strategy of concentrating on the psychopathology of schizophrenia, we decided to look at the premorbid social adjustment and the familial environments. We took as a starting point the evidence emanating from a number of sources, such as those reported by the Lidz group at Yale [9], those associated with Wynne at NIMH [17, 18] and Rodnick and Garmezy at Duke [12] and the work of some of our students at UCLA. This research indicated that the intra-familial environment of schizophrenics is very likely discriminably different from that of other adult forms of psychopathology, although the actual evidence on this point is sketchy and frag-mentary. As suggested in Figure 1, Stage 1, studies on the adult schizophrenic suggest that the specific attributes of this intra-familial environment are probably antecedent to the development of schizophrenic behavior, and not primarily a result of having to cope with the psychotic behavior of the schizophrenic offspring.

Another set of precursor variables which appeared to have significance for the course of development of adult schizophrenia is that of the social competence level prior to the onset of the schizophrenic condition on which Garmezy and Rodnick and their associates [4, 12] had reported, and which has been elaborated by a number of others in recent years.

We decided therefore to identify a cohort of adolescents who might have a high risk for adult psychopathology, including schizo-phrenia, who might be studied intensively without the complication of the presence of overt psychotic behavior. The particular foci in this research standpoint are the attributes of the intrafamilial environment and the social (or interpersonal) competence of the adolescents across a broad domain of functioning. Our concerns here are three-fold: First is there a specificity of intrafamilial environ-ments which relates to different forms of adolescent disturbance? Second what is the relationship between the specificity of the intra-familial environments to the social competence of the adolescents?

And do the attributes of the social competencies and the intrafamilial environments of this cohort of adolescents bear any resemblance to those reported as relevant precursors to the schizophrenic psychosis?

We were well aware of the overwhelming likelihood that vulnerability for schizophrenia is a function of the interaction of a broad array of factors ranging from genetic liability, biochemical and physiological dysfunctions to specific patterns of early learning and social experience which shape both interpersonal competence and the display of psychopathological behavior. If successful, we would be content merely to identify a cohort with greater than random probability of showing schizophreniform behavior as they entered the period of risk for schizophrenia in early adulthood. This leads us to Stage 2 in the research design.

Stage 2.   Identification of an Adolescent Cohort Which May Be High Risk for Schizophrenia

Our problem was to identify a cohort that could be researched intensively. Since we wished to identify a sufficiently large group who might be high risk for contrasting patterns of adult psychopathology, and who were being studied under exactly the same conditions, we had to identify a population where the potentiality for adult pathology was considerably higher than random. Furthermore, both the adolescents and the members of their families were to be studied intensively in interaction with one another. The active cooperation of all of them would be required under conditions in which there had to be considerable self-disclosure to the various members of the research team. This could be achieved best if their needs were being met by the research team.

We decided to achieve a set of conditions by selecting a random sample of adolescents who had been referred to a psychological clinic for difficulties in school, for behavioral maladjustment within the family, or because of pressure from juvenile court or probation authorities. The only restriction we placed on the sample was that the family be intact and that the adolescent and both parents, and in some cases a sibling, come together to the clinic for an assessment period lasting five to six weeks, after which recommendations for treatment or referral elsewhere would be discussed with them.

We were aware of the biased and restricted sample that this

procedure would provoke. On the one hand, it reduced the likelihood of obtaining adolescents with frank psychotic behavior or with significant somatic symptoms, since such patients would tend to be referred to a medically oriented rather than a psychological clinic. From our standpoint this sample restriction was desirable since it reduced the likelihood that any unique intrafamilial reaction patterns we found were derivatives of psychotic behavior or a serious somatic symptom of the adolescent. On the other hand, other attributes of the sample tended to reduce its comparability with other studies of adolescents with high risk for schizophrenia. These are:

1. A clinic on a university campus tends to attract clients biased toward higher educational and social economic levels and away from black and chicano ethnicity.
2. The requirement of family intactness probably resulted in biasing the sample away from some forms of pathology resulting from child neglect and lack of stable parental surrogates, but perhaps toward concentrating the sample on those forms of pathology in which patterns of long-standing familial interaction are significant precursors.
3. The requirement of parental and adolescent cooperation in appearing as a group probably resulted in selecting a sample which favors passivity of adolescent and involvement of the parents.
4. The major restriction on the sample is, of course, the occurrence of behavioral disturbance in adolescents and the desire of members of the family to alleviate the disturbance by psychological means. These families might thus be more prone to interpret and react to interpersonal cues in ways that could differ significantly from those who are seen in a psychiatric hospital or as nonvoluntary clients in a community health center.

We decided to compensate for these sampling biases by comparing with one another various subsamples within the total sample, using as independent variable either patterns of behavioral disturbance of the adolescent or styles of particular intrafamilial interaction.

We decided to explore the interactions within the family by having the various family members interact with one another in roleplaying their actual spontaneous responses to problems which both child and parent had identified as significant issues for either or both of them, and which appeared to be closely related to the reasons bringing them to the clinic for assistance.

We were trying to get at the interior of the interpersonal relations within the family in a relatively short period of time, with some intensity and directness which seemed relevant to the adolescents and their families. But this presented us with a dilemma. We wished to use objective and quantitative measures under sufficiently controlled conditions to permit direct comparisons between groups of families in complex interactions. The temptation at first was to use standardized stimulus situations in controlled environmental contexts, such as had been used by various groups to study the behavior of adult schizophrenics. But since the subjects came for direct assistance, our procedures had to meet their needs, even though we might dawdle somewhat if we felt that it did not exact any psychological cost from our subjects. We also wished to study the interaction under conditions that seemed natural and that could elicit sufficiently intense responses in the various family members, while still keeping them in the situation of being assessed under systematic conditions. We decided therefore to forgo standardized cue situations, or experimental interactions such as we had employed in earlier research with adult psychotics, or the solution of universal problems such as had been used by most investigators working with variants of the Strodbeck [14] procedure.

We decided to use a limited psychological assessment battery specially designed interviews, and direct interaction with one another in response to relevant personalized interpersonal cues which the various members of the family had all identified as key problem issues between adolescent and parents. The interactions were employed under conditions in which each person could serve as both initiator and recipient. The only nonverbal instrumentation we introduced was limited to the recording of skin resistance during the interaction in order to have some direct nonverbal indices of somatic arousal and control.

Without going into any of the details of the procedure, which are described more extensively elsewhere [6], perhaps it will suffice to indicate that the data available to us are psychological assessment test protocols for each of the members of the family, a systematic interview of the adolescent's behavior as seen by child and parents, role-playing cue statements and responses of each family member with each other, and finally dyadic and triadic interactions based on discussions of how they interact with one another in the role-playing phase.

This phase provided our primary data, and a number of reports on various aspects of our findings to date have already been published. We found, taking the presenting behavioral problem which brought the adolescent to the clinic as the independent variable, that distinctive patterns of familial interaction correlated with the various adolescent symptom groups. We found that we could sort our adolescent sample into four groups with satisfactorily high reliability and without undue arbitrariness.

Based primarily on parents' description of the child's problem, we were able to divide our subject sample seen in the clinic into four groups:

Group I: Aggressive and antisocial behavior, characterized by poorly controlled, impulsive, and acting out behavior toward authority in the community.

Group II: Active family conflict, characterized by an overtly defiant stance toward parents.

Group III: Negativism, sullenness, and passive-negative forms of hostility and resistance toward parents and school authority.

Group IV: Withdrawn, passive, and isolated adolescents, characterized by marked social isolation, general uncommunicativeness, and excessive dependence on parents.

The following table indicates the number of families we have studied intensively to date:

| Group | Adolescents | | |
	Male	Female	Total
I	10	8	18
II	8	8	16
III	11	5	16
IV	8	7	15
			65

We have also studied a limited number of families in which the adolescent was hospitalized for schizophrenia or anorexia nervosa at UCLA-Neuropsychiatric Institute.

At the time we started the project we aimed for an analysis of the relationship between familial interaction and pattern of adolescent disturbance. Our objective was to determine whether familial interactions which resemble those reported for schizophrenia are associated with adolescent behavioral disturbances which resemble presumed precursors of schizophrenia. From the beginning of our analyses with the first few cases, we found that there indeed did appear to be some degree of specificity between intrafamilial characteristics and adolescent disturbance in a number of areas of functioning. To date we have reported on the following types of response in interactional situations:

1. Social influence and counterinfluence as revealed by the role-playing cue statements and responses [1].
2. Skin resistance response in various contexts of interaction between parent and child [7].
3. Attribution of familial relations on the TAT [7].
4. Communication of intents in parent and child interactions in triadic and dyadic interaction [10].
5. Comparisons of stimulus-response in triadic and dyadic interaction [11].
6. Parental and child attributes as revealed in parental descriptions of the child's problem [16].

We are in the midst of analyzing the adolescent behavioral attributes as derived from parental and adolescent interviews, as well as the ways in which they evaluate one another. We are also analyzing psychopathology indicators in both parents and adolescents, using methods described by Singer and Wynne [13] and DeVos [3].

Our findings to date have been particularly encouraging. We have found systematic consistencies between familial interaction patterns and adolescent behavior. The schizophreniform behavior seems to covary with intrafamilial communications resembling those reported for schizophrenics. This encouraged us to follow up our adolescents into Stage 3 of our research design.

Stage 3. Follow-Up of High Risk Adolescents into Early Adulthood

As indicated schematically in Figure 1, the next stage in the research program involves the prospective study of the cohort of adolescents through a series of follow-up periods. The follow-up study has two general purposes, to determine first whether any adolescent behavior patterns possess continuity with later schizophrenic development and second whether distinctive patterns of family interaction are particularly associated with schizophrenia development as contrasted with patterns found for other psychopathological conditions. In this type of study the goal is not merely to establish continuities with schizophrenia but to isolate patterns *not* related to that disorder which anticipate other contrasting forms of psychopathology. Thus a wide variety of outcomes provides a more meaningful follow-up study than does a single homogeneous outcome in our cohort.

The initial follow-up period, as indicated in Figure 1, only takes us into the earliest phases of the period of greatest risk for schizophrenia. It is unlikely that a large percentage of our sample, who eventually break down, will do so by age 20–21, but signs of shifts in level of adjustment may be apparent at this developmental transition point. Since this is so, the follow-up data must be broad enough to reveal signs of incipient disorder as well as the full-blown symptoms of psychoses or allied psychopathological conditions.

A major problem in this phase of the research is to establish two classes of measures, one believed to possess continuity with earlier measures obtained during adolescence, which would permit an estimate of rates of change in various aspects of behavior, and a second class which provides a link to the behavioral characteristics of adult schizophrenics. If we can achieve both goals in the same measures, all to the good, but it has been our experience that they may not overlap to the degree desired.

A major assumption of most follow-up studies is that continuity exists between earlier and later estimates of behavior. The assumption is further made that these relationships will involve what Bell's group [2] term *homotypic continuities* in which similar behaviors are continuous over time. We should also be alert to what these investigators term *heterotypic* continuities in which inverse or more complicated relationships exist between variables sampled at different time periods.

This distinction is hardly one of theory alone, since the choice of measures for the follow-up phase of the research may reflect one or the other bias and not permit a test of the other. As one of our former students, Frederic Jones [8] commented on the measurement of social competence at two points, adolescence and early adolescence, "the basic tasks requiring mastery, which function as indices of competence at one level of development, may be quite different from those which function as the indices of competence at the next stage of development. In fact, the developmental tasks during adolescence which are functionally related to successful adult heterosexual behavior may be topographically quite different." Successful marriage may be more readily predictive from indices of social responsibility in adolescence than from indices of heterosexual involvement during that same period.

The lack of continuity found by Jones in one area and the surprising continuity in another is illustrated in Table 1, which presents correlations between global ratings of social competence and perceived family interaction patterns. Here we see that the traditional indices of social competence do not predict the global rating at all. This is true despite the fact that the discrete social competence indices correlate moderately with each other across this five-year period and that these same social competence variables measured in early adulthood correlate significantly with the global evaluation at the same point. The variables that do possess continuity with early adult social competence are measures of family interaction, particularly the degree of perceived closeness among family members

Table 1 Correlation of Adolescent Interview Clusters with Early Adult Global Ratings of Social Competence

Cluster			
Familial		Social Competence	
Constructive relationships		Peer friendship	−.04
within the family	−.46	Dating	.18
Responsibility/autonomy		School achievement	.05
struggles and family		Career ambition	.09
balance	.45	Assertiveness	−.15

and the degree of struggle for autonomy from familial influence shown by the teenager. Thus if there is continuity in social competence between adolescence and early adulthood, it may be based on the mastery of the critical developmental tasks in each period (separation from the family in adolescence and achievement and interpersonal competence in early adulthood), which are not homologs of each other in a manifest behavioral sense. This argues very strongly for the inclusion of a variety of indices of behavior at various points in a follow-up study to permit a test of the nature of continuities and discontinuities between behavior sampled at two time intervals.

We have ignored for the moment the various classes of variables to be measured in a follow-up study of this sort. Most such studies emphasize the need to measure two things, social competence, defined as the ability to master relevant developmental tasks at each period, and psychopathological symptoms or tendencies. In the case of the former, we have previously suggested some of the methodological problems involved in defining indices which bear topographical continuity with one another. With regard to the latter class of measures, we generally search out indices at two levels, treatment records which suggest that the person has manifested symptom patterns of one or another psychopathological disorder, and direct assessment of a case through contact with him and significant others who know him well. In Stage 3 of the research program described in this essay, we are not very far into the period of risk for schizophrenia. Therefore the use of available treatment records is of limited value in measuring psychopathological status. We are forced to rely on direct assessment of the target case to estimate (1) current signs of psychopathological functioning and (2) previous signs based on interview reports of the target case or informant. Further, this assessment must be done with a young person who does not seek you out for treatment and who fears the revelation of failure and psychopathology in the self. This poses technical and ethical problems which are too complicated for this paper to cover—but they cannot be ignored in high risk research.

In the process of direct assessment in Stage 3 of this research program, we have relied upon the following data: (1) an extended, detailed interview with the target case and a separate one with one or both parents; (2) psychological testing of the target case using MMPI,

3-card Rorschach (Zülliger Test), and Word Association Test;
(3) inventories of drug use and sexual experience in the intervening
years between adolescence and early adulthood. Each of the indices
chosen was selected to provide a behavioral bridge between these
data and the signs and symptoms of adult schizophrenia. As suggested
previously, the intermediate level of follow-up present in Stage 3
requires not only the establishment of continuity and discontinuity
into earlier behavior but also with adult manifestations of schizophrenia. Thus the Rorschach Test was utilized in our assessment to
obtain measures of various forms of thought disturbances specified
by Singer and Wynne as common in schizophrenics and their
families. Since we feel that it is unlikely that we will obtain test
protocols indicative of full-blown schizophrenia, we plan to search
for the type of subclinical forms of attentional and thought
disturbance indices outlined by these investigators. This is also the
basis for selection of the Word Association Test, which is particularly
significant because it was also administered five years previously to
the teenager. The MMPI was selected for a number of reasons, but
particularly for the large-scale normative base and the ability of the
test to reveal characterological as well as symptomatic behavior
patterns.

In the direct assessment of the young adult, the interviews with
the parent and the young adult are carried out independently at
different times and in different places. Thus we have observations
from two vantage points on how the target case is doing now and how
he has been doing over the last five years. Naturally, we are
concerned with the relationship between these two sets of data.
Although we have only some preliminary analyses carried out by one
of our students, Bonnie Burstein, comparing the parental interview
(which focuses exclusively on social competence items) and the young
adult interview (which covers both social competence and psychopathology), the relationship varies with the dimensions analyzed.

In one instance the respondent's interview tapes were rated by the
team, and the young adult's were rated by another team. One rating
consisted of the 3-point global social competence scale used by Jones
in his study. In Table 2 we see the relationship between the ratings
of the interview tapes. There are a number of interesting trends in
the table. First, in his own interview, the impression of the young
adult resulted in a wider range of social competence ratings than the

Table 2 Rating of Social Competence of Young Adults from Recorded Interviews

		Young adult interviews			
		1	2	3	
Parent	1	2	0	0	2
	2	4	3	3	10
Interview	3	1	1	4	6
		7	4	7	

1 = marginal competence.
3 = severely incompetent.

reports of the parents who in almost all cases rated their offspring as moderately to severely incompetent in meeting life's demands. Second, except for a few cases where the ratings agree completely, there is considerable discrepancy between the two sets of ratings.

Lest we assume that this is necessarily true for all ratings of the two levels of interview data, let us look in Table 3 at the comparison between the previous ratings of global social competence from the parental tape and ratings on a thought-disturbance scale used with the young adult's tape. This scale ranged from 1 to 8, with 1 indicating normal clear and flexible thought, and 7 and 8 flagrantly schizophrenic thought. Since the latter was rarely seen, the usable scale ranged from 1 to 6, with 6 indicative of attentional and thought-disturbances of the type reported by Wynne and Singer. In Table 3 we see a much sharper relationship between the two sets of data. No case rated reasonably high on the global competence scale receives a rating indicating pathological, schizoid type of thought processes. The modal rating for the intermediate group on the social

Table 3 Comparison of Thought Disturbance Ratings from Young Adult Interview and Global Social Competence Rating from Parental Interview

		Thought Disturbance		
		1–2	3–4	5–6
Global rating	1	1	2	0
of	2	2	6	1
social competence	3	0	2	4

competence scale is in the intermediate range on the thought-disturbance scale and four out of six socially incompetent cases receive ratings of schizoid thought processes.

These two comparisons suggest that the interview with the informant and the target case may be sensitive to different phenotypical manifestations of the same basic process. The respondent may be capable of a more objective view of the actual accomplishments of the young adult, whereas the target case may distort his self-portrait in a more favorable direction. On the other hand, the target case's behavior in the interview and his descriptions of experiences may be uniquely suited to revealing thought processes and coping patterns *not* accessible to parents or inferable from their reports. That they relate to each other suggests further that indices of social competence in young adulthood can be related to the potential for schizophrenic development through the mediating mechanism of disturbances in attention and thought.

We have only begun to utilize the various types of data obtained during the adolescent period to predict early adult adjustment. As indicated previously, Frederic Jones investigated the predictive value of cluster scores obtained from an initial interview with the parents four to five years before follow-up. The cluster relating to perceived family relationships predicted the 3-point criteria of social competence and psychopathology. But since we have expended considerable effort observing actual interactions among the family members, we wished to determine the value of these data in predicting the same outcome criterion. We are currently investigating both the content and the style of these interactions but have completed only predictive studies with some of the stylistic variables. One of our students, Suzanne Wu Bliss, has recently completed a study examining what she terms the "turnover rate" in the intensely emotional interaction confrontation session of the project in which family members discuss personally selected material of a conflictual nature. In the study, turnover rate was defined as the number of times the conversation shifted to another speaker during a fixed period of time. The higher the score, the more times the conversation shifted to another speaker. Bliss found that this index correlated .67 with the 3-point outcome criteria developed by Jones for our first sample of 24 males.

In an effort to determine why a high turnover score correlated with very poor adjustment in early adulthood, Bliss examined other parameters of the interaction protocol. As expected, the rate of interruptions or intrusions into the speech of another family member accounts for a small part of the variation in turnover scores. However, it was not a major factor. Further examination revealed that high turnover rate was accompanied by a family style in which recurrent accusations, criticism, and self-defense followed each other in rapid order. These accusations more often involve statements concerning the fundamental character or value of the listener than criticism of specific behaviors. Paraphrasing Carl Rogers, the families of the most disturbed young adults experience considerable *unconditional negative regard* from each other and a minimum of empathic listening.

These data are based on a small sample and we hope to cross-validate them against our later cases who are just entering the follow-up period. But they do suggest the value of considering measures of familial interaction in evaluating risk for subsequent psychopathology.

Stage 4. Retrospective Analysis of Significant Leads from the Follow-Up Studies

As suggested in Figure 1, the next phase of the research program involves a retrospective study of a cohort of adult schizophrenics. Despite the obvious advantages of prospective studies of schizophrenic development, one need not be limited to a single methodology in which restrospective data are ignored. Once clues arise in prospective studies concerning other behavioral or familial antecedents of schizophrenia, it is possible and valuable to cross-check these trends on samples of adult schizophrenics using careful retrospective methods. This is the logic of Stage 4 in our research program. This stage in high risk research, in which we test trends noted in a prospective study against retrospective data, provides an intermediate test of the validity of findings from high risk research and a guide to the wisdom of carrying on costly and lengthy replication of the original prospective study.

As a result of follow-up data in our prospective study, certain preliminary data indicated that particular adolescent groups, defined on the basis of parental descriptions of the child's behavior problems, had a greater likelihood of severe psychopathology five years later than did others. For example, the withdrawn, socially isolated teenagers uniformly received low ratings as young adults on the global social competence scale developed by Frederic Jones. This was largely true of the active family conflict group as well.

In a recent study Sturzenberger applied the strategy of Stage 4 to attempt to learn whether retrospective parental reports of the adolescent behavior of a cohort of adult schizophrenics resembled these two adolescent groups more than others that have been delineated by our research group [15]. To sharpen the likelihood of finding distinctive patterns, she divided the schizophrenic group into good and poor premorbid subsamples. Each parent was interviewed using the interview form that was used to elicit parental descriptions in the prospective study, supplemented by additional questions. In Table 4 we see the major differences that Sturzenberger found between the good and poor premorbid schizophrenics.

These two patterns of behavior resemble, in certain ways, the patterns found in two of four groups that have been investigated in Stage 2 of the prospective study of disturbed adolescents. These patterns were also based on parental descriptions. The *good* premorbid schizophrenic behaviors are similar to those found in the adolescents of the *active family conflict* group, and those of the *poor* premorbid schizophrenic patients are similar to those of the *withdrawn-socially isolated* adolescents. To appreciate these parallels, the description of each of these adolescent groups follows:

> The *active family conflict* adolescents are characterized by a defiant, disrespectful stance toward parents. They are belligerent and antagonistic in the family setting and often show signs of inner distress or turmoil, such as tension, anxiety, and somatic complaints. They rarely manifest aggression or rebelliousness *outside* the family.
>
> The *withdrawn-socially* isolated adolescents are characterized by marked social isolation, general uncommunicativeness, few or no friends, and excessive dependence upon one or both parents. They often show gross fears and signs of marked anxiety and tension. Much of the unstructured time of these adolescents is spent in solitary pursuits.

Early in our analyses of our findings these two groups were

Table 4 Adolescent Behavior Problems of Good and Poor Premorbid Schizophrenics from Retrospective Study

Good Premorbids	Poor Premorbids
Major Problem Identified: Rebelliousness	
Impulsivity, immaturity, defiance of parental wishes, poor judgment	Withdrawal, social isolation (passivity, apathy/achievement of peer relationships)
Specific Problem Areas	
1. Achievement Orientation and Motivation	
Lacked academic motivation, showed initiative outside school (seeking jobs, etc.)	Conscientious in school, Lacked initiative outside school
2. Sociability	
Displayed confidence and initiative with friends, had many and were adept with them	Extreme lack of confidence with friends, had few and rarely sought them out
3. Response to Parental Frustration	
Active response to parental frustration (yelling, arguing, and active defiance)	Passive response (no visible response, withdrawal, or yielding)
4. Sex and Dating	
Highly active dating pattern displaying self-confidence with opposite sex	No self-confidence with opposite sex, very little dating or continuous relationships

classified as *inside home locus* groups since in both of them the behavioral problems of the adolescent appeared to be restricted largely to relationships within the home. They resemble in many ways the two patterns of preschizophrenic behavior found in the present sample of good and poor premorbid schizophrenics. This suggests that the data from the prospective and retrospective studies confirm and support the trends of each other.

The parallel between the reported adolescent histories of the good and poor premorbid schizophrenics and the inside-home locus groups in the adolescent study suggest the hypothesis that schizophrenia may be particularly common in family settings in which there is an intense but distorted emotional attachment between parents(s) and teenage child. The patterns of coping that characterize the two groups, active family conflict and withdrawal, may represent two very different strategies for achieving some sense of autonomy from these intense attachments without severing them completely.

Overview

The strategy described has some specific advantages for the study of populations at risk for various types of severe adult psychopathology.

The selection of disturbed adolescents permits one to carry out high risk studies utilizing readily available clinical populations who need be followed at only relatively short intervals before entering the period of maximal risk.

The design combines elements of both cross-sectional and longitudinal approaches. The fact that adolescents and members of their families are seen initially at their request provides the opportunity to examine in some detail specific attributes of the interaction between the presenting problem of the adolescent and particular aspects of intrafamilial relationships. These various patterns can also be examined for their prospective value as predictors of variations in adult psychopathology. Thus the study of adolescent behavior in the context of familial interaction is valuable both in the *short* run for understanding the dynamics of problems in adolescent adjustment and in the *long* run for the identification of marker variables useful in the early detection of high risk cohorts.

Since our major interest lies in the identification of precursors of schizophrenia, the research strategy requires additional phases to form a tight network of evidence. The absolute number of potential adult schizophrenics in an adolescent cohort will never be great, and many years will go by before the total sample passes through the full risk period. Therefore we will require some type of intermediate cross-validation technique to assess as they emerge leads which hold promise as precursors of schizophrenia. In our particular research, this phase of the design involves the study of a cohort of young acute schizophrenics who can be studied closely both for attributes of their current pathology and retrospectively regarding adolescent pathology and familial relationships. The concordance of these two phases of the design permits the assessment of the validity of hypotheses regarding adolescent and familial precursors of adult schizophrenia.

The ultimate return of this degree of understanding lies in the extent to which it suggests specific techniques for intervention with adolescents and their families which may prevent the occurrence of disabling psychosis or minimize its disruptive effects if one should occur. The long-range goal of our research program at UCLA has been to contribute to the development of strategies for ameliorating or minimizing adult psychopathology, particularly schizophrenia. Therefore we are currently carrying out pilot studies utilizing the findings and techniques derived from our intensive study of disturbed adolescents and their families to determine effective intervention and, we hope, prevention procedures.

References

1. Alkire, A. A., Goldstein, M. J., Rodnick, E. H., and Judd, L. L. Social influence and counterinfluence within families of four types of disturbed adolescents. *J. Abnorm. Psychol.*, 77 (1971), 32–41.
2. Bell, R. Q., Weller, G. M., and Waldrop, M. D. F. Newborn and preschooler: Organization of behavior and relations between periods. *Monogr. Soc. Res. Child Devel.*, 36 (1971), 1–45.
3. DeVos, G. A quantitative approach to affective symbolism in Rorschach responses. *J. Projective Techniques,* 16 (1952), 133–155.
4. Garmezy, N. and Rodnick, E. H. Premorbid adjustment and performance in schizophrenia: Implications for interpreting heterogeneity in schizophrenia. *J. Nerv. Ment. Dis.*, 129 (1959).
5. Goldstein, M. J., Gould, E. Alkire, A., Rodnick, E. H., and Judd, L. L. Interpersonal themas in the thematic apperception test stories of families of disturbed adolescents. *J. Nerv. Ment. Dis.*, 150 (1970), 354–365.
6. Goldstein, M. J., Judd, L. L., Rodnick, E. H., Alkire, A., and Gould, E. A method for studying social influence and coping patterns within families of disturbed adolescents. *J. Nerv. Ment. Dis.*, 147 (1968), 233–251.
7. Goldstein, M. J., Rodnick, E. H., Judd, L. L., and Gould, E. Galvanic skin reactivity among family groups containing disturbed adolescents. *J. Abnorm. Psychol.*, 75 (1970), 57–67.
8. Jones, F. H. A four-year follow-up of vulnerable adolescents: The prediction of outcomes in early adulthood from measures of social competence, coping style, and overall level of psychopathology. *J. Nerv. Ment. Dis.*, 1973, in press.
9. Lidz, T., Fleck, S., and Corneilson, A. *Schizophrenia and the Family.* International Universities Press, New York, 1965.
10. McPherson, S. Communication of intents among parents and their disturbed adolescent child. *J. Abnorm. Psychol.*, 76 (1970), 98–105.
11. McPherson, S. R., Goldstein, M. J., and Rodnick, E. H. Who listens? Who communicates? How? *Arch. Gen. Psychiat.* 28 (1973), 393–399.
12. Rodnick, E. H. and Garmezy, N. An experimental approach to the study of motivation in schizophrenia, in *Nebraska Symposium on Motivation,* M. R. Jones, Ed. University of Nebraska Press, Lincoln, 1957, pp. 109–184.

13. Singer, M. T. and Wynne, L. D. Differentiating characteristics of parents of childhood schizophrenics, childhood neurotics and young adult schizophrenics. *Amer. J. Psychiat.*, 120 (1963), 234–243.
14. Strodbeck, F. L. Husband and wife interaction over revealed differences. *Amer. Sociol. Rev.*, 16 (1951), 468–473.
15. Sturzenberger, S. C., Goldstein, M. J., and Rodnick, E. H. Adolescent behavioral patterns of good and poor premorbid schizophrenics. Unpublished paper, UCLA, 1973.
16. West, K. L., Rodnick, E. H., and Armstrong, J. R. Parental attributes and the differentiated behavior of disturbed adolescents. Paper presented at the Western Psychological Association meeting, 1972.
17. Wynne, L. C. and Singer, M. T. Thought disorder and the family relations of schizophrenics: I and II. *Arch. Gen. Psychiat.*, 9 (1963), 191–206.
18. Wynne, L. C. and Singer, M. T. Thought disorder and the family relations of schizophrenics: III and IV. *Arch. Gen. Psychiat.*, 12 (1965), 187–212.

EPILOGUE

The Syndrome of the Psychologically Invulnerable Child*

E. James Anthony, M.D. (U.S.A.)

A Preamble on Mythological Invulnerability

The idea of invulnerability, like the idea of immortality, has haunted the human race since the beginning of recorded history and is reflected in much of the mythology of ancient man. The myth-making propensity of our species has conduced to many and varied interpretations of mysteries appertaining to origin and extinction, to the relationship of the natural to the supernatural order, and to the apparent immunity from the disasters of illness and injury granted to certain individuals [7].

The most celebrated of the myths of invulnerability had to do with the warrior Achilles. It was told that when Thetis, his mother, learned of the fatal destiny that awaited her son, she tried to circumvent it by plunging him into the river Styx at birth, thus rendering his whole body invulnerable except for the heel by which she had held him. She was made aware of this significant shortcoming when he reached the age of 9, and the seer Calchas prophesied that he would not only conquer Troy but would also meet his death

* The Lambie-Dew oration at the University of Sydney School of Medicine, October 1973. Research supported by National Institute of Mental Health Grants MH12043 and MH14052.

there. Once again she took evasive action and disguised him as a girl in the palace of Lycomedes, where Achilles was eventually discovered by means of an ingenious trick perpetrated by the crafty Odysseus, and inducted into the army. He died at Troy when his vulnerable heel was pierced by an arrow.

His counterpart in Teutonic mythology was the son of Odin and the goddess Frigg. Balder, it was said, was so beautiful that he shed a radiance around him, and it was enough to see or hear him to love him. It was therefore not surprising that he was the favorite of the gods. However, because his mother had a strong premonition of danger concerning him, she begged all things on earth—fire, metal, water, stone, minerals, plants, trees, beasts, birds, and snakes—to take an oath never to harm her son, and they all undertook this solemn vow. From then on Balder was deemed invulnerable, but, once again, his immunity was not total. His mother had overlooked the mistletoe, a fact cunningly extracted from her by Loki, a god who hated and envied Balder for his privileged status. Loki took advantage of an occasion when the gods in their assembly played a game of testing the celebrated immunity by bombarding Balder with arrows, stones, and weapons to no effect, until Loki persuaded a blind god to hurl the mistletoe branch at Balder, which he did. It pierced him, and the invulnerable one fell dead.

This first group of myths (and there are others) all share certain common features: the invulnerability is fostered primarily by the mother, it is related to her manipulation of the external environment, it is never quite complete, the seemingly invulnerable one eventually succumbs, his downfall is usually inspired by the envy induced by his special status, and the incomplete immunity is always purchased at high psychological cost to both parent and child.

A second group of myths of invulnerability ascribe it to a different etiology. A representative example is Hercules, who throughout his life was menaced recurrently by a series of risks imposed on him by a jealous goddess. He coped with them all successfully *as a result of his own efforts, initiative, strength, and endurance.* As an infant he was attacked by two serpents, sent to kill him, but he grasped them firmly, one in each hand, and wrung their necks. As a youth he exercised regularly and developed his physical prowess, and at 18 he slew a ferocious lion that came to devour him. He was driven insane by Lyssa, Fury of Madness (again at the urging of the jealous goddess), and killed his wife and two children. For this horrendous crime he was directed by the Delphic Oracle to perform a number of superhuman tasks. First he strangled the Nemean lion and made from its skin a garment *that rendered him invulnerable*. He cleaned the Augean stables, conquered the Cretan bull, who had been driven crazy, captured the terrible mares of Diomedes, took possession of the cattle of Geryon, also driven crazy, and recovered the golden apples of the Hesperides. He even struggled successfully with Death itself. Having survived all these ills, Hercules was finally taken up to the skies in a fitting apotheosis, and he became an Immortal.

Common to this legend and others like it from different cultures are the following factors: rather than being overprotected from risk, the hero is constantly exposed to it and seems to gain in both confidence and competence from each encounter; in his endeavors he relies solely on his own capabilities, and he creates his own invulnerability as Hercules did out of the skin of the Nemean lion; and this self-generated immunity is more complete and long lasting. It is of interest too that this self-confident and self-reliant hero is frequently brought face to face with psychosis, either in himself or in others, as a further test of his resilience. This suggests that psychosis, as a testing ground for vulnerability and invulnerability, has had ancient and hallowed precedents.

In the first mythological group, overprotection by the mother gives rise to a pseudo-invulnerability, which induces, in turn, a false sense of security. When the individual leaves the protective ambience and sets out on his own, his latent vulnerability soon demonstrates itself. In the second group strong affection coupled with "benign neglect" on the part of the mother, who exudes a high degree of confidence in the competence of her offspring to take care of himself and his own affairs, tends to produce a truer invulnerability, one that is self-generated and enduring, in spite of overwhelming hazards. Neither invulnerability is absolute, but the autonomous type emerges with a greater propensity than the heteronomous for creating a relative psychological immunity.

Psychological Invulnerability

The clinician will find no difficulty in perceiving analogies between these mythical cases and those seen in everyday clinical

practice. There are, for example, striking similarities between the
first group and the condition of "maternal overprotection" originally
described by Levy [8], in which certain mothers, for different reasons,
attempt to shield their children from possible harm by eliminating
all elements of risk from their lives.

The typical case history of an overprotected child, almost
invariably a boy, would read as follows:

> When he was an infant, his mother could never leave him for an instant,
> and she still feels worried and unhappy when he is out of her sight. She has
> been sleeping with him at night, because he has needed her nursing care
> owing to frequent colds. She breastfed him for 13 months and spoonfed him
> the first 5 years. She dressed him in the morning although he was now 8 and
> watched from the window while he walked to school. When out together, she
> always insisted on holding his hand. She was afraid to let him run upstairs
> since he got out of breath, and he was not allowed to visit in other homes
> because of possible infection. She never allowed him to play with other
> children because they were rough and might hurt him. He was allowed no
> outdoor sport for fear of injury.

Levy remarks that although the overprotected children were taller
and heavier than comparable groups, because of the high degree of
maternal care, and enjoyed a good measure of health, there was a
higher incidence of tonsillectomy, and "despite maternal vigilance,
evidence of superficial injuries was fairly frequent." Mollycoddling
or pampering therefore not only increased the likelihood of certain
minor physical hazards, but they had the additional psychological
disadvantage of making the boy effeminate, timid, shy, self-centered,
demanding, and fearful of being hurt.

Comparable to the second group is a variety of clinical states in
children in which autonomy, independence, and self-reliance are
exaggerated and out of keeping with the expectations of the
developmental period to which the children belong. Common
examples are older siblings acting as parental surrogates in larger
families; only children in one-parent families where the parent works
and the child is left to fend for himself; children with handicapped
parents; parents with physical or mental illnesses. The self-confidence
of the child seems to be directly in proportion to the confidence that
the parent has in him, and this is especially true for the eldest child.
Freud pointed out that the mother's pride and belief in her firstborn
son may furnish him with a resilience that can see him through the

most serious setbacks. "A man," he said, "who has been the indisputable favorite of his mother, keeps for life the feeling of a conqueror, that confidence of success that often induces real success" [13].

Paradoxes of Risk and Vulnerability

There are many inequalities into which children are born in this unfairly constituted world—inequalities of rank, of riches, of opportunities, of basic endowment—all of which have been with us for so long a time that they are more or less taken for granted. One of the most significant inequalities for the future well-being of the individual is the inequality of risk, that is, the uneven distribution of stress through the population of children. This means that for some the world is secure, stable, and predictable; they are born into acceptance, concern, and care; they are planned for, hoped for, and welcomed. For others the reverse is true. Life for them is short, sharp, and brutish. They have parents who hate them from conception, reject them from birth, batter them as infants, neglect them as toddlers, and institutionalize them or have them fostered at the drop of a hat. Nevertheless, two children from the same stock, the same womb, the same propitious or unpropitious environment may end quite differently with one falling psychologically ill and the other apparently blossoming. A superchild may come out of the ghetto and a sad and sorry child from the well-to-do suburbs. Why and how? By what mysterious process of psychological selection is the one destroyed and the other preserved? Admittedly, the two worlds may not be so different beneath the surface; a seemingly indulgent household in a superior neighborhood may camouflage as many cruelties and crudities as an overcrowded tenement apartment. Exposure is clearly not the whole story; vulnerability and mastery also play integral roles in determining the response to stress.

The critical factors to be investigated are those governing susceptibility. Is there a point in life when a "natural selection" begins to operate permitting the fittest to survive and the unfit to succumb, or does a coat of invulnerability gradually build up from repeatedly successful adjustments? Had Achilles been dipped into the magic water at infancy, or was his highly protected upbringing responsible for the eventual immunity? And if there is such an entity as psychological immunity, is it ever complete? Is the Achilles heel always present in some part of the makeup? Is the invulnerable child merely endowed with a higher threshold of sensitivity to stress, and is he as liable to succumb to an overwhelming experience as his more vulnerable brother? If there is immunity, is it permanent, or does the wear-and-tear of everyday existence eventually reduce its efficacy? Is it paid for out of the store of good human characteristics with the subsequent development of insensitivity, detachment, and self-absorption? Does the individual really master fate or is he especially fortunate in being treated benignly by the world in which he lives?

We are still in the process of learning something about this new field of risk, vulnerability, prevention, and mastery, and of recognizing some of the problems relating to it. The investigator must ask himself whether such global concepts are researchable, measurable, and testable; whether the attributes of the invulnerable child can be successfully identified in the laboratory; and whether, having helped him, one can follow him closely, over time, to learn his secret! If all this is possible, then one can claim with some justification that a crucial advance has been made in the field of psychiatric prevention.

Studies in Invulnerability

The researcher in this field tends to approach the less prevalent phenomenon of invulnerability through a consideration of the far more common occurrence of vulnerability. In fact, invulnerability is usually defined in negative terms as an absence of vulnerability, and this is in keeping with the clinical tradition that chooses to regard health as an absence of sickness. Health is largely taken for granted by both physician and patient; it is sickness that is intrusive and troubling.

In several studies it is possible to infer the characteristics of invulnerability from the antitheses of what is found in the vulnerable person. For example, one can conclude from the investigation by Heider [6] that the invulnerable infant is more likely to have a robust physique, a good health record, better than average energy resources, and smooth vegetative functioning. He will also have experienced a trustful and confident relationship with a mother preoccupied with his needs. His environment would, in general, be supportive and "expectable," and a steady observation of his behavior would disclose a harmony between internal and external milieux, stable thresholds that were neither too high nor too low, and an executive competence in dealing with everyday difficulties. The observer would perceive him as active, interested, curious, and eager to explore.

Haggard has chosen to emphasize the importance of congruence between the characteristics of the individual and of his environment, insisting that "the adaptation of the individual, both in terms of his inner life, and the effectiveness of his performance, cannot be considered apart from the parameters of his environmental context" [5]. The individual's adaptation patterns could break down if the environment in which he is placed is very different from that to which he is accustomed. From their responses to a modified Thematic Apperception Test, Haggard considered that the set of character traits associated with resilient individuals included "a superficial need for independence, with a deeper dependence on outside support; frequent unresolved conflict, ambivalence, or fluctuation of aggressive and sexual drives; and a reliance on external stimulation to determine their thoughts, which tend to be specific and concrete rather than elaborate and abstract." Vulnerability therefore, according to Haggard, is not related to certain innate or acquired superiorities in performance but rather to a harmony between internal and external environments and to a capacity to accommodate flexibly to change. If the individual is flexible enough, one would expect a congruence to develop between the self and the environment. Good homeostatic mechanisms (physical and psychological) require, on one level, an independence, a self-reliance, and an autonomy, and on the other, an interdependence, a recognition of the needs of others, and a reciprocity of interchange; an inner psychological environment that remains flexible and open to change; and under conditions of demand, an ability to transpose from abstract to concrete, from theory to practice, and vice versa.

A third set of studies has tried to link invulnerability with coping skills and active mastery. Murphy has carried out careful observational studies on the different ways in which children learn to cope with difficulties in their environment, and she concludes that irrespective of whether the problems arise inside or outside the child, normal children make use of defensive and mastering capacities in

a mutually supportive way, so that sometimes a particular function
may be employed in the service of defense and sometimes offense [10].
If the various functions of the personality are used too exclusively in
defense, a chronically defensive personality structure can result, with
the child perhaps becoming far less flexible and spontaneous. In the
general run of children, normal development is a complex outcome
of interactions between the balance of vulnerabilities and strengths,
and their interaction with stresses and supports from the environment. However, in a certain number of children the fight is carried
strikingly into the heart of the environment. This type of child is on
the offensive, in the best sense of the term, and chooses his actions
and his roles on the basis of what he wants to accomplish for himself
rather than what the environment is expecting of him.

A final set of studies attempts to relate invulnerability to the
concept of competence, a term that is becoming increasingly popular
although its meaning is often diffused beyond usefulness. People
generally have a fairly clear intuitive grasp of what it signifies, but
exact operational definitions are difficult to construct. For instance,
it is unclear whether competence is a global unitary trait or whether
there are many different kinds of competence; the current assumption
leans toward the global point of view: children who possess one or
more attributes of competence are more likely to possess other
attributes and can be specified, in a general way, as either more or
less competent.

The relationship of competence to vulnerability has thus far been
confined largely to performance in a variety of test situations that
attempt to assess social, cognitive, linguistic, and motor skills.

In our own research [1] the concept of competence has been
extended inwardly to include the ability to construct an internal
representation of an external event, that is, a capacity to conceptualize
and order the manifold incoming data so that they become
sufficiently meaningful for the individual to act upon. The executive
competence of the individual child therefore becomes a function of
both representation and performance. One would expect it to relate
to age, to intelligence, and to the functioning of parents, who
constantly provide models of competence. The sex of the child has
some bearing on the issues of competence and vulnerability: on the
physical plane, the figures for infant mortality and morbidity are
almost universally higher for boys; on the psychological level there

are indications that boys and girls, even in preschool years, differ in their response to challenge and frustration. Murphy [10] found that little girls were more likely to respond passively when under pressure, whereas little boys were more inclined to actively express opposition, and that girls tended to show physical inmobility under stress, whereas boys manifested emotional and social unresponsiveness. This may be the reason why some researchers have found fewer behavioral indices of competence for girls than for boys.

The use of the male child as exemplar in so many illustrations is deliberate; in this true category of invulnerability few of the children appear to be girls, and the reasons for this are only now being explored. Studies are currently being carried out as to what effect traditional modes of upbringing may have on the competence of the female child. Further, the fact that women, in larger numbers, are becoming active participants in achievement-oriented cultures is reflected in the current searching for satisfaction, status, and self-esteem other than those stemming from child rearing. Birnbaum [3] has shown that girls more frequently have the wish to be of the opposite sex than boys do, and that before the birth of a child parents overwhelmingly prefer to have a boy. In cases where girl children are preferred, they are found to be viewed as less noisy and dirty and more obedient and helpful around the house and therefore more desirable. Through the process of identification, these deficiencies in autonomy and self-esteem are passed on from generation to generation.

It is also no longer surprising that the invulnerable ones in classical mythology are always the favored sons of doting mothers.

It therefore seems that whereas risk is a function of the actual physical and psychological environment, vulnerability and invulnerability are states of mind induced in the child by exposure to these risks, and mastery is a force generated in the individual that leads him to test his strength constantly against that of the environment, and to assert himself even against overwhelming odds.

A challenge and response formulation would appear to provide an adequate explanatory framework within which to test various aspects of mastery [1]. When faced with unusual stresses such as the loss or illness of a parent, which is at the heart of his security, the child may resort to "sick" behavior that may be short lived or long term and may perceive himself thereafter as a passive and helpless victim of fate. In his fantasies there is often a magical expectation that some powerful person will one day appear to rescue him.

Another type of child (a much smaller group) responds to similar stresses with the development of new modes of behavior not previously displayed and characterized by qualities of creativity, originality, drive, and resourcefulness that seem to lift the child out of his predicament and into a new world of functioning. Mastery therefore belongs as an attribute to the true invulnerable.

It is now possible for us to construct a two-way table correlating high and low risk with high and low vulnerability, and correlating both to the possibility of disorder (see Table 1). When high risk is coupled with high vulnerability the prospect for disorder is high, and one can, with some measure of confidence, predict this outcome in late childhood, adolescence, or early maturity. Low risk, linked with low vulnerability, is characteristic of the "normal control" in whom one would not predict the development of disorder. This could be termed the average child's invulnerability.[1] It is not striking because the risks are low and normal behavior generally is taken for granted.

The "invulnerability syndrome" is associated with the coexistence of high risk with low vulnerability. One is surprised at the absence

Table 1 Relationship of Risk, Vulnerability, and Disturbance

	High Risk	Low Risk			High Risk	Low Risk
High Vulnerability	(1) HR, HV	(3) LR, HV		Disturbed	(1) HR, D	(3) LR, D
Low Vulnerability	(2) HR, LV	(4) LR, LV		Nondisturbed	(2) HR, ND	(4) LR, ND

	High Vulnerability	*Low* Vulnerability
Disturbed	(1) HV, D	(3) LV, D
Nondisturbed	(2) HV, ND	(4) LV, ND

[1] In the Robins follow-up study, the control subjects were strikingly different from the antisocial referrals in terms of alcoholism, imprisonment, and divorce [12].

of disorder in the presence of appalling living conditions, horrifying experiences, chronic physical ailments, and disruptive development. In the presence of all this, an individual emerges who is energetic, well balanced, and normally active and reactive.

Finally there is the individual with a good endowment, benign experiences, and a comfortable environment, but he is hypersensitive in the test situation and unable to construct a meaningful model of himself in relation to his surroundings. He cannot integrate what he is with where he is, and this lack of congruence makes him stand out like a sore thumb in an otherwise good set of circumstances. This has sometimes been described as the suburban syndrome since it affects the children of the elite, who are overprotected, overprivileged, and very disturbed.[2] Low risk conditions may create false expectations that the child is invulnerable, but he is invulnerable only in the sense that he has never been tested or tried in the fire of experience, and sooner or later the mistletoe may strike him or an arrow find his heel. There is much more to invulnerability than low risk.

Invulnerability and Parental Psychosis

The ideas set forth in this presentation are mainly derived from ongoing research, over the past eight years, into the risks and vulnerabilities associated with being offspring of psychotic or physically ill parents.

The research material is rich in documenting the syndrome of invulnerability because the investigators are constantly haunted by the "fine metallic sounds" given out by the "steel doll."[3] It has been growing clearer to us that invulnerability is also a function of time: the individual who seems invulnerable throughout childhood may develop vulnerabilities during adolescence and early adult life. A number of research questions suggest themselves. Is it possible to distinguish between the early and late invulnerables and between the true and false invulnerables? Do the invulnerables (true or false) pay a price for their immunity? And finally, if so, in what kind and what degree are males more likely to develop psychological invulner-

---

[2] See Sociopsychological Aspects of the Vulnerable Child, Risk and Mastery: Children of the Modern Elite in Nigeria, by T. Asuni in this volume.
[3] See A Risk-Vulnerability Intervention Model for Children of Psychotic Parents, by the author, in this volume.

ability than females? In our own data there is a striking paucity of females among the true invulnerables, although the sexes are equally distributed among the false invulnerables. Related to this is the fact that female children seemed to identify more closely and more intensely with a sick mother and to assimilate more of her "sick" characteristics than do boys with regard to either sick fathers or sick mothers.

What seemed to characterize the true invulnerables in our sample were the following factors: a seemingly stubborn resistance to the process of being engulfed by the illness; a curiosity in studying the etiology, diagnosis, symptoms, and treatment of the illness reaching to a level of knowledge that is quite surprising; a capacity to develop an objective, realistic, somewhat distant and yet distinctly compassionate approach to the parental illness, neither retreating from it nor being intimidated by it, but viewing it as something needing to be fully understood; an exposure to the stressful experience only after immunity has had time to build up; and support, encouragement, and candor from an adequately functioning other parent. The invulnerable child not only speaks well for himself, but he speaks well for his family and well also for the sick parent. He understands illness both as a personal experience invading his life and as a phenomenon to be investigated and treated. Of all the children in our sample, these true invulnerables were among the most collaborative and proffered us the greatest amount of information.

The interplay of defense and coping was always in evidence, but offense in the positive sense was equally prominent. At times we felt that the price paid might be in terms of future love relationships; the distance imposed in the relationship with the sick parent appeared to carry over into other relationships and set restrictions.

What we are emphasizing here is that although true invulnerability is usually associated with other indications of satisfactory family life rather than with the individual protection afforded a particular child by a particular parent as in false invulnerability, true invulnerability can have some important shortcomings.

We have had examples of creative outbursts and originality of ideas in about 10 percent of our sample of children of schizophrenic parents, whom we refer to as "superphrenics." We are not suggesting that true invulnerability is invariably linked with creativity, but that as a result of the development of invulnerability, creativity may emerge. In one genetic study [16] the author presented extensive pedigrees on an Icelandic kindred whose complete genealogy could be traced back for seven generations. Schizophrenia was first encountered in a woman born in 1735, and psychosis occurred in each subsequent generation, usually transmitted through non-psychotic members. Many gifted persons belonged to this kindred, including scholars, political leaders, and successful community officials. Five different groups were isolated in the population, designated normophrenic (79 percent), tensiphrenic (15 percent), schizophrenic (1 percent), retarded or autistic (0.1 to 0.01 percent), and superphrenic (5 percent). The superphrenic is defined as a healthy person who is known to have a psychotic parent or a psychotic sibling as well as having himself produced a psychotic child. He would be a gene carrier and would be likely to show "thought disorder" on specific object sorting tests. He is often highly productive, tending to assume leadership in cultural or social affairs, and is altogether more gifted than the ordinary person.

In another study [15] a follow-up of 47 children born to schizophrenic mothers but reared in foster homes revealed the existence of several gifted persons, whereas no individuals of superior performance were encountered in a control group consisting of 50 foster-reared persons born to nonschizophrenic mothers.

It therefore seems that a good case can be made for the existence of genetic factors in the syndrome of psychological invulnerability.

Conclusions

Instead of aiming at making children absolutely invulnerable, which sounds like a mythological ideal, one might consider some of the steps that could make them relatively invulnerable to the stresses and strains of contemporary existence.

First we should undoubtedly take a leaf from the studies of invulnerability and discover from the source itself how the immune mechanisms are generated and how they work. The parents of the invulnerable child are not less protective, but less anxious, than average parents and more likely to leave matters to the child himself even to the extent of taxing his immaturity. Confidence and competence go hand in hand. The parents of the invulnerable child are not less loving, but less possessive, than the average and more likely to allow the child his own territorial imperatives in which he can operate fairly autonomously. This fostering of autonomy is based on a realistic appreciation of what the child can do when extended and in no way constitutes an excuse to shed parental responsibility. The extent to which he is inquisitive and exploratory in his attitudes also indicates that the invulnerable individual is short on conformity, and there should be evidence to indicate that authoritarian parents are less prone to generate invulnerability.

How does one go about decreasing risk without going as far as some of the mythological mothers of invulnerable children. Today many of the hazards are becoming better understood and ameliorated. Genetic risks, although still largely obscure in relation to malfunctioning behavior, have made some response to genetic counseling. Obstetrical risks (prenatal damage to the central nervous system, perinatal damage during delivery, prematurity and intrauterine growth retardations, together with socioeconomic factors and the more subtle factors of the mother-infant relationships) are also beginning to be treated in more concerted ways by national authorities. The idea that the pregnant woman should be seen by an obstetrician at least once or twice during her pregnancy is still a hopeless ideal in most parts of the world. This is equally true of the care that women in parturition receive, and it has been suggested that at least half the cases of perinatal brain lesions at the time of the delivery of the full-term infant are caused by the improper management of labor, which means that all through the world hundreds of thousands of handicapped children are being produced by poor obstetrical procedures [9].[4]

Continuous electronic fetal monitoring is now recognized as providing an excellent alarm system of fetal distress during labor, but only a few countries can afford the luxury of such well-equipped intensive care units. Yet until these obstetrical precautions are taken on a larger scale, incidence of central nervous system damage will remain high, and our invulnerables will come from a smaller population of survivors. By definition, the psychologically invulnerable child has an intact central nervous system. The substandard environment as the ecologist would view it (polluted air, dirty water,

[4] See Obstetrical Risk in the Genesis of Vulnerability in this volume.

overcrowding, lack of recreational facilities, poor schooling, and inadequate medical and psychological services) is a political question that gets kicked around by politicians to the exasperation of ecologists and social scientists, but while conditions remain substandard throughout the world, it becomes hard for the truly invulnerable child to rise above some of the filth and fumes and futility that beset his dark world. There is such a thing as too much challenge even for the most willing child.

We know today about the effect of large institutions in the development of children, and very gradually they are being cut down to size, but even when we achieve this physical miracle, we will be left the idea of selling the very precious interpersonal commodity to administrators. The psychologically invulnerable child obtains warm, satisfying, one-to-one relationships to set him off in life. Without such relationships, or something very much like them, any child has less hope of surviving psychologically into healthy adult life.

How does one go about decreasing vulnerability? We have been trying to do this now for a number of years at our research center for high risk children. We can say at once that it is not easy to undo the cumulative susceptibilities built up over many years. We have taken the line of attempting to give the child a corrective experience of what the environment and the people in it are really like shorn of their unpredictable attitudes and behaviors induced by disease and disturbance. We offer the experience of trustful, supportive relationships, based on the deliberate non-use of reproachful and guilt-provoking techniques, on relationships geared to reality and rationality, on communications that are single-minded and unequivocal, and on feelings that correlate directly with experience and are not incongruous with it. In all, to the children who are living in the milieu of psychotic unreality, we have been attempting to offer an "average expectable environment" populated by individuals who interact in a fairly reasonable and predictable fashion.

Like the natural parents of the truly invulnerable, we tend to leave a great deal to the children and to foster the idea that it is up to them and that, as far as we are concerned, they are the masters of their own fate. We will crew for them and always be around when they really need us, but the really hard battles may need to be fought alone. This may sound like a tough philosophy for child rearing, but

we are talking about producing a relatively invulnerable child to live
in a relatively tough world, and we have to find ways of toughening
him while at the same time preserving his normal characteristics.
In some instances we may be doing too much and in others too little;
we still need to find the right prescription.

References

1. Anthony, E. J. The mutative impact on family life of serious mental and
   physical illness in a parent. *Canad. Psychiat. Assoc. J.*, 14 (1969).
2. Anthony, E. J. A risk-vulnerability intervention model in operation. In this
   volume.
3. Birnbaum, J. Life patterns, personality style and self-esteem in gifted
   family-oriented and career-committed women. Doctoral dissertation, Ann
   Arbor, University of Michigan, 1971.
4. Haggard, E. Isolation and personality, in *Personality Change*, P. Worchel
   and D. Byrne, Eds. John Wiley & Sons, New York, pp. 433–469.
5. Haggard, E. Some effects of geographic and social isolation in natural
   settings, in *Man in Isolation and Confinement*, J. Rasmussen, Ed. Aldine,.
   Chicago, 1973.
6. Heider, G. M. Vulnerability in infants and young children: A pilot study.
   Genet. Psychol. Monogr., 73 (1966), 1–216.
7. *Larousse Encyclopedia of Mythology*. Prometheus Press, New York, 1959.
8. Levy, D. M. *Maternal Overprotection*. Columbia University Press, New York,
   1943.
9. Minkowski, A. and Amiel-Tison, E. Obstetrical risk in the genesis of
   vulnerability. In this volume.
10. Murphy, L. B. et al. The problem of defense and the concept of coping,
    in *The Child and His Family*. E. J. Anthony and C. Koupernik, Eds. John
    Wiley & Sons, New York, 1970.
11. Murphy, L. B. et al. *The Widening World of Childhood: Paths toward
    Mastery*. Basic Books, New York, 1962.
12. Robins, L. *Deviant Children Grown Up*. Williams and Wilkins, Baltimore,
    1966.
13. Jones, E. *Sigmund Freud: Life and Work*. Vol. 1. Hogarth Press, London,
    1953.
14. Ogilvie, D. M. and Shapiro, B. Social behaviors of competent and
    incompetent three- to six-year-old children. Mimeographed paper,
    Cambridge, Harvard University, February 1969.
15. Heston, L. L. Psychiatric disorders in foster home reared children of
    schizophrenic mothers. *Brit. J. Psychiat.*, 112 (1966), 819–825.
16. Karlsson, J. L. Genealogic studies of schizophrenia, in *The Transmission of
    Schizophrenia*. D. Rosenthal and S. Kety, Eds. Pergamon Press,
    Oxford, 1968.

Index